Retail Strategies to Support Healthy Eating

Retail Strategies to Support Healthy Eating

Editors

Alyssa Moran
Christina Roberto

MDPI • Basel • Beijing • Wuhan • Barcelona • Belgrade • Manchester • Tokyo • Cluj • Tianjin

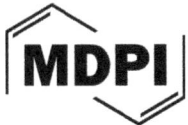

Editors

Alyssa Moran
Johns Hopkins University
USA

Christina Roberto
University of Pennsylvania
USA

Editorial Office
MDPI
St. Alban-Anlage 66
4052 Basel, Switzerland

This is a reprint of articles from the Special Issue published online in the open access journal *International Journal of Environmental Research and Public Health* (ISSN 1660-4601) (available at: https://www.mdpi.com/journal/ijerph/special_issues/Retail_Strateg_Support_Health_Eat).

For citation purposes, cite each article independently as indicated on the article page online and as indicated below:

LastName, A.A.; LastName, B.B.; LastName, C.C. Article Title. *Journal Name* **Year**, *Volume Number*, Page Range.

ISBN 978-3-0365-0052-2 (Hbk)
ISBN 978-3-0365-0053-9 (PDF)

© 2020 by the authors. Articles in this book are Open Access and distributed under the Creative Commons Attribution (CC BY) license, which allows users to download, copy and build upon published articles, as long as the author and publisher are properly credited, which ensures maximum dissemination and a wider impact of our publications.

The book as a whole is distributed by MDPI under the terms and conditions of the Creative Commons license CC BY-NC-ND.

Contents

About the Editors vii

Alyssa Moran and Christina Roberto
The Retail Food Environment: Time for a Change
Reprinted from: *Int. J. Environ. Res. Public Health* **2020**, *17*, 8846, doi:10.3390/ijerph17238846 . . . 1

Neha Khandpur, Laura Y. Zatz, Sara N. Bleich, Lindsey Smith Taillie, Jennifer A. Orr, Eric B. Rimm and Alyssa J. Moran
Supermarkets in Cyberspace: A Conceptual Framework to Capture the Influence of Online Food Retail Environments on Consumer Behavior
Reprinted from: *Int. J. Environ. Res. Public Health* **2020**, *17*, 8639, doi:10.3390/ijerph17228639 . . . 5

Amelie A. Hecht, Megan M. Lott, Kirsten Arm, Mary T. Story, Emily Snyder, Margo G. Wootan and Alyssa J. Moran
Developing a National Research Agenda to Support Healthy Food Retail
Reprinted from: *Int. J. Environ. Res. Public Health* **2020**, *17*, 8141, doi:10.3390/ijerph17218141 . . . 21

Allison Lacko, Shu Wen Ng and Barry Popkin
Urban vs. Rural Socioeconomic Differences in the Nutritional Quality of Household Packaged Food Purchases by Store Type
Reprinted from: *Int. J. Environ. Res. Public Health* **2020**, *17*, 7637, doi:10.3390/ijerph17207637 . . 39

Megan R. Winkler, Shannon N. Zenk, Barbara Baquero, Elizabeth Anderson Steeves, Sheila E. Fleischhacker, Joel Gittelsohn, Lucia A Leone and Elizabeth F. Racine
A Model Depicting the Retail Food Environment and Customer Interactions: Components, Outcomes, and Future Directions
Reprinted from: *Int. J. Environ. Res. Public Health* **2020**, *17*, 7591, doi:10.3390/ijerph17207591 . . . 57

Lucia A. Leone, Sheila Fleischhacker, Betsy Anderson-Steeves, Kaitlyn Harper, Megan Winkler, Elizabeth Racine, Barbara Baquero and Joel Gittelsohn
Healthy Food Retail during the COVID-19 Pandemic: Challenges and Future Directions
Reprinted from: *Int. J. Environ. Res. Public Health* **2020**, *17*, 7397, doi:10.3390/ijerph17207397 - . . 79

Chelsea R. Singleton, Megan Winkler, Bailey Houghtaling, Oluwafikayo S. Adeyemi, Alexandra M. Roehll, JJ Pionke and Elizabeth Anderson Steeves
Understanding the Intersection of Race/Ethnicity, Socioeconomic Status, and Geographic Location: A Scoping Review of U.S. Consumer Food Purchasing
Reprinted from: *Int. J. Environ. Res. Public Health* **2020**, *17*, 7677, doi:10.3390/ijerph17207677 . . . 93

Allison Karpyn, Kathleen McCallops, Henry Wolgast and Karen Glanz
Improving Consumption and Purchases of Healthier Foods in Retail Environments: A Systematic Review
Reprinted from: *Int. J. Environ. Res. Public Health* **2020**, *17*, 7524, doi:10.3390/ijerph17207524 . . . 119

Alyssa J. Moran, Yuxuan Gu, Sasha Clynes, Attia Goheer, Christina A. Roberto and Anne Palmer
Associations between Governmental Policies to Improve the Nutritional Quality of Supermarket Purchases and Individual, Retailer, and Community Health Outcomes: An Integrative Review
Reprinted from: *Int. J. Environ. Res. Public Health* **2020**, *17*, 7493, doi:10.3390/ijerph17207493 . . . 147

Amelie A. Hecht, Crystal L. Perez, Michele Polacsek, Anne N. Thorndike, Rebecca L. Franckle and Alyssa J. Moran
Influence of Food and Beverage Companies on Retailer Marketing Strategies and Consumer Behavior
Reprinted from: *Int. J. Environ. Res. Public Health* **2020**, *17*, 7381, doi:10.3390/ijerph17207381 . . **171**

About the Editors

Alyssa Moran is an Assistant Professor in the Department of Health Policy and Management and Core Faculty within the Institute for Health and Social Policy and Bloomberg American Health Initiative at the Johns Hopkins Bloomberg School of Public Health. Dr. Moran earned her ScD in Nutrition from the Harvard T.H. Chan School of Public Health in 2018 and her MPH/RDN from the New York University Global Institute of Public Health in 2011. Her research and teaching center on the identification and adoption of effective public health policies to promote equitable access to healthful food, reduce food insecurity, and prevent diet-related diseases. Before coming to the Bloomberg School of Public Health, Dr. Moran worked in the Nutrition Strategy Program at the New York City Department of Health & Mental Hygiene, where she implemented and evaluated New York City's Healthy Hospital Food Initiative. She enjoys collaborating with government agencies on nutrition programs and policies, and she has consulted on several projects, including the New York City Food Standards, the New York State Prevention Agenda, and the National Salt and Sugar Reduction Initiative.

Christina Roberto, Ph.D., is the Mitchell J. Blutt and Margo Krody Blutt Presidential Associate Professor of Health Policy at the Perelman School of Medicine at the University of Pennsylvania. She is also an Associate Director of the Center for Health Incentives and Behavioral Economics at Penn. Dr. Roberto is a psychologist and epidemiologist whose research aims to identify and understand factors that promote unhealthy eating behaviors and design interventions to improve eating habits. In her work, she draws upon the fields of psychology, behavioral economics, epidemiology, and public health to answer research questions that can provide policymakers and institutions with science-based guidance. Dr. Roberto has an undergraduate degree in Psychology from Princeton University where she graduated magna cum laude. She earned a joint-PhD at Yale University in clinical psychology and chronic disease epidemiology. Dr. Roberto completed her clinical internship at the Yale School of Medicine and was a Robert Wood Johnson Foundation Health and Society Scholar at the Harvard T.H. Chan School of Public Health.

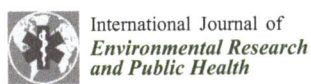

Editorial

The Retail Food Environment: Time for a Change

Alyssa Moran [1,*] and Christina Roberto [2]

1. Department of Health Policy and Management, Johns Hopkins Bloomberg School of Public Health, Baltimore, MD 21205, USA
2. Department of Health Policy and Medical Ethics, Perelman School of Medicine at the University of Pennsylvania, Philadelphia, PA 19104, USA; croberto@pennmedicine.penn.edu
* Correspondence: amoran10@jhu.edu; Tel.: +1-410-614-0256

Received: 24 November 2020; Accepted: 26 November 2020; Published: 28 November 2020

1. Introduction

Food retailers, manufacturers, and distributors exert powerful influence on our food choices through decisions about stocking, pricing, marketing, and promotional practices [1]. Such practices often encourage selection and consumption of foods and beverages that are nutritionally poor [2] and may exacerbate the global burden of obesity and diet-related chronic diseases [3]. Interventions that alter the retail food environment to support healthy eating are urgently needed. In the United States, this is particularly pressing in communities of color, rural areas, and low-income neighborhoods, where unhealthy food marketing is highly prevalent [4]. In this Special Issue, we summarize the current evidence on the links between the food retail environment and health behaviors and outcomes and identify future research priorities.

This Special Issue was borne out of a convening held in January 2020, sponsored by Center for Science in the Public Interest, The Food Trust, the Johns Hopkins Bloomberg School of Public Health, and Healthy Eating Research (HER), a national program of the Robert Wood Johnson Foundation. Recognizing that sustainable interventions require cross-sector and multidisciplinary collaboration, meeting attendees included food industry representatives, non-profit organizations, and researchers spanning a wide range of disciplines relevant to healthy food retail. The objective of the convening was to develop a national healthy retail research agenda, which aimed to identify effective retail interventions to support nutritious food choices, with an intentional focus on reducing disparities in food marketing and access. This Special Issue includes research commissioned for or resulting from the meeting, including one paper describing the research agenda, one communication, three empirical papers, and four reviews. Papers are organized into four sections: (1) the retail food environment and industry practices; (2) consumer food shopping patterns; (3) effectiveness of retail interventions to support healthy eating; and (4) the future of food retail research.

2. The Retail Food Environment and Industry Practices

Relationships between the retail food environment and consumer food and beverage choices are complex. Prior conceptual frameworks do not fully capture factors influencing where retailers locate, which products they choose to sell, how products are marketed or merchandised in the store, and how these decisions interact with other factors to influence consumer selection. To fill this gap, Hecht and colleagues [5] review industry and academic literature to catalogue trade promotion practices used by manufacturers and distributors to influence retail food marketing strategies and to examine the effects of these practices on consumer purchases. The authors identify four categories of trade promotion practices—category management, cooperative advertising, price discounts, and slotting allowances—which influence pricing, placement, and promotion of products by retailers.

The categories of promotional practices catalogued by Hecht and colleagues are incorporated into two new conceptual frameworks describing the influence of the retail food environment on consumer behaviors. The Retail Food Environment and Customer Interaction Model, put forth by Winkler and colleagues [6], conceptualizes the retail food environment as a complex dynamic system, including reciprocal relationships between characteristics of retailers (sources, actors, business models) and customers (individual, interpersonal, and household factors), as well as macro-level contexts, such as policies and economic systems, that influence these relationships. The authors contend that interactions between these factors can influence important population outcomes, which include health, but also food security, environmental sustainability, business sustainability, and food sovereignty, equity, and justice. A second conceptual framework, developed by Khandpur and colleagues [7], takes a closer look at the online food retail environment. This framework, which is nested in the socioecological model, identifies both consumer- and retailer-level influences along the online path-to-purchase, including consumer demographic characteristics, preferences, and past behaviors, as well as equity and transparency of retailer policies and practices, which interact to influence decision-making. The framework draws from multiple disciplines, emphasizing the dynamic nature of personalized marketing by retailers and customizable website content, which separates food marketing in the online setting from that within the brick-and-mortar store.

3. Consumer Food Shopping Patterns

This Special Issue includes research designed to better understand consumer food shopping patterns, particularly across understudied populations. Original research by Lacko and colleagues [8] updates and extends prior work examining trends in grocery sales since 2012. The authors document the top sources of calories across different retail store types, break this down by urban or rural household residence and household income, and then examine the interaction between household income and urbanicity. Their research reveals differences in nutritional quality of packaged foods purchased across store types, with purchases of lower nutritional quality made at dollar stores and convenience stores compared to club stores and supermarkets. They find that rural shoppers purchase more calories per person per day from mass merchandisers and dollar stores compared to urban households. The paper reports little influence of urbanicity or household income on food purchases within store type.

The new empirical data presented by Lacko and colleagues is complemented by a systematic review by Singleton and colleagues [9] that was designed to summarize studies examining the influence of intersectionality—interactions between race/ethnicity, socioeconomic status, and geographic location—on consumer food purchasing. The paper reviews literature describing differences in food purchases within attributes like socioeconomic status but reveals a dearth of studies examining how sociodemographic factors interact. In their paper, they propose areas where future work is needed to address these major gaps to better inform efforts to implement healthy food retail strategies in underserved, low-resourced, and marginalized communities.

4. Effectiveness of Retail Interventions to Support Healthy Eating

This Special Issue includes two systematic reviews examining effects of interventions to support healthy eating. Karpyn and colleagues [10] review 64 in-store marketing studies published between 2010 and 2019 intending to promote nutritious food choices. The authors find that in-store interventions are often multi-component, including changes to in-store promotions (e.g., signage or shelf labels), pricing (e.g., discounts or subsidies), placement (e.g., product prominence or display); and/or product (e.g., availability within the store). Most interventions are associated with at least one positive outcome related to dietary behaviors; however, few studies have used strong experimental or quasi-experimental designs or objective outcome measures.

A systematic review written by Moran and colleagues [11] complements the work of Karpyn and colleagues by examining the effects of government policy interventions. The paper reviews 147 academic papers describing associations between governmental policies intended to promote healthy food and beverage choices in supermarkets and a wide range of individual, retailer, and community health outcomes. Findings show positive associations between three policies and dietary behaviors: financial incentives for fruits and vegetables provided to low-income households, revisions to the USDA Special Supplemental Nutrition Program for Women, Infants, and Children food package, and sugary drink excise taxes. Two policies—increases in Supplemental Nutrition Assistance Program (SNAP) benefits and incentives for supermarkets to open in underserved areas—show limited effects on dietary intake and food purchasing, but may improve food security. The paper identifies significant gaps in knowledge about children, rural populations, and people living in the Midwestern and Southern United States.

5. The Future of Food Retail Research

The final full-length paper in the series by Hecht and colleagues [12] describes the scope of the healthy retail research agenda, which includes ten priority areas designed to understand current food retail environments and their influence on consumer behavior and effectiveness of interventions to create healthier retail environments. The paper also details the agenda-setting process, and recommendations from expert stakeholders on healthy retail research approaches, data sources, and areas of future research.

The series is then completed with a timely communication from Leone and colleagues [13] that reflects on the impact COVID-19 has had on food systems and environments in the U.S. Using Winkler and colleagues' Retail Food Environment and Customer Interaction Model, the authors describe how COVID-19 has impacted policies, retailers, and customer experiences and dietary intake. The commentary also discusses how the COVID-19 pandemic has further exacerbated long-standing inequities in food insecurity, food access, and health across race, ethnicity, class and geography. The authors then identify a series of research priorities that are needed to create a more just and equitable retail food environment and improve the country's emergency preparedness.

6. Conclusions

Taken together, these papers advance our understanding of the complex relationships between the retail food environment, dietary behaviors, and the public's health. This Special Issue highlights substantial gaps in our knowledge of consumer food purchasing patterns and impacts of healthy retail interventions by race, ethnicity, class and geography—research that is critical for addressing health inequities. The culminating healthy retail research agenda synthesizes this work and details a path forward, describing partnerships, data sources, research methods, and priority questions for advancing the field.

Author Contributions: A.M. and C.R. co-conceived and co-wrote the paper. All authors have read and agreed to the published version of the manuscript.

Funding: Publication fees were supported by Healthy Eating Research, a national program of the Robert Wood Johnson Foundation.

Acknowledgments: The authors would like to thank the Healthy Eating Research team, particularly Kirsten Arm, Megan Lott, Lauren Dawson, and Mary Story, for their support in creating this Special Issue.

Conflicts of Interest: The authors declare no conflict of interest.

References

1. Glanz, K.; Bader, M.D.M.; Iyer, S. Retail grocery store marketing strategies and obesity. *Am. J. Prev. Med.* **2012**, *42*, 503–512. [CrossRef] [PubMed]
2. Rivlin, G. *Rigged: Supermarket Shelves for Sale*; Center for Science in the Public Interest: Washington, DC, USA, 2016. Available online: https://cspinet.org/sites/default/files/attachment/Rigged%20report_0.pdf (accessed on 27 November 2020).
3. Gortmaker, S.L.; Swinburn, B.; Levy, D.; Carter, R.; Mabry, P.L.; Finegood, D.; Huang, T.; Marsh, T.; Moodie, M.L. Changing the future of obesity: Science, policy, and action. *Lancet* **2011**, *378*, 838–847. [CrossRef]

4. Berkeley Media Studies Group. *The 4 PS of Marketing: Selling Junk Food to Communities of Color*; Berkeley Media Studies Group: Berkeley, CA, USA, 2019. Available online: http://www.bmsg.org/resources/publications/place-the-4-ps-of-marketing-selling-junk-food-to-communities-of-color/ (accessed on 27 November 2020).
5. Hecht, A.A.; Perez, C.L.; Polacsek, M.; Thorndike, A.N.; Franckle, R.L.; Moran, A.J. Influence of food and beverage companies on retailer marketing strategies and consumer behavior. *Int. J. Environ. Res. Public Health* **2020**, *17*, 7381. [CrossRef] [PubMed]
6. Winkler, M.R.; Zenk, S.N.; Baquero, B.; Anderson Steeves, E.; Fleischhacker, S.E.; Gittelsohn, J.; Leone, L.A.; Racine, E.F. A model depicting the retail food environment and customer interactions: Components, outcomes, and future directions. *Int. J. Environ. Res. Public Health* **2020**, *17*, 7591. [CrossRef] [PubMed]
7. Khandpur, N.; Zatz, L.Y.; Bleich, S.N.; Taillie, L.S.; Orr, J.A.; Rimm, E.B.; Moran, A.J. Supermarkets in cyberspace: A conceptual framework to capture the influence of online food retail environments on consumer behavior. *Int. J. Environ. Res. Public Health* **2020**, *17*, 8639. [CrossRef] [PubMed]
8. Lacko, A.; Ng, S.W.; Popkin, B. Urban vs. rural socioeconomic differences in the nutritional quality of household packaged food purchases by store type. *Int. J. Environ. Res. Public Health* **2020**, *17*, 7637. [CrossRef] [PubMed]
9. Singleton, C.R.; Winkler, M.; Houghtaling, B.; Adeyemi, O.S.; Roehll, A.M.; Pionke, J.J.; Anderson Steeves, E. Understanding the intersection of race/ethnicity, socioeconomic status, and geographic location: A scoping review of U.S. consumer food purchasing. *Int. J. Environ. Res. Public Health* **2020**, *17*, 7677. [CrossRef] [PubMed]
10. Karpyn, A.; McCallops, K.; Wolgast, H.; Glanz, K. Improving consumption and purchases of healthier foods in retail environments: A systematic review. *Int. J. Environ. Res. Public Health* **2020**, *17*, 7524. [CrossRef]
11. Moran, A.J.; Gu, Y.; Clynes, S.; Goheer, A.; Roberto, C.A.; Palmer, A. Associations between governmental policies to improve the nutritional quality of supermarket purchases and individual, retailer, and community health outcomes: An integrative review. *Int. J. Environ. Res. Public Health* **2020**, *17*, 7493. [CrossRef] [PubMed]
12. Hecht, A.A.; Lott, M.M.; Arm, K.; Story, M.T.; Snyder, E.; Wootan, M.G.; Moran, A.J. Developing a national research agenda to support healthy food retail. *Int. J. Environ. Res. Public Health* **2020**, *17*, 8141. [CrossRef] [PubMed]
13. Leone, L.A.; Fleischhacker, S.; Anderson-Steeves, B.; Harper, K.; Winkler, M.; Racine, E.F.; Baquero, B.; Gittelsohn, J. Healthy food retail during the COVID-19 pandemic: Challenges and future directions. *Int. J. Environ. Res. Public Health* **2020**, *17*, 7397. [CrossRef] [PubMed]

Publisher's Note: MDPI stays neutral with regard to jurisdictional claims in published maps and institutional affiliations.

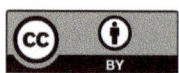

© 2020 by the authors. Licensee MDPI, Basel, Switzerland. This article is an open access article distributed under the terms and conditions of the Creative Commons Attribution (CC BY) license (http://creativecommons.org/licenses/by/4.0/).

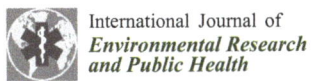

Article

Supermarkets in Cyberspace: A Conceptual Framework to Capture the Influence of Online Food Retail Environments on Consumer Behavior

Neha Khandpur [1,2,*], Laura Y. Zatz [2], Sara N. Bleich [2], Lindsey Smith Taillie [3], Jennifer A. Orr [4], Eric B. Rimm [2] and Alyssa J. Moran [5]

1. University of São Paulo, Av. Dr. Arnaldo, 715 Cerqueira César, São Paulo SP 01246-904, Brazil
2. Harvard T.H. Chan School of Public Health, Harvard University, 677 Huntington Ave, Boston, MA 02115, USA; laz491@mail.harvard.edu (L.Y.Z.); sbleich@hsph.harvard.edu (S.N.B.); erimm@hsph.harvard.edu (E.B.R.)
3. Gillings School of Global Public Health, University of North Carolina at Chapel Hill, 135 Dauer Dr, Chapel Hill, NC 27599, USA; taillie@unc.edu
4. University of Pennsylvania, 423 Guardian Drive, Philadelphia, PA 19104-6021, USA; Jennifer.Orr@pennmedicine.upenn.edu
5. Bloomberg School of Public Health, Johns Hopkins University, Baltimore, MD 21218, USA; amoran10@jhu.edu
* Correspondence: neha.khandpur@usp.br or nek564@mail.harvard.edu

Received: 27 October 2020; Accepted: 16 November 2020; Published: 20 November 2020

Abstract: The rapid increase in online shopping and the extension of online food purchase and delivery services to federal nutrition program participants highlight the need for a conceptual framework capturing the influence of online food retail environments on consumer behaviors. This study aims to develop such a conceptual framework. To achieve this, mixed methods were used, including: (1) a literature review and development of an initial framework; (2) key informant interviews; (3) pilot testing and refinement of the draft framework; and (4) a group discussion with experts to establish content validity. The resulting framework captures both consumer- and retailer-level influences across the entire shopping journey, as well as the broader social, community, and policy context. It identifies important factors such as consumer demographic characteristics, preferences, past behaviors, and retailer policies and practices. The framework also emphasizes the dynamic nature of personalized marketing by retailers and customizable website content, and captures equity and transparency in retailer policies and practices. The framework draws from multiple disciplines, providing a foundation for understanding the impact of online food retail on dietary behaviors. It can be utilized to inform public health interventions, retailer practices, and governmental policies for creating healthy and equitable online food retail environments.

Keywords: online food retail; conceptual framework; consumer behavior; food choices; online shopping; retailer policies

1. Introduction

Online food retail is an increasingly popular means of acquiring food and is expected to grow rapidly over the coming decade. In 2017, online food retail represented $13 billion in sales [1] and was projected to increase to $100 billion [2], reaching 70% of U.S. shoppers by 2025 [3]. The 2019 coronavirus (COVID-19) pandemic has accelerated this growth and served as a catalyst for retailers to increase investments in their online food retail infrastructure and services. In April 2020, U.S. shoppers spent $5.3 billion on online food purchases, an increase of 37% from the previous month [4,5]. Based on this recent surge, revised growth projections estimate a nine-fold increase in online grocery purchases between 2017 and 2023 [6].

Online food retail has also emerged as an important avenue to improve food access. In 2018, the United States Department of Agriculture (USDA) selected 10 retailers in 9 states for a two-year Online Purchasing Pilot ("online Electronic Benefits Transfer (EBT)") to test the use of Supplemental Nutrition Assistance Program (SNAP) benefits as payment for online food purchases [7]. The affordability, access, and delivery inequities, as well as the disproportionate food security challenges faced by low-income communities have been brought to the fore during the pandemic [8], prompting the USDA to expand online EBT both geographically and across a wider range of retailers. At the time of writing, at least 40 states had been approved to participate in online EBT, with several others in the planning stage [9]. The Special Supplemental Nutrition Program for Women, Infants, and Children (WIC) is also considering how to offer online food purchasing options to its participants [10].

These shifts in consumer food purchase behaviors, the increasing investment in online infrastructure, and the expansion of online food purchasing to participants in federal programs, highlight the need for an assessment of the online food retail environment. A substantial and growing body of evidence captures the influence of in-store food marketing on consumer purchases [11,12]. In comparison, little is known about the relationship between the online food retail environment and consumer food choices. Some evidence supports the influence of social, contextual, and demographic factors on consumers' use of online platforms for food purchases [13–15]. Retailer-level factors like credibility, product freshness, product quality and price have also been shown to predict online purchasing [16]. However, there is a dearth of information about factors influencing the spectrum of online consumer behaviors which is important for understanding how online food retailers influence consumer food purchases and subsequent dietary intake and health outcomes.

What is currently lacking is an integrated framework capturing both consumer- and retailer-level factors and their interaction that influence consumer behaviors within online environments. The few existing frameworks focus on specific consumer determinants like their attitudes, privacy concerns, social influences, facilitating conditions, hedonic motivations, and perceived risk or satisfaction with the online experience [17–19]. Retailer influence is incompletely captured or mentioned briefly [20]. The models do not illustrate the interactive and dynamic nature of online food retail platforms or the active and responsive role that consumers play in shaping their food purchase experience. Existing frameworks are also explicitly geared towards retaining and expanding the consumer base or maximizing profits [21]; they are not designed to study the effects these platforms have on dietary behaviors or health. Perhaps most revealing is the concentration of this literature in the fields of marketing, retail, decision sciences, and informatics; studies are largely absent in the public health domain.

In the absence of a comprehensive conceptual framework that looks at consumer grocery purchase behaviors it becomes impossible to systematically study the effect of food retail environments on food choices. Such a framework is crucial for informing public health interventions, guidelines, retailer practices, and governmental policies to create healthy and equitable online food retail environments. To address this gap in the literature, the present study aims to develop and refine a conceptual framework capturing factors that influence consumer food purchase behaviors within online food retail environments. For the purposes of this study, online food retail environments were described as websites providing click-and-collect (i.e., order online and pick up at the store) or food delivery services. 'Retailers' include e-commerce platforms hosted by the retailer themselves or by a third-party vendor (e.g., Instacart).

2. Materials and Methods

The development and refinement of the conceptual framework was guided by the approach suggested by Jabareen, 2009 [22], and involved extensive reading and categorizing of data; identifying concepts; deconstructing, categorizing, synthesizing, and integrating concepts; and validating the final framework. To achieve this, mixed methods were used, including:

1. A literature review and development of an initial framework
2. Key informant interviews
3. Pilot testing and refinement of the draft framework
4. Group discussion with experts to establish content validity

The study methodology was reviewed and determined to be non-human subjects research by the Institutional Review Board at the Johns Hopkins Bloomberg School of Public Health.

2.1. Literature Review

A scoping review was undertaken between April and June of 2019 to identify peer-reviewed and grey literature, in English, on the attributes, preferences, and shopping behaviors of consumers that make purchases online, consumer interaction with and acceptance of technology, online and in-store food marketing and merchandising, and design of online retail environments. Databases were searched from January 2009 to May 2019 (ProQuest, PubMed, and Thomson ONE) using combinations of the keywords *food, grocer*, supermarket*, retail*, shop*, store*, purchas*, buy*, online, ecommerce (or e-commerce), internet,* and *web*. Search results were supplemented with health agency reports, trade publications, and industry reports from 2015 to 2019. Reference lists from peer-reviewed publications were also scanned. While peer-reviewed literature was not restricted by geographic location, only US-focused analyst reports and trade publications were included to ensure contextual relevance. Paper titles and abstracts were screened. A total of 136 industry reports and 97 peer-reviewed papers informed the development of the draft framework.

2.2. Key Informant Interviews

We interviewed seven experts in grocery merchandizing and marketing, e-commerce and online retail, behavioral psychology, public policy, computer science and data privacy and digital marketing. Experts were identified through a combination of known contacts, through their published work, or were referred to by other experts during interviews. The interviews were conducted in person or via teleconference by a member of the research team and lasted 45–60 min.

The interview began with an overview of the objectives of the study. Experts were presented with the draft framework and asked: (i) for their feedback on the extent to which it captured their understanding of factors influencing consumer food choices when shopping online; (ii) to identify constructs that could be improved or simplified; and (iii) for additional constructs that should be included. Follow-up questions were tailored to each key informant's area of expertise. For example, an expert in computer science and engineering was asked an additional question about when and how personal data are collected from consumers along the path to purchase. Experts in food retail marketing were asked how personal data are used to adapt online marketing practices to specific consumers. Insights were requested on how the key domains influenced one another. Suggestions were incorporated, and the framework was refined after each interview.

2.3. Pilot Testing

Study researchers (A.J.M., N.K.) independently tested the internal consistency of the conceptual framework by using it to guide a mock shopping exercise. This was done to identify additional concepts that may have been missed during the literature review and the key informant interview, but not with the aim of formally testing the framework. An online shopping account was created at two U.S. online food retailers. Researchers navigated each store's website, browsed through their departments, added three grocery items to the shopping cart, and proceeded to the checkout. The applicability of the conceptual framework to the experience of a consumer searching for and selecting food was discussed in detail. Revisions to the framework were incorporated as necessary.

2.4. Expert Discussion

A teleconference discussion was convened with six members of the Healthy Food Retail Working Group to determine the content validity of the conceptual framework. This group is a collaborative effort of the Robert Wood Johnson Foundation's Healthy Eating Research program and the Centers for Disease Control and Prevention's Nutrition and Obesity Policy Research and Evaluation Network. Members include researchers and technical experts working on healthy food retail and related areas.

To engage fully with the framework, members of the Working Group were asked to undertake a mock shopping exercise, similar to the one conducted by the study authors, two weeks prior to the call. A Qualtrics form was created to guide the sequence of product searching and selection activities and to record feedback. After selecting an online food retailer from a list of 21 options, members navigated to the grocery department homepage, the breakfast cereal department page, and the product pages of two specific brands of bread and canned fish. They documented marketing strategies, customizable features, tools, options, and multimedia content on each of these webpages. Members also recorded ease of navigation and site policies. Their feedback from this exercise was discussed in the teleconference, during which the purpose of the research was clarified, and a draft of the conceptual framework (including what the concepts represent and how they relate to each other) was presented. Members were asked whether the current framework captured their understanding of the range of factors influencing consumer behavior in the online store and for ideas for improvement. Notes from the discussion were recorded, and relevant revisions were incorporated into the framework.

3. Results

3.1. Evolution of the Conceptual Framework

Insights from the literature review informed the development of a draft framework that captured the influence of consumer characteristics, online food marketing, and retailer and website characteristics on online grocery shopping intention. Feedback from the key informant interviews added further detail by delineating the different stages of the online shopping process, the sequence of online consumer behaviors, the key role of personalized marketing, relationships between online retailers and manufacturers, disclosure of sponsored content, factors influencing site design, and the use of personal information in customizing the platform.

The pilot test provided additional insights into retailer characteristics related to membership and loyalty programs, privacy and data use, and order payment, fulfillment, and collection. This exercise also differentiated the static versus the dynamic elements of the online platform (i.e., attributes of the site that are consistent for all consumers versus those that can be personalized by the retailer or customized by the consumer), differences in site functionality as viewed by an anonymous shopper versus a registered shopper, and marketing strategies employed at checkout.

Healthy Food Retail Working Group members acknowledged the detail and clarity of the current version of the framework and agreed that it captured relevant constructs that influence consumer food choice in online environments. Their feedback focused on the applicability of the conceptual framework to specific subgroups of consumers (e.g., SNAP and WIC beneficiaries), retailers (e.g., small stores), and online formats (e.g., mobile applications). These ideas were discussed, and relevant constructs in the framework were added or made more salient.

The final framework combined elements of the Technology Acceptance Model, consumer behavior and decision-making frameworks, brick-and-mortar marketing categories (product, price, placement, and promotion) [11,23], key themes from the data privacy and e-commerce literature, and constructs described in existing food environment measures (e.g., Nutrition Environment Measures in Stores) [18,20,24–30].

3.2. Description of the Conceptual Framework

3.2.1. Path to Purchase

Central to the conceptual framework is the sequence of consumer behaviors involved in online grocery shopping. This Path to Purchase consists of four stages—Pre-Shop, Online Shopping, Pick-Up or Delivery, and Post-Shop—encompassing six behaviors. Under Pre-Shop behaviors, the consumer selects an online retailer. He/she then searches for or discovers, selects, and purchases food (Online Shopping). The consumer receives the order (Pick-Up or Delivery) and prepares and consumes the food or/and discards it (Post-Shop). The quality of the consumer's experience engaging in each of these behaviors determines their overall satisfaction with the retailer and likelihood of shopping again.

Consumer behaviors are influenced by consumer- and retailer-level attributes, presented above and below the Path to Purchase in Figure 1. Attributes presented in solid outline are not likely to change over the shopping journey (static domains). Attributes presented in dashed outline are likely to change over the duration of a single shopping visit (dynamic domains). The cross-cutting themes of Equity and Transparency influence retailer-level factors, while Social, Community, and Policy Context influences both retailer- and consumer-level factors.

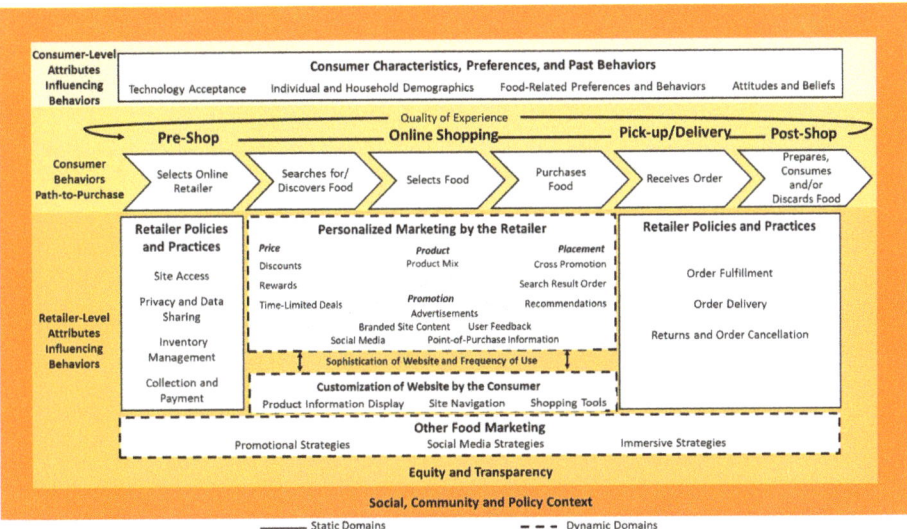

Figure 1. Consumer behavior in the online food retail environment.

3.2.2. Consumer-Level Attributes

Consumer Characteristics, Preferences, and Past Behaviors: this domain encompasses consumers' Technology Acceptance, Individual and Household Demographics, Food-Related Preferences and Behaviors, and Attitudes and Beliefs (detailed in Table 1). These attributes may influence decision-making at each stage of food selection and purchase. For instance, consumers with positive experiences with e-commerce and online food retail may be more likely to select an online retailer. Individual and demographic characteristics such as age, education, income, household composition (e.g., having young children) and location also influence the likelihood of shopping online, the platform selected, the foods purchased, and their preparation and consumption.

3.2.3. Retailer-Level Attributes

Retailer Policies and Practices: they include static attributes of online retailers that may influence retailer selection, food receipt, and food preparation and consumption. During retailer selection, Site Access policies include information required to purchase groceries online, retailer incentives offered to first-time users (e.g., free trials), membership requirements prior to shopping, and delivery service areas (e.g., zip codes served). Privacy and Data Sharing policies include the terms and conditions that govern the collection, tracking, storage, use, and sharing of personal information by the retailer. Policies on Inventory Management guide the availability of products and brands, pricing strategy, and accuracy of inventory tracking, while policies on Collection and Payment determine the payment options accepted by the retailer (e.g., SNAP), the integration of loyalty and reward programs, fees for delivery and restocking, and delivery options (e.g., availability of click and collect or delivery).

Table 1. Description of consumer- and retailer-level domains and constructs that influence consumer behavior in the online food retail environment. EBT, Electronic Benefits Transfer, GMO, genetically modified organism.

Consumer-Level Attributes		
Domain *Stage of Path to Purchase* (Static vs. Dynamic)	Construct	Description and Examples
Consumer Characteristics Preferences and Past Behaviors *Pre-Shop Online Shopping Pick-up/Delivery Post-Shop* (Static)	Technology Acceptance	Associated factors include familiarity with internet technology, perceived ease of use, risks associated with online food retail, concerns with web security and privacy of personal and financial information, past exposure to online food retail, safe and reliable access to the internet
	Individual and Household Demographics	Factors include age, sex, income, education level, employment, disability, injuries resulting from accidents, urban/rural residence, geographic location, distance from physical store, price sensitivity, marital status, family culture, household size, and social class
	Food-Related Preferences and Behaviors	Associated factors include familiarity with product, health consciousness, perceived need to inspect item or assess sensory properties prior to purchase, dietary preferences and allergies, perceived safety of delivered foods, perceived costs, and value of online versus in-store products
	Attitudes and Beliefs	These encompass consumer beliefs about the online retailer's brand image, online service quality, perceived importance of social contact while grocery shopping, time savings, convenience, perceived cognitive effort versus gain, perceived comparative advantage compared to brick-and-mortar stores

Table 1. Cont.

Domain Stage of Path to Purchase (Static vs. Dynamic)	Construct	Description and Examples
Retailer Policies and Practices *Pre-Shop* (Static)	Site Access	Associated policies include ease of initiating and terminating grocery purchase services (online sign-up policies, membership cancellation procedures), referral schemes and incentives that allow risk-free trial of the online platform, multi-channel presence to help streamline access to food retailer services through mobile applications, websites, and the physical store
	Privacy and Data Sharing	These policies determine how consumer data on purchase patterns, personal demographic information, etc., are stored, protected, and used by the retailer and/or shared with third parties
	Inventory Management	Associated practices encompass product availability, assortment and variety of fresh and packaged goods, variety among the brands stocked, similarity in online–offline assortment, product price point, dynamic pricing strategies, similarity in online–offline pricing and promotions
	Collection and Payment	Policies cover consumer-friendly pick-up, delivery, and payment (no cost delivery, pick-up options, waiver of fees for purchases over a designated value or those made at a certain frequency, etc.), multi-option payment channels, acceptance of EBT, loyalty programs linked to redeemable rewards
Retailer Policies and Practices *Pick-up/Delivery* *Post-Shop* (Static)	Order Fulfillment	Policies determine the concordance between items delivered compared to items ordered, item quantity, freshness, and the physical condition in which the grocery items arrive, packaging of products, handling of stock-outs, and appropriateness and price of product substitutions
	Order Delivery	Policies cover flexibility in choosing type of collection (click-and-collect versus delivery), availability of delivery slots, length of delivery slot, delivery coordination, the ability to track the real-time location of the groceries purchased, convenient and safe drop-off location options (doorstep delivery, key locations within the community)

Table 1. *Cont.*

Retailer-Level Attributes		
Domain *Stage of Path to Purchase* (Static vs. Dynamic)	**Construct**	**Description and Examples**
	Returns and Order Cancellation	Associated policies address unsatisfactory deliveries, incorrect orders, cancelled orders, and requests for refunds or store credit
Personalized Marketing by Retailers *Online Shopping* (Dynamic)	Product—Product Mix	These include the variety, brands, and assortment of products the consumer can view on the online platform
	Price—Discounts	Examples include lower prices on targeted products (discounts, two-for-one deals, cost-saving strategies) which may be open to all customers or exclusive to members of loyalty programs
	Price—Rewards	Rewards include links to coupons, loyalty programs, membership rewards, and other redeemable rewards
	Price—Time-Limited Deals	These include special deals that are valid for a set period (24 h, 3 h, etc.) or weekly flyers meant to incentivize food purchase within a specific period of time
	Placement—Cross-Promotions	Examples include marketing of complementary products anchored to a previous search or to items already in the shopping cart (milk and eggs suggested on a search results page for bread or milk suggested at checkout when cereal is in the shopping cart)
	Placement—Search Result Order	Examples include non-random presentation of products (search results ordered by the most expensive products or display of sponsored products before other items)
	Placement—Recommendations	Examples include seasonal products, popular items, recently viewed products, suggestions based on past purchases, recommended product/brand swaps, or impulse buys (cookies or candy recommended at checkout)
	Promotions—Advertisements	These include products on paid banner advertisements or title cards (large panel of images or text at the top of a page) displayed on the website that link to a separate landing page featuring the sponsored product

Table 1. Cont.

Domain Stage of Path to Purchase (Static vs. Dynamic)	Construct	Description and Examples
	Retailer-Level Attributes	
	Promotions—Branded Site Content	Examples include branded products integrated into the existing site content, like department images (branded cereal displayed to indicate the breakfast cereal department), branded recipes or meal solutions (branded marinara sauce depicted in a lasagna recipe), promoted product swaps, and retailer-generated shopping lists
	Promotions—User Feedback	This includes highlighting consumer product reviews and ratings to promote the selection of certain products
	Promotions—Social Media	Examples include links to the retailer's Instagram, Facebook, or other social media pages promoting specific brands or products and opportunities for consumers to share purchased products through personal social media accounts
	Promotions—Point-of-purchase Information	These include labels, nutrient and health claims (non-GMO, whole-grain), and other product descriptors (product source, organic) that may be personalized to promote the selection of certain products
Customization of Website by Consumer *Online Shopping* (Dynamic)	Product Information Display	Functional features on the webpage may allow consumers to filter products based on pre-selected information about their allergens, ingredients, nutrition facts, nutrition rating systems, country of origin, product reviews, and ratings based on their preferences
	Site Navigation	Examples include tools and tutorials to help consumers navigate the website, browse through departments, engage with available features to customize the 'look and feel' of their online shopping interface (change display size, image size, orientation)
	Shopping Tools	These tools increase the convenience of product search and selection by allowing consumers to choose their preferred setting to create and save shopping lists, notes and wish lists, and allow for product/brand comparisons

Table 1. Cont.

Domain Stage of Path to Purchase (Static vs. Dynamic)	Retailer-Level Attributes	
	Construct	Description and Examples
Other Food Marketing Pre-Shop Online Shopping Pick-up/Delivery Post-Shop (Dynamic)	Promotional Strategies	Examples include advertisements, sponsorship, endorsements, search result optimization
	Social Media Strategies	These include strategies that utilize social media content, podcasts, videos, or user-generated content
	Immersive Strategies	These include strategies like advergames, interactive advertisements to increase the marketing that the consumer is exposed to, while increasing consumer site engagement

The Pick-Up and Post-Shop behaviors are likely to be determined by Retailer Policies and Practices that govern Order Fulfillment, Order Delivery, and Returns and Order Cancellation. Policies on Order Fulfillment include the price and appropriateness of product substitutions during stock-outs and the quality of the food received. The availability of convenient time slots, delivery coordination (e.g., text message communication, online order tracking), and the availability of secure delivery options are examples of policies associated with Order Delivery. Policies determining the ease of cancelling incomplete or incorrect orders of items purchased online (e.g., store credit, vouchers, full refund) relate to Returns and Order Cancellation.

Personalized Marketing by Retailers: a consumer's search, selection and purchase of food are influenced by factors within the dynamic domain of Personalized Marketing. These marketing strategies are based on personal information provided by the consumer when registering with the online platform and from past purchases and browsing history. They may also be based on consumer data purchased by the retailer, shared by third parties, or automatically collected upon visiting the site (e.g., IP address, operating system). The consumer, either knowingly (by actively agreeing to) or unknowingly (by using the site, by signing-up for an account or a loyalty card that activates implicit agreements) or without full knowledge of the implications, allows retailers to use various sources of information to create a tailored experience.

Personalized Marketing maps onto the marketing mix of Product, Price, Placement, and Promotion ("the 4Ps"), but manifests differently in the online food retail environment than in brick-and-mortar stores [11]. Product-related personalized marketing includes Product Mix or the range and variety of products the consumer can view and explore. In the online space, this may include personalized storefronts created for the consumer which display products aligning with the consumer's revealed preferences (e.g., vegan, gluten-free). Product Price relates to different types of Discounts, Rewards, or Time-Limited Special Deals offered. These strategies can be personalized (e.g., the discounted products or discount amount is tailored) and often interact with Placement or Promotional strategies (e.g., recommended products may also be discounted). Under Placement, Cross-Promotion describes suggested complementary products, Search Result Ordering describes the default appearance of products (e.g., higher cost or sponsored products may appear before other options), and Recommendations captures the strategies used to increase exposure to featured, seasonal, or popular products on the site—all of which can be personalized to the consumer's preferences. Promotion refers to personalized marketing to increase consumer exposure to or visibility of sponsored products through Advertisements (e.g., title cards or banner advertisements), Branded Site Content, User Feedback (e.g., product ratings and reviews), links to Social Media, and other Point-of-Purchase Information (e.g., product labels).

These strategies are frequently used in combination to influence product discovery, selection and purchase on the website homepage, search results page, product page, or at checkout.

Customization of the Website by the Consumer: this is the other dynamic domain that influences the search, selection, and purchase of food and includes Product Information Display, Site Navigation, and Shopping Tools. These attributes allow consumers to change what nutrition information they see (Product Information Display), filter products based on preferred attributes, save shopping lists, or request certain product comparisons (Shopping Tools). Combined with tools and tutorials to ease website navigation (Site Navigation), website customization features can increase the convenience of product searches, enhance consumer engagement with the product catalogue and improve the quality of the food purchase experience.

Other Food Marketing: this dynamic domain includes Promotional Strategies, Social Media Strategies, and Immersive Strategies, recognizing that exposure to marketing in other settings (brick-and-mortar stores), through direct-to-consumer promotions, product endorsements, and sponsorships, and targeted marketing through social media platforms will affect food choices made online.

Sophistication of Website and Frequency of Use: technological progress in interface design, communications, and data security is likely to improve consumer trust and increase the volume and frequency of purchases made online. Advancements in personal data collection, advertising technology, purchase data analytics, and consumers' increased involvement in the co-creation of food retail platforms will allow retailers to better profile customers and more efficiently match them to products and promotions, increasing engagement. In this way, more sophisticated online platforms and frequent consumer visits will ensure greater personalization of retailer marketing strategies and a more customized website.

3.2.4. Cross-Cutting Domains

Equity and Transparency are fundamental to retailer engagement with the consumer. Equity refers to the differential impact of retailer policies and practices on the food behaviors and privacy of underserved populations (e.g., individuals and communities of Color, low-income households, older adults, people with disabilities, households in rural areas). For example, a consumer's ability to utilize online services may be affected by the retail service area, availability of convenient delivery slots, or accepted payment methods. A retailer's targeted and personalized marketing strategies may trigger impulse purchases or increase the basket size, differentially impacting low-income consumers, especially if the promoted products are of inferior nutritional quality. Transparency in policies and practices captures the retailer's clear and upfront disclosure of data collection, storage and use of data, surveillance methods, marketing, sponsorships, etc., that may consciously or unconsciously influence the consumer's choices along the Path to Purchase. For instance, disclosure of fees and hidden costs and collection of personal data prior to checkout may affect a consumer's choice of retailer. Disclosure of product sponsorship at point of purchase may affect product selection.

Social, Community, and Policy Context: this conceptual framework is nested in the socio-ecological model [31]. Consumer and Retailer-Level attributes are likely influenced by the social context (e.g., social norms, endorsements from trusted members of society) and the structural factors (community, institutional, and policy contexts) in which they are embedded. The surge in online grocery purchases resulting from the physical distancing measures implemented in 2020 is an example of how contextual factors can affect consumers behaviors. Similarly, the acceptance of SNAP benefits for online food purchases would first require a favorable state-level policy context (e.g., states need approval for use of EBT test cards) [7], before retailer policies can be implemented. In this way, the provision of certain services by retailers is very much dependent on the broader political context.

4. Discussion

This study presents a conceptual framework that captures factors influencing consumer behavior within online food retail environments. It also details the methodology for framework development and refinement—a process that identified and integrated evidence across multiple fields of study. The conceptual framework captures both consumer- and retailer-level influences across the entire Path to Purchase as well as the broader social, community, and policy context. Important static attributes of retailer policies and practices and consumer characteristics, preferences, and past behaviors are captured. The framework also emphasizes the dynamic attributes of the online platform, including those of personalized marketing by retailers, customization of the website content, navigation by the consumer, and the two-way interaction between these domains that enables a variety of online food retail interfaces uniquely tailored to consumer preferences.

This conceptual framework makes an important contribution to our understanding of the burgeoning field of online food retail. It serves as a foundation for a deeper study into the influences on consumer food purchase behaviors within online platforms and the interactions between them. To our knowledge, this is the first time that the relatively under-studied domains of personalization and customization of the online food retail environment or the domains of equity and transparency or the social, community, and the policy context, have been considered in any framework. Further investigation is certainly warranted. Future studies could use the framework to compare brick-and-mortar retailers and their online platforms to identify the convergence and divergence of consumer behaviors and retailer responses within these settings. The conceptual framework itself could be empirically tested to support its validity and better establish a hierarchy between attributes. Previous work has used structural equation modelling techniques to examine the hypothesized relationships between constructs in a proposed model and identify possible causal relationships between them [32]. While online retail platforms seem largely similar across contexts, a multi-country investigation of the framework's domains and their interactions would help confirm its applicability to different settings. Testing the framework among a diverse group of consumers to ensure that it adequately captures their selection and purchase experiences is also warranted.

The conceptual framework provides a foundation for understanding how a lack of transparency within online retail platforms could impact health equity. Indeed, if an equity lens is not applied in the development and implementation of retailer policies, online platforms may unintentionally widen disparities in healthy food access, affordability, and diet quality for vulnerable groups [33]. For instance, lack of transparency around membership fees, costs associated with platform access or delivery, accepted forms of payment, or inappropriate product substitutions for SNAP beneficiaries, may be more detrimental to a household with scarce resources to spend on food than to a household with greater financial resources. Concerns have also been raised about the surveillance practices, data collection, use, storage, sharing, and privacy measures of online retailers [34]. Current practices leverage digital tools to capture sensitive data on consumer purchases, location, and preferences or require people to share personal information to avail of savings [34]. This may facilitate targeted marketing on the basis of race, ethnicity, or socioeconomic status. Although targeted marketing is not harmful in and of itself, it may exacerbate existing disparities in diet-related chronic diseases if used to disproportionately advertise unhealthy products.

The framework may help to study the effect of predatory marketing tactics, similar to those employed across other digital media where communities of color are targeted with the least nutritious products [35]. Indeed, several forms of discriminatory and disparate advertising to vulnerable groups have been identified [34], exposure to which is likely to encourage unhealthy purchases. More research to identify and address these equity gaps is crucial to safeguarding the sub-groups that are disproportionately affected by adverse health outcomes and those that stand to benefit most from policy, systems, and environmental interventions that promote healthy eating.

Finally, the conceptual framework could be used to inform and evaluate public health interventions aimed at improving consumer food choices in the online food environment. On the policy and practice front, the framework could inform: (i) recommendations and standards for best practices related to online food marketing; (ii) specific guidance for online retailers to ensure policy transparency, equitable access, and assurance of privacy; (iii) tailored educational content for consumers unfamiliar with online grocery retail; and (iv) personalized nutrition education and communication. For example, nutrition interventions delivered via the online retail platform could offer personalized healthy shopping lists that draw on information about consumer preferences and budget constraints, offer personalized healthy recipes or meal solutions, or develop a personalized labeling campaign that makes specific nutritional attributes of a product more salient at the point of purchase. SNAP-Ed—SNAP's voluntary nutrition education program—could partner with online retailers to allow participants to interact with a registered dietitian in real time while food shopping. Local WIC agencies could work with online retailers to create a WIC-friendly web interface with WIC-eligible products, label products as being part of WIC food packages, and allow only WIC-approved substitutions in case of stock-outs.

This study does have its limitations. Despite a comprehensive approach to development, the resulting conceptual framework may not have captured all the elements of the online food retail environment. The descriptions of the constructs in the framework serve as examples and are not exhaustive. The literature reviewed was almost entirely from the US and Europe. Pilot testing and content validity were established for the US context. Therefore, it is possible that the framework may not adequately capture the online environments in other contexts and would need further testing to gauge applicability in different settings, including its applicability to food purchases made via mobile applications. Advances in technology will result in new and innovative features that will need to be incorporated into the evolving conceptual framework.

This study has several strengths. It leveraged multiple methods in the development and refinement of the framework, including key informant interviews, comprehensive systematic literature reviews, mock shopping exercises and group discussions, improving its validity. The framework development drew from multiple disciplines and benefited greatly from the insights of experts across different fields, allowing for an in-depth understanding of the factors influencing consumer purchases and underscoring the need for the public health community to collaborate with scientists and policymakers from non-traditional public health disciplines to map the influence of the online food environment. Finally, applying a public health perspective to the development of the framework expanded its utility in informing future interventions in this field.

5. Conclusions

This paper integrated multiple perspectives across a wide range of fields to develop a framework capturing both consumer- and retailer-level factors influencing consumer purchases in the online food retail environment, as well as the broader social, community, and policy context. It identifies important static factors and emphasizes the dynamic nature of personalized marketing by retailers and customizable website content. Equity and transparency in retailer policies and practices are also captured. Researchers, retailers, advocates and policymakers are encouraged to utilize the framework to guide the development and evaluation of interventions, policies, and practices in the online food retail space.

Author Contributions: Conceptualization—N.K., A.J.M.; methodological design—N.K., A.J.M., L.Y.Z.; data collection—L.Y.Z., J.A.O., N.K., A.J.M.; analysis—L.Y.Z., J.A.O., N.K., A.J.M.; interpretation—N.K., L.Y.Z., S.N.B., L.S.T., E.B.R., A.J.M.; original draft preparation—N.K., A.J.M.; review and editing—N.K., L.Y.Z., S.N.B., L.S.T., E.B.R., A.J.M.; project administration—A.J.M.; funding acquisition—A.J.M. All authors have read and agreed to the published version of the manuscript.

Funding: This research was supported by Healthy Eating Research, a national program of the Robert Wood Johnson Foundation.

Acknowledgments: The authors would like to acknowledge the contributions of members of the Healthy Food Retail Working Group (Lucia Leone, Diana Grigsby-Toussaint, Pasquale Rummo, Jared McGuirt, Alice Ammerman, Betsy Anderson Steeves, Stephanie Jilcott Pitts) in the development of the conceptual framework.

Conflicts of Interest: The authors declare no conflict of interest.

References

1. Business Insider. Online Grocery Shopping Report 2020: Market Stats and Delivery Trends for Ecommerce Groceries. 2020. Available online: https://www.businessinsider.com/online-grocery-report (accessed on 28 April 2020).
2. The Nielsen Company & Food Marketing Institute. The Digitally Engaged Food Shopper. 2017. Available online: www.fmi.org/digital-shopper (accessed on 20 April 2020).
3. Nielsen Company & Food Marketing Institute: 70% of Consumers will be Grocery Shopping Online by 2024. 2018. Available online: https://www.nielsen.com/us/en/press-releases/2018/fmi-and-nielsen-online-grocery-shopping-is-quickly-approaching-saturation/ (accessed on 29 April 2020).
4. Grocery Drive. Online Grocery Reaches New Heights in April. 2020. Available online: https://www.grocerydive.com/news/online-grocery-reaches-new-heights-in-april/576993/ (accessed on 30 April 2020).
5. Food Navigator. Online Grocery Sales Surge 37% in April to $5.3bn, Finds Brick Meets Click. 2020. Available online: https://www.foodnavigator-usa.com/Article/2020/05/05/US-online-grocery-sales-surge-37-to-5.3bn-in-April-finds-Brick-Meets-Click# (accessed on 30 April 2020).
6. Superfood. Online Grocery Shopping Statistics: Pre and Post Covid-19. 2020. Available online: https://superfood.digital/online-grocery-store-ecommerce-statistics/ (accessed on 30 April 2020).
7. USDA. Supplemental Nutrition Assistance Program Online Purchasing Pilot. 2020. Available online: https://www.fns.usda.gov/snap/online-purchasing-pilot (accessed on 28 April 2020).
8. Brookings. For Millions of Low-Income Seniors, Coronavirus Is a Food-Security Issue. 2020. Available online: https://www.brookings.edu/blog/the-avenue/2020/03/16/for-millions-of-low-income-seniors-coronavirus-is-a-food-security-issue/ (accessed on 28 April 2020).
9. USDA. SNAP Online Purchasing to Cover 90% of Households. 2020. Available online: https://www.usda.gov/media/press-releases/2020/05/20/snap-online-purchasing-cover-90-households (accessed on 28 April 2020).
10. National WIC Association. WIC/EWIC Pickup and Delivery Options. 2020. Available online: https://s3.amazonaws.com/aws.upl/nwica.org/fy20_nwa_factsheet_pickup-and-delivery-requirements_phase-1.pdf (accessed on 26 July 2020).
11. Glanz, K.; Bader, M.D.; Iyer, S. Retail grocery store marketing strategies and obesity: An integrative review. *Am. J. Prev. Med.* **2012**, *42*, 503–512. [CrossRef] [PubMed]
12. Dawson, J. Retailer activity in shaping food choice. *Food Qual. Pref.* **2013**, *28*, 339–347. [CrossRef]
13. Hand, C.; Riley, F.D.O.; Harris, P.; Singh, J.; Rettie, R. Online grocery shopping: The influence of situational factors. *Eur. J. Mark.* **2009**, *43*, 1205–1219. [CrossRef]
14. Hansen, T. Consumer adoption of online grocery buying: A discriminant analysis. *Int. J. Retail Distrib. Manag.* **2005**, *33*, 101–121. [CrossRef]
15. Cetina, I.; Munthiu, M.-C.; Radulescu, V. Psychological and social factors that influence online consumer behavior. *Soc. Behav. Sci.* **2012**, *62*, 184–188. [CrossRef]
16. Zheng, Q.; Chen, J.; Zhang, R.; Wang, H.H. What factors affect Chinese consumers' online grocery shopping? Product attributes, e-vendor characteristics and consumer perceptions. *China Agric. Econ. Rev.* **2020**, *12*, 193–213. [CrossRef]
17. Inman, J.J.; Nikolova, H. Shopper-facing retail technology: A retailer adoption decision framework incorporating shopper attitudes and privacy concerns. *J. Retail.* **2017**, *93*, 7–28. [CrossRef]
18. Pauzi, S.F.F.; Thoo, A.C.; Tan, L.C.; Muharam, F.M.; Talib, N.A. Factors influencing consumers intention for online grocery shopping—A proposed framework. *IOP Conf. Ser. Mater. Sci. Eng.* **2017**, *215*, 012013. [CrossRef]
19. Esbjerg, L.; Jensen, B.B.; Bech-Larsen, T.; de Barcellos, M.D.; Boztug, Y.; Grunert, K.G. An integrative conceptual framework for analyzing customer satisfaction with shopping trip experiences in grocery retailing. *J. Retail. Cons. Serv.* **2012**, *19*, 445–456. [CrossRef]
20. Darley, W.K.; Blankson, C.; Luethge, D.J. Toward an integrated framework for online consumer behavior and decision-making process. A review. *Psychol. Mark.* **2010**, *27*, 94–116. [CrossRef]
21. Nguyen, D.H.; de Leeuw, S.; Dullaert, W.E. Consumer behaviour and order fulfilment in online retailing: A systematic review. *Int. J. Manag. Rev.* **2018**, *20*, 255–276. [CrossRef]
22. Jabareen, Y. Building a conceptual framework: Philosophy, definitions, and procedure. *Int. J. Qual. Methods* **2009**, *8*, 49–62. [CrossRef]

23. Armstrong, G.; Adam, S.; Denize, S.; Kotler, P. *Principles of Marketing*; Pearson: Melbourne, Australia, 2014.
24. Dominici, G. From marketing mix to e-marketing mix: A literature overview and classification. *Int. J. Bus. Manag.* **2009**, *4*, 17–24. [CrossRef]
25. Davis, F.D. Perceived usefulness, perceived ease of use, and user acceptance of information technology. *MIS Q.* **1989**, *13*, 319–340. [CrossRef]
26. Cheung, C.M.; Chan, G.W.; Limayem, M. A critical review of online consumer behavior: Empirical research. *J. Electron. Commerce Org.* **2005**, *3*, 1–19. [CrossRef]
27. Marreiros, C.; Ness, M. *A Conceptual Framework of Consumer Food Choice Behaviour*; Working Paper; University of Evora, CEFAGE-UE: Évora, Portugal, 2009.
28. Penim, J.M.C.D.S. Online Grocery Shopping: An Exploratory Study of Consumer Decision Making Processes. Masters's Thesis, Universiade Catholica Portuguesa, Porto, Portugal, 2013.
29. Kurnia, S.; Chien, J.A.W. The Acceptance of The Online Grocery Shopping. In Proceedings of the 16th Bled Electronic Commerce Conference, Bled, Slovenia, 9–11 June 2003.
30. Glanz, K.; Johnson, L.; Yaroch, A.L.; Phillips, M.; Ayala, G.X.; Davis, E.L. Measures of retail food store environments and sales: Review and implications for healthy eating initiatives. *J. Nutr. Ed. Behav.* **2016**, *48*, 280–288. [CrossRef] [PubMed]
31. Bronfenbrenner, U. *The Ecology of Human Development*; Harvard University Press: Boston, MA, USA, 1979.
32. Choi, Y.A. Structural Equation Model of the Determinants of Repeat Purchase Behaviour of Online Grocery Shoppers in the UK. Ph.D. Thesis, Newcastle University, Newcastle Upon Tyne, UK, 2013.
33. Kumanyika, S.K. A framework for increasing equity impact in obesity prevention. *Am. J. Public Health* **2019**, *109*, 1350–1357. [CrossRef] [PubMed]
34. Center for Digital Democracy. USDA Online Buying Program for Snap Participants Threatens Their Privacy and Can Exacerbate Racial and Health Inequities, Says New Report. 2020. Available online: https://www.democraticmedia.org/article/usda-online-buying-program-snap-participants-threatens-their-privacy-and-can-exacerbate (accessed on 26 July 2020).
35. The Rudd Centre for Food Policy and Obesity. Increasing Disparities in Unhealthy Food Advertising Targeted to Hispanic and Black Youth. 2019. Available online: http://uconnruddcenter.org/files/Pdfs/TargetedMarketingReport2019.pdf (accessed on 28 April 2020).

Publisher's Note: MDPI stays neutral with regard to jurisdictional claims in published maps and institutional affiliations.

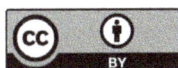

© 2020 by the authors. Licensee MDPI, Basel, Switzerland. This article is an open access article distributed under the terms and conditions of the Creative Commons Attribution (CC BY) license (http://creativecommons.org/licenses/by/4.0/).

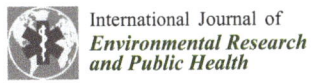

Article

Developing a National Research Agenda to Support Healthy Food Retail

Amelie A. Hecht [1,*], Megan M. Lott [2], Kirsten Arm [2], Mary T. Story [2], Emily Snyder [3,†], Margo G. Wootan [3,‡] and Alyssa J. Moran [1]

[1] Department of Health Policy and Management, Johns Hopkins Bloomberg School of Public Health, Baltimore, MD 21205, USA; AMoran10@jhu.edu
[2] Healthy Eating Research, Duke Global Health Institute, Duke University, Durham, NC 27708, USA; megan.lott@duke.edu (M.M.L.); kirsten.arm@duke.edu (K.A.); mary.story@duke.edu (M.T.S.)
[3] Center for Science in the Public Interest, Washington, DC 20005, USA; esnyder@cspinet.org (E.S.); mwootan@mxgstrategies.com (M.G.W.)
* Correspondence: AHecht3@jhu.edu
† Deceased.
‡ Affilicated to the Center for Science in the Public Interest at the time of the study.

Received: 28 August 2020; Accepted: 2 November 2020; Published: 4 November 2020

Abstract: The food retail environment is an important driver of dietary choices. This article presents a national agenda for research in food retail, with the goal of identifying policies and corporate practices that effectively promote healthy food and beverage purchases and decrease unhealthy purchases. The research agenda was developed through a multi-step process that included (1) convening a scientific advisory committee; (2) commissioned research; (3) in-person expert convening; (4) thematic analysis of meeting notes and refining research questions; (5) follow-up survey of convening participants; and (6) refining the final research agenda. Public health researchers, advocates, food and beverage retailers, and funders participated in the agenda setting process. A total of 37 research questions grouped into ten priority areas emerged. Five priority areas focus on understanding the current food retail environment and consumer behavior and five focus on assessing implementation and effectiveness of interventions and policies to attain healthier retail. Priority topics include how frequency, duration, and impact of retailer promotion practices differ by community characteristics and how to leverage federal nutrition assistance programs to support healthy eating. To improve feasibility, researchers should explore partnerships with retailers and advocacy groups, identify novel data sources, and use a variety of study designs. This agenda can serve as a guide for researchers, food retailers, funders, government agencies, and advocacy organizations.

Keywords: food and beverage; grocery retail; supermarket; marketing; policy; research agenda; healthy food retail; food environment

1. Introduction

The food retail environment is an important driver of dietary choices in the U.S. Components of the food retail environment, including access to food retail, availability and price of healthy products in stores, and presence of in-store marketing, all play a role in shaping dietary patterns [1,2]. Food and beverage manufacturers spend billions of dollars annually to ensure retailers stock, prominently place, and promote their products [3]. Unhealthy products are promoted more often than healthy products, and evidence suggests that promotion of unhealthy products shapes consumer purchasing more than promotion of healthy products [4,5].

Current dietary patterns, which, compared to the *2015–2020 Dietary Guidelines for Americans*, are low in fruits and vegetables, whole grains, and lean protein, and high in sodium, added sugars, and saturated fat, put many Americans at elevated risk of chronic health conditions, including obesity and diabetes [6,7]. Low-income and racial/ethnic communities, who experience greater prevalence of diet-related chronic diseases, may also be more likely to be targeted by marketing of unhealthy foods and beverages [8–10]. For example, in-store marketing of unhealthy beverages has been shown to increase at the time of month when Supplemental Nutrition Assistance Program (SNAP) benefits are distributed, particularly in neighborhoods with high SNAP participation [10].

As national attention toward health disparities and diet-related chronic diseases has increased in recent years, researchers, advocates, and policymakers have recognized the need to improve the food retail environment. In 2010, the Robert Wood Johnson Foundation (RWJF) and The Food Trust convened researchers, public health advocates, food retailers, manufacturers, and marketing professionals to discuss strategies to promote healthy retail, with a particular focus on children in low-income communities. The report that followed, *Harnessing the Power of Supermarkets to Help Reverse Childhood Obesity*, recommended marketing tactics to promote healthier purchases that jointly benefited consumers, retailers, and manufacturers [11]. In the intervening years, progress has been made toward identifying retail practices that undermine healthy eating and designing interventions that promote healthy eating in the retail food environment. At the same time, the retail food landscape has evolved: grocery store chains have consolidated, dollar stores have gained market share, and some consumers have shifted their purchases online. Research to fill remaining and emerging gaps in the food retail literature is needed.

This article outlines a national research agenda to support healthy food retail developed by Healthy Eating Research (HER; a national program of RWJF), the Center for Science in the Public Interest (CSPI), The Food Trust, and other researchers. This is the first national research agenda focused on healthy food retail. Research agendas have been developed to guide work on a variety of other public health topics [12,13]. Agenda-setting helps to identify important gaps in knowledge and to build consensus and support to fill those gaps among funders, advocates, and researchers. This agenda describes key areas for research to better understand current food retail practices and consumer behaviors and potential retail strategies to promote healthy eating while addressing racial and income disparities in diet quality and related disease. Research in these domains can inform policy strategies and corporate practices to improve the food retail environment and promote health equity. This article describes the collaborative and iterative methods used to develop the research agenda and the results generated at each step of the process. It then presents a final set of research questions in a comprehensive research agenda, key considerations for how to conduct that research, and ways in which the research agenda can be used to advance the field and public health.

2. Methods

The research agenda was developed through an iterative process between October 2019 and July 2020 that included the following steps: (1) convening a scientific advisory committee; (2) commissioning five systematic literature reviews and one original research project on food retail practices and interventions; (3) in-person convening of expert stakeholders; (4) thematic analysis of meeting notes and refining research questions; (5) follow-up survey of convening participants; and (6) developing the final research agenda (Figure 1). The scientific advisory committee provided input at each stage of the process. This agenda-setting process was based on methods used by Duffy et al. [12].

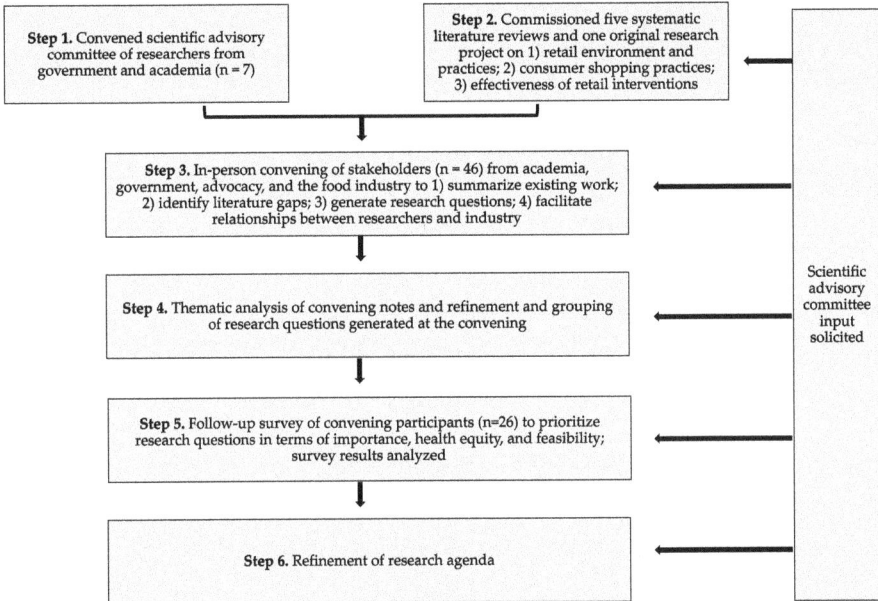

Figure 1. Flow chart depicting the process of developing the national healthy retail research agenda.

The research agenda was developed with an emphasis on health equity and the demographic groups that are at highest risk for poor health, especially nutrition and weight-related health disparities. These priority populations, identified by HER, include Non-Hispanic Black, Hispanic/Latinx, Asian American, Native Hawaiian/Pacific Islander, American Indian/Alaska Native, and rural children and their families [14].

2.1. Convening a Scientific Advisory Committee

A scientific advisory committee was formed and included seven researchers from government, academia, and nonprofit organizations, representing a variety of substantive areas related to psychology, nutrition, health behavior, anthropology, and public policy. The committee was selected based on prior work in the field, leadership in related working groups and professional organizations, and experience working with HER's priority populations. The committee provided input on topics for commissioned research, the in-person convening agenda and guest list, and content of the follow-up survey and final research agenda. Committee members also took notes and guided small group discussions at the in-person convening.

2.2. Commissioned Research

Five literature reviews and one original research project were commissioned for the in-person convening and were conducted by experts in the field. (Five of these papers are published jointly with this special issue.) These works aimed to provide an overview of previous research on key topics and guide convening discussion. Commissioned papers were organized into three themes: (1) retailer and manufacturer marketing practices, (2) consumer food purchasing trends by race/ethnicity, socioeconomic status, and geographic location, and (3) effectiveness of government- and researcher-led retail interventions to increase healthy food access and purchases. The original research paper used Nielsen Homescan Consumer Panel data from 2008–2018 to assess how packaged food purchases differ by store type and consumer demographics (urban vs. rural, high vs. low income).

2.3. In-Person Convening of Expert Stakeholders

The goals of the in-person convening were to (1) summarize previous research on healthy food retail, (2) identify gaps in the literature, (3) generate and prioritize questions for future research, (4) highlight best practices for research collaboration with the food industry, and (5) facilitate relationships between retailers and researchers to implement and evaluate healthy retail interventions. The full-day event was held in Washington, DC on 29 January 2020 and was organized by staff from HER, CSPI, and The Food Trust and the scientific advisory committee. Forty-six expert stakeholders from academia, government, advocacy, and the food industry participated.

In advance of the meeting, participants were asked to read six brief reports with the preliminary findings from the five commissioned systematic reviews and one original research project. At the convening, academic researchers presented key findings from each of the commissioned projects. Presentations were grouped according to the three themes discussed in Section 2.2 (two presentations per theme). After each pair of presentations, scientific advisory committee members facilitated small group breakout discussions. In breakout groups, participants discussed findings from the presentations and research gaps related to the theme, including understudied populations. Participants were asked to brainstorm new research methods, data sources, and study designs to facilitate future evaluation.

Meeting organizers also facilitated a large group discussion during which participants were asked where they would recommend directing intervention research over the next ten years to have the greatest impact on population health and equity. Subsequently, a panel of industry representatives discussed best practices for researchers seeking to partner with retailers and food manufacturers on healthy retail research. Finally, in small groups, participants were asked prioritize research questions identified throughout the day that would help fill knowledge gaps.

After each small and large group discussion, participants were asked to write research questions that emerged on sticky notes. Sticky notes were placed on walls throughout the meeting room according to the theme. At the end of the convening, participants were asked to walk around the room and place dots next to the research questions they thought were most important for advancing health equity.

2.4. Thematic Analysis of Notes and Refinement of Research Questions

Notes taken by the scientific advisory committee at the convening and sticky notes generated by convening participants were thematically analyzed and grouped by three authors collaboratively (A.A.H., M.G.W., A.J.M.). The list of research questions was collated and refined by deleting duplicate questions, questions that were too vague or specific, and questions outside the scope of the research agenda. Cross-cutting considerations related to study design, setting, data sources, and partnerships raised during group discussions were also refined.

2.5. Follow-Up Participant Survey

An online follow-up survey was sent via email to convening participants in May 2020. The survey was developed by the authors with feedback from the scientific advisory committee. The survey was first entered into Qualtrics and tested for functionality and length. Respondents were asked to complete the survey within two weeks, during which time two reminder emails were sent.

A total of 40 research questions generated at the in-person convening were included in the follow-up survey. Survey respondents were asked to rank each research question on a scale from 1 (lowest) to 5 (highest) in terms of feasibility, equity, and importance (defined in Table 1). For each research question, average scores for each domain and composite scores were calculated using Microsoft Excel. Research questions that received low composite scores (<3) or low scores in all three domains (<3.5) were removed. This allowed research questions that received low scores in one domain but high scores in one or both of the remaining domains to be preserved (for example, a question that received a score of 2.0 for feasibility but a score of 3.7 for importance and 3.5 for health equity would be preserved). Respondents were asked to list any missing research questions. Finally, respondents were provided a list of data sources for healthy retail research identified at the convening and provided an opportunity to list additional data sources.

Table 1. Definitions of domains used to rank healthy retail research questions in a follow-up survey sent to experts who previously participated in an in-person healthy retail research convening (n = 46).

Term	Definition
Feasibility	What is the likelihood that this research can be conducted successfully and produce valid and reliable results?
Importance	How important is this research to help inform policy, programs, or retailer practice, given the state of the current evidence?
Health equity	How impactful might the results of this research be in ensuring that all people have a fair and just opportunity to be as healthy as possible?

2.6. Developing a Final Research Agenda

The final research agenda was developed based on findings from steps 2–5 (see Figure 1) and with critical input from the scientific advisory committee and select members of the Healthy Food Retail Working Group, which is supported by HER and the Centers for Disease Control and Prevention's (CDC) Nutrition and Obesity Policy Research and Evaluation Network (NOPREN). The final research questions (selected based on follow-up survey results) and the cross-cutting considerations for research were grouped into key themes.

3. Results

3.1. Commissioned Research Findings

Key findings from the commissioned research papers, including research gaps, are discussed briefly here; five of the commissioned papers are also published in this special issue.

Two commissioned systematic reviews focused on retailer and manufacturer marketing practices. The first identified four key strategies that food and beverage manufacturers use to influence retailer marketing practices, but called for further research to understand the role that financial incentives from manufacturers play in shaping the retail environment, including analyses using proprietary data from retailers and manufacturers [15]. The review also found evidence that retailer marketing strategies, including price discounts and prominent store placement, are associated with increased product sales, but concluded that other in-store promotional strategies, such as signs and displays, are understudied. A second commissioned paper assessed marketing-mix and choice-architecture (MMCA) strategies used to promote and sell sugar-sweetened beverages (SSBs) in U.S. food stores and found that SSBs were widely available and price reductions and promotions were used often to boost sales. The authors found that targeted MMCA strategies may be used to influence SSB purchases among at-risk consumers on the basis of income or race/ethnicity, for example, and that MMCA strategies may vary by retail format. They noted that most studies were not designed to capture such differences, representing a need for future investigation to inform practice and policy approaches to mitigate health disparities [16].

Two additional commissioned papers focused on differences in consumer shopping patterns by race/ethnicity, socioeconomic status, and geographic location (urban vs. rural). In one systematic review, the authors called for more research that examines how these three factors intersect to influence U.S. consumer food purchasing [17]. In particular, they found a small proportion of included studies examined purchasing at the intersection of two factors (race/ethnicity and socioeconomic status), and no studies examined purchasing at the intersection of all three factors or assessed geographic differences in purchasing. The other paper, an original research project using household packaged food purchase panel data from 2008–2018, identified heterogeneity in the type and nutritional quality of packaged foods and beverages purchased by urban versus rural households and low- versus high-income households in different retail formats [18]. The authors called for research to examine why these differences exist—for example, why rural households tend to buy more packaged foods from mass merchandisers and dollar stores, which offer foods of poorer nutritional quality.

The final two commissioned systematic reviews examined the impact of retail interventions on consumers and retailers. One review synthesized 148 evaluations of governmental policies designed to increase healthy food purchases in supermarkets and found that sweetened beverage taxes, revisions to the Special Supplemental Nutrition Program for Women, Infants and Children (WIC) food packages, and financial incentives for fruits and vegetables were associated with improvements in dietary behaviors [19]. Providing financial incentives to supermarkets to open in underserved areas and increases in SNAP benefits were not associated with changes in diet quality but may improve food security. The authors called for more research to understand the effects of calorie labeling in supermarkets and online SNAP purchasing on consumer purchasing and consumption. The second paper reviewed 64 in-store marketing studies conducted between 2009–2019 and found that the majority of interventions identified at least one positive effect related to healthier food purchasing, consumption, or sales. Promotion was the most commonly studied marketing strategy for single-component interventions, while changing promotion, placement, and product together were the most common for multi-component interventions. The quality of research, however, precluded definitive conclusions, as fewer than 36% of studies used experimental designs. The review called for more research to understand what combinations of strategies work best by product category and retail format [20].

3.2. In-Person Convening Findings

Research questions generated at the meeting (n = 147) were initially grouped according to the three meeting agenda themes (retailer and manufacturer marketing practices; consumer food purchasing trends; and effectiveness of retail interventions). (Figure 2) Forty-nine questions fell under the retailer and manufacturer marketing practices theme, 59 under the consumer food purchasing trends theme, and 39 under the effectiveness of retail interventions. These questions were refined and reorganized prior to inclusion in the follow-up survey. Two themes—retailer and manufacturer marketing practices and consumer food purchasing trends—were condensed due to overlap between research questions in these categories. In total, 40 questions representing two themes were included in the follow-up survey.

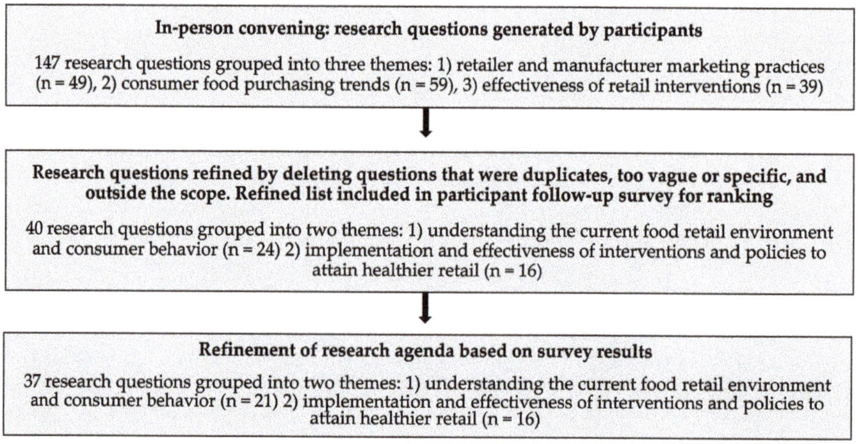

In-person convening: research questions generated by participants

147 research questions grouped into three themes: 1) retailer and manufacturer marketing practices (n = 49), 2) consumer food purchasing trends (n = 59), 3) effectiveness of retail interventions (n = 39)

↓

Research questions refined by deleting questions that were duplicates, too vague or specific, and outside the scope. Refined list included in participant follow-up survey for ranking

40 research questions grouped into two themes: 1) understanding the current food retail environment and consumer behavior (n = 24) 2) implementation and effectiveness of interventions and policies to attain healthier retail (n = 16)

↓

Refinement of research agenda based on survey results

37 research questions grouped into two themes: 1) understanding the current food retail environment and consumer behavior (n = 21) 2) implementation and effectiveness of interventions and policies to attain healthier retail (n = 16)

Figure 2. Flow chart depicting how research questions were generated and refined through the agenda-setting process.

3.3. Follow-Up Survey Findings

Twenty-six convening attendees completed the follow-up survey (response rate 57%). Three research questions were eliminated due to low scores: one question earned a low composite score (<3), and two questions earned low scores across all three domains (<3.5) (Table A1).

Research questions that received the highest composite scores focused on describing how frequency, duration, and impact of retailer promotion practices differed by community characteristics and how to leverage SNAP benefits to support healthy eating behaviors. (Figure 3) Research questions that received the highest scores for importance and equity focused on (1) evaluating the impact of retailer marketing practices on consumer health, (2) understanding the optimal retail design to promote healthy and reduce unhealthy purchases, and (3) evaluating the impact of healthy retail policies to address the social determinants of health. These questions, however, received lower scores for feasibility. Research questions that received the highest scores for feasibility focused on describing the current retail environment, including assessing the healthfulness of products currently available and promoted in stores, and describing the factors that influence consumer decision-making.

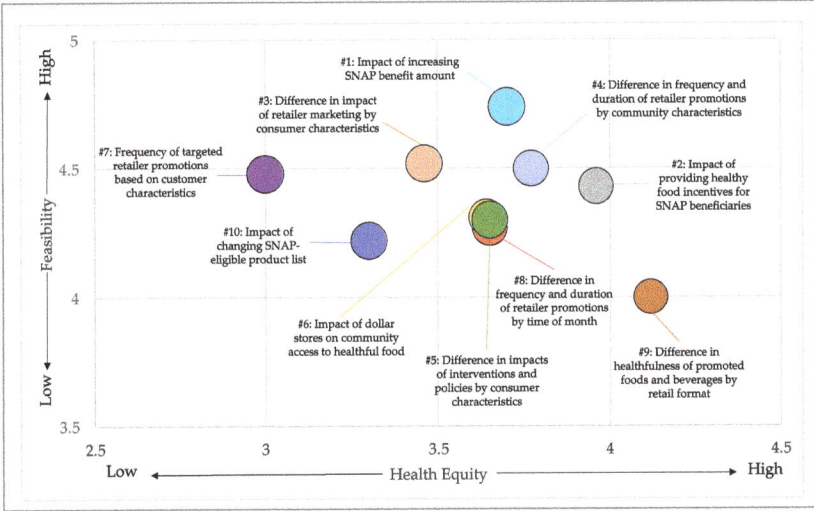

Figure 3. Research questions with the 10 highest composite scores from the follow-up survey. Numbers listed before questions represent ranking from 1–10 by composite score. Research questions were ranked on a 5-point Likert scale in terms of feasibility (y-axis) and health equity (x-axis). Ratings for importance are not displayed due to low variation (3.8–4.5) among the top ten questions. SNAP is the Supplemental Nutrition Assistance Program.

In the open-ended portion of the survey, several participants suggested additional research questions related to the COVID-19 pandemic. The research questions that participants were asked to rank were generated at the January convening, before widespread awareness of COVID-19 pandemic in the U.S., but the survey was conducted in May during the pandemic. A few participants indicated an interest in evaluating how COVID-19, generally, and the U.S. Department of Agriculture (USDA) waivers during the pandemic for SNAP and WIC statutory and regulatory requirements, specifically, affected food supply, retailer marketing, and consumer purchasing. Another participant called for research on how expansion of the SNAP Online Purchasing Pilot Program (a federal program to test the feasibility and impact of allowing online food retailers to accept SNAP benefits [21]) affects small and independent grocers.

Survey respondents identified several additional data sources for healthy retail research in the open-ended section portion of the survey. See Table 2 for a full list of data sources identified through the convening and follow-up survey.

Table 2. Data sources for healthy retail research identified at the in-person convening and through the follow-up survey.

Data Source	Accessibility
Store visitor data using cell phone geolocation information from companies such as SafeGraph	Fee
Sales and customer demographic data from companies such as Nielsen and Information Resources Inc. (IRI)	Fee
Sales and loyalty card data from independent or chain retailers	Through partnerships
Prepared food purchase data from university cafeterias	Through partnerships
State electronic benefit transfer redemption data	Through partnerships
Farmers market sales and customer demographic data through the Farmers Register Portal	Free, coming soon
Data collected by federal agencies • Customer Expenditure Survey (Bureau of Labor Statistics) • National Household Food Acquisition and Purchase Survey (U.S. Department of Agriculture) • National Health and Nutrition Examination Survey (Centers for Disease Control and Prevention)	Free, public use, and restricted datasets

3.4. Research Agenda Findings

Based on the information gathered in steps 2–5 (see Figure 1), a total of 37 research questions, grouped into ten key issue areas, emerged as priorities for future research (Table 3). Five of these issue areas focus on understanding the current food retail environment and consumer behavior and five focus on assessing implementation and effectiveness of interventions and policies to attain healthier retail.

Table 3. National research agenda questions.

Key Issue Area	Research Question
Understanding the Current Food Retail Environment and Consumer Behavior	
Understanding and describing the retail food marketing environment	How does the healthfulness of foods and beverages available in retail outlets differ by retail format?
	How does the healthfulness of foods and beverages promoted in retail outlets differ by retail format?
	What are the effects of manufacturer trade promotion practices on retailer practices?
	How do frequency and duration of retailer promotions differ by: • community characteristics (e.g., race/ethnicity, socioeconomic status)? • time of month (e.g., when SNAP benefits are issued)? • product characteristics (e.g., healthfulness, category)? • retail format (e.g., supermarkets vs. convenience stores)? • retail ordering platform (e.g., brick-and-mortar vs. online)? • geography (e.g., urban vs. rural)?

Table 3. Cont.

Key Issue Area	Research Question
Understanding the Current Food Retail Environment and Consumer Behavior	
Understanding consumer shopping behavior	Which factors influence consumer decision-making at the point of purchase?
	Which factors influence where consumers shop (e.g., shopping at a dollar store vs. supermarket)?
Impact of retailer marketing strategies	What are the impacts of retailer marketing strategies on: • consumer behaviors (e.g., purchasing, impulse buying, stockpiling)? • consumer health (e.g., diet quality, body mass index, overweight/obesity)? • outcomes of importance to retailers (e.g., sales, profitability, brand loyalty)?
	How do the impacts of retailer marketing strategies differ by: • consumer characteristics (e.g., race/ethnicity, socioeconomic status, participation in federal nutrition programs)? • time of month (e.g., when SNAP benefits are issued)? • product characteristics (e.g., healthfulness, category)? • geography (e.g., urban vs. rural)?
Understanding targeted food marketing	To what extent do retailers create targeted promotions based on customer characteristics (e.g., race/ethnicity, socioeconomic status, participation in federal nutrition programs)?
	Which food or beverage manufacturers and food categories have deceptive marketing or front-of-package claims?
Role of emerging retail formats in supporting healthy food access	How do dollar stores affect a community's access to healthful food?
Implementation and Effectiveness of Interventions and Policies to Attain Healthier Retail	
Supporting healthy purchases and reducing unhealthy purchases	What is the optimal design of a retail environment to support healthy eating?
	What changes to retailer marketing strategies improve the healthfulness of food purchases?
	What changes to product packaging, labeling, and/or portion size improve the healthfulness of food purchases?
	What are effective digital strategies to improve the healthfulness of food purchases?
Leveraging SNAP to support healthy eating	What is the impact of increasing the SNAP benefit amount?
	What is the impact of changing the frequency and/or timing of SNAP distribution (e.g., benefits issued twice per month or benefits issued on different days of the month)?
	What is the impact of changing the list of products eligible for purchase with SNAP (e.g., sugar-sweetened beverages)?
	What is the impact of offering produce boxes to SNAP beneficiaries?
	What is the impact of providing incentives for healthy foods for SNAP beneficiaries (e.g., discounts or matching dollars for purchases of whole grains, fruits and vegetables)?
Limiting unhealthy food establishments	How do zoning restrictions for unhealthy food retailers impact access to healthy food in the community?
Addressing social determinants of health	How do interventions or policies that address social determinants of health (e.g., universal basic income, increased minimum wage) impact food and beverage purchasing and consumption?
Assessing differential impacts	How do the impacts of interventions and policies differ by: • consumer characteristics (e.g., race/ethnicity, socioeconomic status, participation in federal nutrition programs)? • product characteristics (e.g., healthfulness, category)? • retail format (e.g., supermarkets vs. convenience stores)? • retail ordering platform (e.g., brick-and-mortar vs. online)? • geography (e.g., urban vs. rural)?

Through small and large group discussions at the in-person convening, several cross-cutting considerations for future research emerged and were grouped into three themes: potential research partners, data sources, and study designs and settings (Table 4).

Table 4. Cross-cutting considerations for future research on healthy food retail discussed by in-person convening participants.

Theme	Consideration
Research partnerships	Build long-term relationships with retailers and manufacturers to facilitate the implementation and evaluation of in-store interventions and access to proprietary data
	Collaborate with nontraditional partners, including trade associations, growers and distributors, marketing firms, business schools, advocacy groups, and retailers connected to academic research institutions (e.g., university hospitals, cafeterias, campus stores)
Data sources	Increase access to federal data sources (e.g., SNAP redemption data)
	Make data accessible and affordable to researchers through programs modeled after RWJF Health Data for Action, which serves as a conduit between data owners and researchers [22]
Study design and setting	Study nontraditional retailers, including supercenters, dollar stores, and online retailers
	Use a variety of study designs (e.g., laboratory experiments, pilot programs, randomized controlled trials, longitudinal evaluations)
	Draw lessons from interventions or policies abroad Promote innovative data collection approaches, such as investigative journalism or federally or congressionally commissioned investigations

4. Discussion

This article is the first to present a national agenda for research to support healthy food retail, developed iteratively and collaboratively by experts in public health research, advocacy, and food retail and marketing. This research agenda builds on the 2011 *Harnessing the Power of Supermarkets to Help Reverse Childhood Obesity* report, which proposed in-store marketing strategies developed collaboratively by retailers, researchers, manufacturers, and marketing professionals to encourage the purchase of healthy products while maintaining or improving retailers' bottom lines [11]. This research agenda reflects advancements in research that have occurred in the intervening years and outlines key areas for future research.

Thirty-seven key research questions, grouped into ten overarching themes, were identified. Priority topics include how frequency, duration, and impact of retailer promotion practices differ by community characteristics and how to leverage federal nutrition assistance programs to support healthy eating. Many of the research questions that received the highest scores in the follow-up survey for importance or health equity received low scores for feasibility, underscoring the need to address barriers to evaluation. Identified strategies to address these barriers include partnerships with retailers, government agencies, business schools, advocacy organizations, and others to implement and evaluate pilot programs and policies, as well as exploration of new study designs and data sharing opportunities.

Of the ten key research themes that emerged, half centered around describing the current food retail environment and how environmental factors shape consumer behavior. Considering that an estimated three-quarters of purchase decisions are made while shopping, a nuanced understanding of marketing strategies used by manufacturers and retailers and how those strategies drive behavior can guide targeted interventions [23]. Additionally, most research to-date has focused on grocery stores, but changes in the food retail environment, including growth in online retail and proliferation of dollar-stores in low-income and rural areas, point to a need for research on nontraditional retail outlets [24–26].

The other five key research themes focused on evaluating interventions designed to improve the retail environment and access to nutritious food. The commissioned reviews highlighted evidence of retailer-, researcher- and government-initiated interventions that have led to increased healthy purchases, including fresh fruit and vegetable prescriptions, revisions to the WIC packages, and financial incentives for healthy purchases using SNAP [19,27,28]. Yet, additional research is warranted to evaluate these interventions at a larger scale, in other settings, and over longer periods of time. Evaluation of novel policies through natural experimentation at the state and local level is also needed. As one step toward facilitating such policy evaluation, federal agencies should provide states greater flexibility to innovate. For example, the USDA could approve state or local waiver applications to remove SSBs from eligible SNAP purchases [29]. Considering SNAP serves as an important source of revenue for many retailers, changes in SNAP and other federal nutrition assistance programs could shift the broader food landscape [30].

4.1. Implications for Research and Practice

The agenda-setting process centered around promoting health equity, and the research questions identified account for and aim to address health disparities. As researchers and practitioners pursue the policy, systems, and environmental change strategies identified in this agenda, the Equity-Oriented Obesity Prevention Framework developed by Kumanyika can serve as a guide to ensure equity issues continue to be prioritized [31]. Specifically, Kumanyika calls for designing and evaluating interventions using an explicit equity lens that acknowledges the realities of social inequities, incorporates a "people perspective", and prioritizes community engagement.

This research agenda can serve as a resource for researchers writing grant applications, retailers seeking to conduct healthy retail pilots on their own or with researchers or advocates, funders drafting requests for proposals, and advocates engaging in organizational strategic planning. In particular, private foundations and federal agencies including the USDA, CDC, and the National Institutes of Health (NIH) should integrate the research themes outlined in this agenda into their strategic plans, ongoing initiatives, and funding priorities.

While federal agencies have made progress toward recognizing the importance of the food environment and healthy retail as a strategy to reduce disease and disparities, much work remains. For example, in the *National Nutrition Research Roadmap for 2016-2021*, the federal Interagency Committee on Human Nutrition Research, which includes representatives from USDA and the U.S. Department of Health and Human Services, identified research on food retail as an area of interest [32]. The CDC has acknowledged the importance of the food retail environment in multiple reports and, in 2015, published *Healthier Food Retail: An Action Guide for Public Health Practitioners* [33,34]. The CDC also promotes healthier retail among small, independent retailers through cooperative purchasing initiatives and communities of practice in the High Obesity Program and Racial and Ethnic Approaches to Community Health program. The NIH, between 1975 and 2018, funded more than 200 grants related to healthy food retail, and the *2020–2030 Strategic Plan for NIH Nutrition Research* recognized the important role of the food environment in shaping dietary behavior [35,36]. At the same time, the *Strategic Plan for NIH Obesity Research* only briefly mentions the food environment and does not mention retail [37]. Similarly, healthy retail is missing from the *USDA Science Blueprint* [38].

As federal departments and agencies use this research agenda to guide future funding priorities, coordination and harmonization across these entities are needed to ensure existing efforts are leveraged and amplified and that critical areas are not overlooked. Drawing on recent recommendations from Fleischhacker et al., creation of a new authority for cross-governmental coordination of nutrition research and policy, as well as strengthened authority, coordination, and investment for nutrition research within the NIH and USDA could help to catalyze new science and partnerships [39].

Research on healthy retail requires collaboration across sectors and disciplines, including relationship-building and data sharing between researchers and retailers. Research institutions and funders should provide financial and technical support to advance these efforts without expectation of immediate research deliverables. For example, to improve accessibility and affordability of data, foundations could serve as a conduit between researchers and industry, following the model of the RWJF Health Data for Action program [22]. Another potential model is the Johns Hopkins Bloomberg American Health Initiative, which provides funding to researchers engaged in consultancies and special projects that facilitate cross-sector partnerships [40].

Progress toward meeting the research goals outlined herein should be monitored. In five years, key stakeholders should be re-convened to discuss achievements and remaining gaps. In the intervening years, researchers, retailers, manufacturers, funders, and advocates should convene periodically to foster partnerships and data sharing.

4.2. Strengths and Limitations

This study has limitations. First, the list of attendees for the in-person convening was developed with the aim of bringing together groups across research and practice with a mutual interest in promoting health; thus, some interested parties such as manufacturers and trade associations may have been excluded, and the research questions and other ideas generated at the convening may be subject to bias. Additionally, 43 percent of meeting participants did not complete the follow-up survey; therefore, survey results may be impacted by self-selection bias. Finally, the food retail landscape is rapidly evolving, and this agenda reflects priorities identified at a specific period in time. For example, research questions were generated at an in-person convening in January 2020, before widespread awareness of COVID-19 in the U.S. The pandemic brought about important changes in how people in the U.S. purchase groceries and inspired new research questions (e.g., what are the impacts of increased online grocery purchasing; increased at-home food preparation; expansion of the SNAP Online Purchasing Pilot Program?) [21,41].

The methods used in this study, however, are strong. This study used a multi-step, iterative approach to develop the final research agenda. A range of stakeholders who represented diverse disciplines and organizations, including retailers, were engaged in this process. Finally, a focus on health equity was incorporated in every stage of the retail research agenda-setting process, increasing the likelihood that the research questions identified as part of this process will help address disparities in health.

5. Conclusions

The food retail environment presents an ideal setting for intervention to improve diet quality and reduce the prevalence of chronic disease and health disparities. The collaborative agenda-setting process, which included representatives from academic, government, advocacy, funding organizations, and industry, built consensus around key research gaps. The research questions identified through this process aim to inform policies and corporate practices that improve the food retail environment, and, ultimately, public health. This agenda can serve as a guide for researchers, funders, and advocates, ensuring that future work fills critical knowledge gaps, promotes equity, and advances policy and practice.

Author Contributions: Conceptualization and methodology: A.A.H., M.M.L., K.A., M.T.S., M.G.W., A.J.M. Formal analysis and investigation: A.A.H., M.G.W., A.J.M. Writing—original draft preparation: A.A.H., E.S., M.G.W., A.J.M. Writing—reviewing and editing: all. Project administration and funding acquisition: A.J.M., M.M.L., K.A., M.T.S., M.G.W. All authors have read and agreed to the published version of the manuscript.

Funding: This research was supported by Healthy Eating Research (a national program of the Robert Wood Johnson Foundation), the Johns Hopkins University Center for a Livable Future, the Institute for Health and Social Policy at the Johns Hopkins Bloomberg School of Public Health, the Bloomberg American Health Initiative of the Johns Hopkins Bloomberg School of Public Health, and the Center for Science in the Public Interest.

Acknowledgments: The authors would like to express their gratitude and appreciation to the attendees of the January 2020 Healthy Retail Research Convening, members of the Scientific Advisory Committee (Joel Gittelsohn, Karen Glanz, Lisa Harnack, Allison Karpyn, Anne Palmer, Kate Reddy, Christina Roberto, Shannon Zenk), and other expert reviewers (Betsy Anderson Steeves, Sheila Fleischhacker, Lucia Leone) who were instrumental in shaping this research agenda. The authors would also like to thank staff of HER, The Food Trust, and Center for Science in the Public Interest for their valuable guidance in planning and executing the research convening, especially Darya Minovi, Julia McCarthy, and Julia Koprak.

Conflicts of Interest: The authors (A.A.H., E.S., M.G.W., A.J.M.) declare no conflict of interest. One funder (H.E.R.) did contribute significantly to the design of the study and in the collection of the data at the convening; however, the affiliated authors (M.M.L., K.A., M.T.S.) did not play a role in the analysis or interpretation of the data.

Appendix A

Table A1. Follow-up survey participant (n = 26) mean rankings of research questions in terms of feasibility, equity, and importance.

Key Issue Area	Research Question	Feasibility	Equity	Importance	Composite
Understanding the Current Food Retail Environment and Consumer Behavior					
Understanding and describing the retail food marketing environment	How does the healthfulness of foods and beverages available in retail outlets differ by retail format?	4.35	3.62	3.35	3.77
	How does the healthfulness of foods and beverages promoted in retail outlets differ by retail format?	4.12	4.00	3.81	3.97
	What are the effects of manufacturer trade promotion practices on retailer practices?	2.52	3.60	3.88	3.36
	How important is revenue from trade promotion to retailers? (e.g., what proportion of total revenue comes from trade promotion?) *	2.26	3.04	3.44	2.93
	How do frequency and duration of retailer promotions differ by ...				
	community characteristics (e.g., race/ethnicity, socioeconomic status)?	3.77	4.50	4.15	4.14
	time of month (e.g., when SNAP benefits are issued)?	3.65	4.27	4.08	4.00
	product characteristics (e.g., healthfulness, category)?	3.92	3.40	3.36	3.56
	retail format (e.g., supermarkets vs. convenience stores)?	3.72	3.36	3.08	3.39
	retail ordering platform (e.g., brick-and-mortar vs. online)?	3.48	3.31	3.50	3.43
	geography (e.g., urban vs. rural)?	3.88	3.85	3.54	3.76
Understanding consumer shopping behavior	Which factors influence consumer decision-making at the point of purchase?	4.04	3.62	3.73	3.79
	Which factors influence where consumers shop (e.g., shopping at a dollar store vs. supermarket)?	4.00	3.81	3.46	3.76

Table A1. Cont.

Key Issue Area	Research Question	Feasibility	Equity	Importance	Composite
Impact of retailer marketing strategies	What are the impacts of retailer marketing strategies on …				
	consumer behaviors (e.g., purchasing, impulse buying, stockpiling)?	3.50	3.69	4.04	3.74
	consumer health (e.g., diet quality, body mass index, overweight/obesity)?	2.54	3.88	4.31	3.58
	outcomes of importance to retailers (e.g., sales, profitability, brand loyalty)?	2.92	2.85	3.80	3.18
	How do the impacts of retailer marketing strategies differ by …				
	consumer characteristics (e.g., race/ethnicity, socioeconomic status, participation in federal nutrition programs)?	3.46	4.52	4.40	4.14
	time of month (e.g., when SNAP benefits are issued)?	3.52	4.12	4.12	3.92
	product characteristics (e.g., healthfulness, category)?	3.60	3.20	3.36	3.39
	retail format (e.g., supermarkets vs. convenience stores)? *	3.40	3.08	2.96	3.15
	retail ordering platform (e.g., brick-and-mortar vs. online)? *	3.29	2.84	3.40	3.18
	geography (e.g., urban vs. rural)?	3.22	3.70	3.48	3.46
Understanding targeted food marketing	To what extent do retailers create targeted promotions based on customer characteristics (e.g., race/ethnicity, socioeconomic status, participation in federal nutrition programs)?	3.00	4.48	4.52	4.01
	Which food or beverage manufacturers and food categories have deceptive marketing or front-of-package claims?	4.00	3.32	3.52	3.61
Role of emerging retail formats in supporting healthy food access	How do dollar stores affect a community's access to healthful food?	3.64	4.31	4.08	4.01
Implementation and Effectiveness of Interventions and Policies to Attain Healthier Retail					
Supporting healthy purchases and reducing unhealthy purchases	What is the optimal design of a retail environment to support healthy eating?	2.74	3.74	4.30	3.59
	What changes to retailer marketing strategies improve the healthfulness of food purchases?	3.09	3.91	4.22	3.74
	What changes to product packaging, labeling, and/or portion size improve the healthfulness of food purchases?	3.26	3.52	3.78	3.52
	What are effective digital strategies to improve the healthfulness of food purchases?	3.61	3.61	3.91	3.71

Table A1. Cont.

Key Issue Area	Research Question	Feasibility	Equity	Importance	Composite
Leveraging SNAP to support healthy eating	What is the impact of increasing the SNAP benefit amount?	3.70	4.74	4.52	4.32
	What is the impact of changing the frequency and/or timing of SNAP distribution (e.g., benefits issued twice per month or benefits issued on different days of the month)?	3.35	4.17	3.83	3.78
	What is the impact of changing the list of products eligible for purchase with SNAP (e.g., sugar-sweetened beverages)?	3.30	4.22	4.35	3.96
	What is the impact of offering produce boxes to SNAP beneficiaries?	3.48	3.74	3.43	3.55
	What is the impact of providing incentives for healthy foods for SNAP beneficiaries (e.g., discounts or matching dollars for purchases of whole grains, fruits and vegetables)?	3.96	4.43	4.09	4.16
Limiting unhealthy food establishments	How do zoning restrictions for unhealthy food retailers impact access to healthy food in the community?	2.61	3.83	3.70	3.38
Addressing social determinants of health	How do interventions or policies that address social determinants of health (e.g., universal basic income, increased minimum wage) impact food and beverage purchasing and consumption?	2.52	4.73	4.59	3.93
Assessing differential impacts	How do the impacts of interventions and policies differ by ...				
	consumer characteristics (e.g., race/ethnicity, socioeconomic status, participation in federal nutrition programs)?	3.65	4.30	4.30	4.09
	product characteristics (e.g., healthfulness, category)?	3.70	3.00	3.26	3.32
	retail format (e.g., supermarkets vs. convenience stores)?	3.78	3.26	3.30	3.45
	retail ordering platform (e.g., brick-and-mortar vs. online)?	3.36	3.26	3.57	3.40
	geography (e.g., urban vs. rural)?	3.70	4.00	3.78	3.83

* Indicates question was eliminated due to low composite score or low score for equity or importance (<3).

References

1. Story, M.; Kaphingst, K.M.; Robinson-O'Brien, R.; Glanz, K. Creating healthy food and eating environments: Policy and environmental approaches. *Annu. Rev. Public Health* **2008**, *29*, 253–272. [CrossRef] [PubMed]
2. Mattioni, D.; Loconto, A.M.; Brunori, G. Healthy diets and the retail food environment: A sociological approach. *Health Place* **2020**, *61*, 102244. [CrossRef] [PubMed]
3. Rivlin, G. *Rigged: Supermarket Shelves for Sale*; Center for Science in the Public Interest: Washington, DC, USA, 2016.
4. Bennett, R.; Zorbas, C.; Huse, O.; Peeters, A.; Cameron, A.J.; Sacks, G.; Backholer, K. Prevalence of healthy and unhealthy food and beverage price promotions and their potential influence on shopper purchasing behaviour: A systematic review of the literature. *Obes. Rev.* **2019**, *21*, e12948. [CrossRef] [PubMed]
5. Glanz, K.; Bader, M.D.; Iyer, S. Retail grocery store marketing strategies and obesity: An integrative review. *Am. J. Prev. Med.* **2012**, *42*, 503–512. [CrossRef] [PubMed]

6. National Heart, Lung, and Blood Institute. *Managing Overweight and Obesity in Adults: Systematic Evidence Review from the Obesity Expert Panel*; National Heart, Lung and Blood Institute, Bethesda: Rockville, MD, USA, 2013.
7. US Department of Health and Human Services; US Department of Agriculture. *2015–2020 Dietary Guidelines for Americans: Current Eating Patterns in the United States*; US Department of Health and Human Services and US Department of Agriculture: Washington, DC, USA, 2015.
8. Krueger, P.M.; Reither, E.N. Mind the gap: Race/ethnic and socioeconomic disparities in obesity. *Curr. Diabetes Rep.* **2015**, *15*, 95. [CrossRef]
9. Grier, S.A.; Kumanyika, S.K. The context for choice: Health implications of targeted food and beverage marketing to African Americans. *Am. J. Public Health* **2008**, *98*, 1616–1629. [CrossRef] [PubMed]
10. Moran, A.J.; Musicus, A.; Findling, M.T.G.; Brissette, I.F.; Lowenfels, A.A.; Subramanian, S.; Roberto, C.A. Increases in sugary drink marketing during supplemental nutrition assistance program benefit issuance in New York. *Am. J. Prev. Med.* **2018**, *55*, 55–62. [CrossRef] [PubMed]
11. The Food Trust. *Harnessing the Power of Supermarkets to Help Reverse Childhood Obesity*; The Food Trust: Philadelphia, PA, USA, 2011.
12. Duffy, E.W.; Lott, M.M.; Johnson, E.J.; Story, M.T. Developing a national research agenda to reduce consumption of sugar-sweetened beverages and increase safe water access and consumption among 0- to 5-year-olds: A mixed methods approach. *Public Health Nutr.* **2020**, *23*, 22–33. [CrossRef] [PubMed]
13. Johnson, D.B.; Quinn, E.L.; Sitaker, M.; Ammerman, A.; Byker, C.; Dean, W.; Fleischhacker, S.E.; Morgan, E.; Pinard, C.A.; Pitts, S.J.; et al. Developing an agenda for research about policies to improve access to healthy foods in rural communities: A concept mapping study. *BMC Public Health* **2014**, *14*, 550–572. [CrossRef] [PubMed]
14. Healthy Eating Research. *A National Research Agenda to Reduce Consumption of Sugar-Sweetened Beverages and Increase Safe Water Access and Consumption among Zero- to Five-Year-Old*; Healthy Eating Research: Durham, NC, USA, 2018.
15. Hecht, A.A.; Perez, C.L.; Polascek, M.; Thorndike, A.N.; Franckle, R.L.; Moran, A.J. Influence of food and beverage companies on retailer marketing strategies and consumer behavior. *Int. J. Environ. Res. Public Health* **2020**, *17*, 7381. [CrossRef] [PubMed]
16. Houghtaling, B.; Holston, D.; Szocs, C.; Qi, D.; Penn, J.; Hedrick, V. Current Practices in the Stocking and Marketing of Sugar-Sweetened Beverages in United States Food Stores: A Rapid Review. Under review.
17. Singleton, C.R.; Winkler, M.; Houghtaling, B.; Adeyemi, O.S.; Roehl, A.; Pionke, J.J.; Anderson Steeves, E. Understanding the Intersection of Race/Ethnicity, Socioeconomic Status, and Geographic Location: A Scoping Review of U.S. Consumer Food Purchasing. *Int. J. Environ. Res. Public Health* **2020**, *17*, 7677. [CrossRef] [PubMed]
18. Lacko, A.; Ng, S.W.; Popkin, B. Urban vs. rural socioeconomic differences in the nutritional quality of household packaged food purchases by store type. *Int. J. Environ. Res. Public Health* **2020**, *17*, 7637. [CrossRef] [PubMed]
19. Moran, A.J.; Gu, Y.; Clynes, S.; Goheer, A.; Roberto, C.A.; Palmer, A. Associations between Governmental Policies to Improve the Nutritional Quality of Supermarket Purchases and Individual, Retailer, and Community Health Outcomes: An Integrative Review. *Int. J. Environ. Res. Public Health* **2020**, *17*, 7493. [CrossRef] [PubMed]
20. Karpyn, A.; McCallops, K.; Wolgast, H.; Glanz, K. Improving consumption and purchases of healthier foods in retail environments: A systematic review. *Int. J. Environ. Res. Public Health* **2020**, *17*, 7524. [CrossRef] [PubMed]
21. US Department of Agriculture FNS Launches the Online Purchasing Pilot. Available online: https://www.fns.usda.gov/snap/online-purchasing-pilot (accessed on 2 July 2020).
22. AcademyHealth Health Data for Action. Available online: https://www.academyhealth.org/about/programs/health-data-for-action (accessed on 21 July 2020).
23. Point of Purchase Advertising International. *2012 Shopper Engagement Study Media Topline Report*; Point of Purchase Advertising International: Alexandria, VA, USA, 2012.
24. Donahue, M.; Mitchell, S. *Dollar Stores are Targeting Struggling Urban Neighborhoods and Small Towns. One Community is Showing How to Fight Back; Institute for Local Self-Reliance*; Institute for Local Self Reliance: Washington, DC, USA, 2018.

25. Volpe, R.; Kuhns, A.; Jaenicke, T. *Store Formats and Patterns in Household Grocery Purchases*; United States Department of Agriculture Economic Research Service: Washington, DC, USA, 2017.
26. Dollar Stores Are Taking over the Grocery Business, and It's Bad News for Public Health and Local Economies. Available online: https://civileats.com/2018/12/17/dollar-stores-are-taking-over-the-grocery-business-and-its-bad-news-for-public-health-and-local-economies/ (accessed on 18 May 2020).
27. Olsho, L.E.; Klerman, J.A.; Wilde, P.E.; Bartlett, S. Financial incentives increase fruit and vegetable intake among Supplemental Nutrition Assistance Program participants: A randomized controlled trial of the USDA Healthy Incentives Pilot. *Am. J. Clin. Nutr.* **2016**, *104*, 423–435. [CrossRef] [PubMed]
28. Ridberg, R.A.; Bell, J.F.; Merritt, K.E.; Harris, D.M.; Young, H.M.; Tancredi, D. Effect of a fruit and vegetable prescription program on children's fruit and vegetable consumption. *Prev. Chronic Dis.* **2019**, *16*, E73. [CrossRef] [PubMed]
29. Negowetti, N. The snap sugar-sweetened beverage debate: Restricting purchases to improve health outcomes of low-income Americans. *Food Policy* **2018**, *14*, 83.
30. United States Department of Agriculture. *SNAP Retailer Data: 2019 Year End Summary*; US Department of Agriculture: Washington, DC, USA, 2019.
31. Kumanyika, S.K. A framework for increasing equity impact in obesity prevention. *Am. J. Public Health* **2019**, *109*, 1350–1357. [CrossRef] [PubMed]
32. Interagency Committee on Human Nutrition Research. *National Nutrition Research Roadmap 2016-2021: Advancing Nutrition Research to Improve and Sustain Health*; Interagency Committee on Human Nutrition Research: Washington, DC, USA, 2016.
33. Centers for Disease Control and Prevention. *Healthier Food Retail: An Action Guide for Public Health Practitioners*; U.S. Department of Health and Human Services: Atlanta, GA, USA, 2014.
34. Centers for Disease Control and Prevention. *Strategies to Prevent Obesity and Other Chronic Diseases: The CDC Guide to Strategies to Increase the Consumption of Fruits and Vegetables*; U.S. Department of Health and Human Services: Atlanta, GA, USA, 2011.
35. Fleischhacker, S.; Ballard, R.; Hunter, C.; Reedy, J.; Kuczmarski, R.; Esposito, L.; Krebs-Smith, J. Trends in Research on Environmental and Policy Interventions Targeting Improvements in the Retail Food Environment Supported by the National Institutes of Health. In Proceedings of the Annual Grantee Meeting of Healthy Eating Research, a national program of the Robert Wood Johnson Foundation, St. Paul, MN, USA, 19 April 2017.
36. National Institute of Diabetes and Digestive and Kidney Diseases. *2020–2030 Strategic Plan for NIH Nutrition Research*; National Institutes of Health: Washington, DC, USA, 2020.
37. NIH Obesity Research Task Force. *Strategic Plan for NIH Obesity Research*; National Institutes of Health: Washington, DC, USA, 2011.
38. United States Department of Agriculture. *USDA Science Blueprint*; United States Department of Agriculture: Washington, DC, USA, 2020.
39. Fleischhacker, S.; Woteki, C.E.; Coates, P.M.; Hubbard, V.S.; Flaherty, G.E.; Glickman, D.R.; Harkin, T.R.; Kessler, D.; Li, W.W.; Loscalzo, J.; et al. Strengthening national nutrition research: Rationale and options for a new coordinated federal research effort and authority. *Am. J. Clin. Nutr.* **2020**, *112*, 721–769. [CrossRef] [PubMed]
40. Bloomberg American Health Initiative Obesity and the Food System. Available online: https://americanhealth.jhu.edu/issue/obesity-food-system (accessed on 21 July 2020).
41. Redman, R. Online Grocery Sales to Grow 40% in 2020. Available online: https://www.supermarketnews.com/online-retail/online-grocery-sales-grow-40-2020 (accessed on 18 May 2020).

Publisher's Note: MDPI stays neutral with regard to jurisdictional claims in published maps and institutional affiliations.

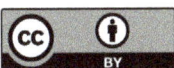

© 2020 by the authors. Licensee MDPI, Basel, Switzerland. This article is an open access article distributed under the terms and conditions of the Creative Commons Attribution (CC BY) license (http://creativecommons.org/licenses/by/4.0/).

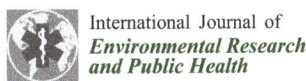

Article

Urban vs. Rural Socioeconomic Differences in the Nutritional Quality of Household Packaged Food Purchases by Store Type

Allison Lacko *, Shu Wen Ng and Barry Popkin

The Carolina Population Center, University of North Carolina at Chapel Hill, Chapel Hill, NC 27516, USA; shuwen@unc.edu (S.W.N.); popkin@unc.edu (B.P.)
* Correspondence: ALacko@frac.org; Tel.: +1-908-625-6323

Received: 1 September 2020; Accepted: 16 October 2020; Published: 20 October 2020

Abstract: The U.S. food system is rapidly changing, including the growth of mass merchandisers and dollar stores, which may impact the quality of packaged food purchases (PFPs). Furthermore, diet-related disparities exist by socioeconomic status (SES) and rural residence. We use data from the 2010–2018 Nielsen Homescan Panel to describe the nutritional profiles of PFPs by store type and to assess whether these vary by household urbanicity and SES. Store types include grocery stores, mass merchandisers, club stores, online shopping, dollar stores, and convenience/drug stores. Food and beverage groups contributing the most calories at each store type are estimated using survey-weighted means, while the associations of urbanicity and SES with nutritional quality are estimated using multivariate regression. We find that households that are customers at particular store types purchase the same quality of food regardless of urbanicity or SES. However, we find differences in the quality of foods between store types and that the quantity of calories purchased at each store type varies according to household urbanicity and SES. Rural shoppers tend to shop more at mass merchandisers and dollar stores with less healthful PFPs. We discuss implications for the types of store interventions most relevant for improving the quality of PFPs.

Keywords: diet quality; nutrition; diet disparities; urban; rural; socioeconomic; income disparities; consumer packaged goods; packaged foods

---

1. Introduction

Public health efforts to improve food retail have focused on increased access to grocery stores under the assumption that the food available is healthier than smaller convenience stores [1]. However, research examining trends in household packaged food purchases (PFPs) found that the share of purchases from grocery stores decreased from 2000 to 2012 and that the PFPs that were the top sources of calories for US households did not vary meaningfully by store type from 2000 to 2012 [2]. Further research is needed to determine whether these trends have continued to the present day and whether national trends by store type differ among sociodemographic subpopulations.

Specifically, there may be differences in the nutritional quality of PFPs between urban and rural households. Residents of rural areas have been found to depend more on smaller convenience and dollar stores, which have limited and more expensive food items compared to other store types [3,4] as well as compared to small convenience stores in urban areas [5]. The cost of healthy food in larger grocery stores has also been found to be higher in rural areas [6]. Furthermore, diet-related disparities by socioeconomic status (SES) may be exacerbated in rural versus urban food deserts, where lower income individuals have fewer transportation options (e.g., money for gas or lack of public transportation) to access retail stores with a larger variety of food and/or more affordable prices [7,8]. While many studies focus only on food access and purchases among either the urban poor or rural poor [9], no research exists that studies the intersection of urban/rural residence and SES as it relates to store use and the healthfulness of food purchases. As rural individuals are at higher risk of poorly treated diet-related diseases compared to urban residents [10,11], it is important to understand how the healthfulness of food purchases varies by urbanicity.

This comparative research is urgently needed in a rapidly changing U.S. food system, which includes the growth of mass merchandisers (e.g., Walmart), small dollar stores, and online shopping. For example, dollar stores (Dollar General, Dollar Tree, and Family Dollar) have nearly doubled in the past decade [12]. Their expansion into poor rural towns hurts local grocery stores, often driving them out of business [13–16]. In poor urban areas that lack traditional grocers, dollar stores tend to cluster, as their small retail footprint allows them to bypass zoning restrictions faced by larger supermarkets [14]. The proliferation of dollar stores in rural and urban low-income neighborhoods makes it especially important to consider the intersection of urbanicity and SES to understand purchasing patterns [17]. Lastly, the COVID-19 outbreak rapidly increased demand for groceries, particularly through online shopping [18]. Therefore, it is important to understand how the quality of online grocery purchases compares to in-store purchases.

PFPs are foods with universal barcodes (e.g., a bag of onions, frozen entrees) and contribute significantly to the healthfulness of the whole diet. Store-bought foods make up most of the U.S. diet [19], and about 70% of calories from store-bought foods come from PFPs (the remainder comes from random weight foods, e.g., loose produce, deli meat) [20]. This has important implications for public health, as packaged foods tend to be highly processed [21] and the intake of highly processed foods is associated with both poor diet quality [21,22] and weight gain [23].

The objectives of this research are as follows: first, determine whether trends in the types of stores households shop at and the nutrient profiles and types of foods/beverages purchased at different store types has changed since 2012; second, investigate whether residence in an urban or rural county is associated with the types of stores shopped at and the nutrient profiles of PFPs within store type; third, understand whether socioeconomic differences in the types of stores shopped at or in the nutritional quality of PFPs varies by urban or rural county of residence. Our analysis uses six store types: grocery stores, mass merchandisers, club stores, online purchases from any store, dollar stores, and other convenience stores. We examine trends beginning in 2010 to provide three years of overlap with prior research (2010–2012).

2. Materials and Methods

2.1. Data

We used 2010–2018 data from the U.S. Nielsen Homescan Consumer Panel [24,25], where participants track their purchases by scanning food and beverage barcodes and recording the store of purchase. Data from each purchase occasion were aggregated at the annual level for each household to create household-year observations. To be included in Homescan, households must participate for at least ten months each year (n = 555,085 household-year observations). We further excluded households if they did not purchase a minimum amount of food and beverages for all quarters in a calendar year or had an incorrect county FIPS code (federal five-digit identifier) (n = 3026, 0.5%) for a final analytic sample of 552,059 household-year observations.

Nielsen Homescan is a panel that uses an open cohort study design, where households may exit any time and new households are enrolled to replace dropouts based on demographic and geographic targets. Households in our final sample participated in Nielsen for an average of 4 years. Households are sampled from 52 metropolitan and 24 non-metropolitan markets across the contiguous US and are weighted to be nationally representative. Homescan's large sample size (about 60,000 households/year) provides a rich demographic and geographic variation of household characteristics which allows for the comparison of urban and rural trends and epidemiological analysis to understand differences by socioeconomic groups.

2.2. Store Type

Store type is based on Nielsen's classification of stores, which is based on store size, annual sales/revenue, and the relative quantity of goods the store carries. Seven non-overlapping categories of stores were analyzed: (1) warehouse clubs (e.g., Costco, Sam's Club); (2) mass merchandisers–supercenters (e.g., Walmart, Target); (3) grocery stores (e.g., Kroger, Safeway, Whole Foods); (4) dollar stores (e.g., Dollar General, Family Dollar); (5) convenience and drug stores (e.g., CVS, gas stations); (6) online shopping from any store type (e.g., Shoprite.com, Walmart.com); (7) other stores (e.g., non-food retail stores such as Best Buy, liquor stores). Since categories are mutually exclusive, purchases made from a mass merchandiser's website (e.g., Target.com, Walmart.com) would be categorized as "online shopping" and not as "mass merchandiser".

2.3. Demographic Data

Nielsen provides data on a household's county of residence, which is updated annually. Following the U.S. Department of Agriculture's Economic Research Service, counties were categorized as urban or rural using the 2013 Office of Management and Budget "metro" and "nonmetro" delineations [26,27].

Household income was used as a proxy for socioeconomic status. To account for differences in the cost of living across the country, self-reported household income was adjusted using Regional Price Parities from the Bureau of Economic Analysis [28]. Then, income was recalculated as a percent of the Federal Poverty Level (FPL) [29], which accounts for household size, and finally divided into tertiles. Household income tertiles were recalculated each year to reflect changes in household composition and income, Regional Price Parities, and the FPL.

Demographic covariates included education, which was defined as the highest self-reported educational attainment of a head of household and categorized into high school or less, some college, college graduate, or post college graduate; race/ethnicity, which was self-reported for one head of household and was categorized as Hispanic, non-Hispanic (NH) White, NH Black, NH Asian, or NH Other; and household composition, which was based on the self-reported age of each household member and included as a series of count variables for the number of individuals in different age groups (0–1, 2–5, 6–11, 19–64, 65 and older).

2.4. Outcomes

Unique barcodes in the Nielsen dataset have been linked to Nutrition Facts Panel data as described elsewhere [30,31]. There is no single measure available to summarize the nutritional quality of packaged foods and beverages (compared to the Healthy Eating Index for overall diet quality [32] or the Grocery Purchase Quality Index, which requires all random-weight and packaged food purchases and excludes mixed dishes [33]). Therefore, a series of outcomes was used to assess the nutritional quality of PFPs. Nutrients of concern included saturated fat, total sugar, and sodium. In addition, we evaluated calories per capita per day from food groups of public health interest (fruits, non-starchy vegetables, processed meats and seafood, mixed dishes, sugar-sweetened beverages (SSBs), and junk foods). The public health relevance for each outcome is detailed in Table 1. In addition, we also examined trends in grains, not as an indicator of nutritional quality but rather because they were a top contributor of calories across store types in prior research [2]. These categories were derived by classifying all products into 27 mutually exclusive food and beverage categories based on Nielsen's product classifications. Mixed dishes include products such as canned soups and frozen entrees, while junk foods include all salty snacks, grain-based desserts, candy, and sweeteners.

Table 1. Public health relevance of nutritional outcomes.

NUTRITIONAL OUTCOMES (UNITS)	RATIONALE
Percent of calories from sugar, percent of calories from saturated fat; grams of sugar, grams of saturated fat, mg of sodium (per capita per day)	• Overconsumed in the US [34] • Diets high in sugar are associated with cancer, metabolic syndrome, and obesity [35] • Replacement of saturated fat with polyunsaturated fat reduces cardiovascular disease risk [36] • Salt intake associated with cancer [35] and cardiovascular disease [37]
Total calories (per capita per day)	Provide context for calories from select food groups below
Calories from healthy food groups: fruit, non-starchy (NS) vegetables (kcal per capita per day)	• Important sources of vitamins and fiber • High consumption associated with lower cardiovascular disease risk [38] • Underconsumed in the US [34]
Calories from unhealthy food groups: processed meats, sugar-sweetened beverages (SSBs), junk foods (kcal per capita per day)	• Large contributors of total energy, sugar, saturated fat, and sodium in US diet [21] • The consumption of processed meat is classified as "carcinogenic to humans" by the International Agency for Research on Cancer [39] possibly due to nitrates, higher salt content, and other chemical preservatives [35,40] • SSBs independently linked to chronic diseases [41]
Calories from grains (kcal per capita per day)	Provide additional context, as grains were the top contributor of calories across store types from 2000 to 2012 [2]

Except for the percent of calories from sugar and saturated fat, all outcomes measured at the household-year level were normalized from annual purchases to daily per capita values. First, we divided annual totals by the number of reliable reporting days that the household participated in the panel. We identified households as "reliable food reporters" if they purchased a minimum amount of food and beverages every three months ($45 for a single-person household and $135 for households with two or more people). Data from reliable reporting quarters within a calendar year were summed to calculate average daily purchases at the household level. Next, daily values were normalized by the number of people in the household in the corresponding year. The proportion of adults and children was later accounted for by adjusting for household composition as a series of covariates.

2.5. Statistical Methods

Statistical analysis was conducted using STATA version 15 [42]. To assess trends in purchases from different store types for our first objective, we calculated the percent volume of household PFPs by store type and year by regressing percent volume on the interaction of store type and year. We tested for statistically significant differences between 2010 and 2018 within the same store type. Similarly, to identify the food groups that were the top contributors of calories, we calculated the share of calories for each food group by regressing each food group on the interaction of store type and year.

Average values for each year and store type were generated using predictive margins. For top food and beverage groups, we tested for statistically significant differences between stores within the same year, including a global F test for between store comparisons, and between 2010 and 2018 within the same store type.

For our second and third objectives, we used multivariate regression to assess urban and rural differences. We use the standardized nutritional outcomes as detailed in Table 1. For all food group outcomes, a two-part regression was estimated using a probit model and a generalized linear model (GLM) with a gamma distribution and log link. All nutrient outcomes were estimated using only a GLM also with a gamma distribution and log link. To estimate urban and rural differences, STATA's margins command was used to estimate predicted values by stratifying predictions into urban and rural populations (margins, over(urban)). To assess a potential interaction with socioeconomic status, an interaction term was added between the urbanicity and household income tertile. All regression models were adjusted for income tertile, education, race/ethnicity, household composition, and year.

For all three objectives, we used STATA's "svy" command to account for survey design (sampling within market strata) and for repeated measurements for those households that participate in the panel for multiple years [43]. While all household-year observations were retained in each model for the correct calculation of standard errors, models were stratified by store type. This was accomplished by using "svy, subpop ():" to limit the analytic subpopulation to those household-years where the household was a reliable reporter and had purchased at least one item from the store type being analyzed.

3. Results

Household demographic characteristics by store type are shown in Table 2. Although most households resided in urban counties, Nielsen sampled at least one household from 93.6% of counties in the contiguous U.S. between 2010 and 2018 (90.4% of rural counties and 98.5% of urban counties). Adjusting for the cost of living slightly increased the proportion of low and middle-income households.

Table 2. Sample characteristics by store type, 2010–2018.

	Club Stores	Mass Merchandisers	Grocery Stores	Online Shopping	Dollar Stores	Convenience Stores	Other Stores
Household-years excluded [1]	265,050	60,748	12,560	497,906	262,351	185,641	160,444
Analytic Sample	290,035	494,337	542,525	57,179	292,734	369,444	394,641
Demographics: % = Survey-Weighted Proportion (n = Household-Year Observations)							
County of Residence							
Urban	91.0% (261,579)	84.7% (417,186)	85.8% (463,604)	85.5% (48,510)	81.7% (238,636)	86.5% (318,196)	86.3% (338,807)
Rural	9.0% (28,456)	15.3% (77,151)	14.2% (78,921)	14.5% (8669)	18.3% (54,098)	13.5% (51,248)	13.7% (55,834)
Household Income after Adjustment for Cost-of-Living and FPL [2]							
Low Income (<185% FPL)	20.9% (41,827)	28.1% (97,521)	28.0% (106,065)	29.0% (11,760)	35.5% (71,792)	28.6% (72,673)	26.8% (73,417)
Middle Income (185–400%)	38.5% (122,639)	38.1% (213,942)	37.4% (231,893)	37.2% (24,408)	37.9% (130,612)	37.2% (157,778)	37.1% (166,796)
High Income (>400% FPL)	40.6% (125,569)	33.8% (182,874)	34.6% (204,567)	33.8% (21,011)	26.7% (90,330)	34.2% (138,993)	36.1% (154,428)

[1] Household-years were excluded from all analyses if the household was a poor food reporter. For both analysis of top contributors of calories and for multivariate regression models, additional household-years were excluded if the household purchased zero packaged food or beverage items from a given store type in that year. Therefore, proportions only include those household-years during which a household shopped at a store type at least once. [2] For analysis, household income was adjusted for cost of living, normalized to the Federal Poverty Level (FPL), and then classified into tertiles. Household income is categorized relative to the FPL for ease of comparison in this table. Nielsen disclaimer: Authors' calculations based in part on data reported by Nielsen through its Homescan Services for all food categories, including beverages and alcohol for the 2008–2018 periods across the U.S. market. The Nielsen Company, 2015. Nielsen is not responsible for and had no role in preparing the results reported herein.

3.1. Trends in Store Type from 2010 to 2018

We find small but significant changes ($p < 0.001$) between 2010 and 2018 in the volume share of purchases from each store type, except for online shopping. Grocery stores constitute the largest share of volume purchased (57.7% in 2010 and 54.3% in 2018), followed by mass merchandisers (23.2% to 25.6%), club stores (9.3% to 11.0%), convenience and drug stores (3.5% to 2.4%), dollar stores (1.8% to 2.6%), and online shopping (0.7% to 0.8%).

Among households who shopped at each store type, the top food and beverage groups were similar across store types and years (Table 3). Top food groups included grains, salty snacks, desserts, mixed dishes, and candy as the average share of total calories purchased across households. Top beverages included SSBs, plain milk, alcohol, and juice (2010 only). In comparison, fruits and non-starchy vegetables made up a small percent of calories purchased by households. Although the top categories of foods and beverages were the same across store type and time, the relative proportion of calories from each group varied widely by store type (p-value < 0.0001 for the F test for each food/beverage group). There were also significant differences between most store pairs using grocery stores as the referent ($p < 0.0001$), with few exceptions (e.g., between grocery stores and mass merchandisers for mixed dishes, SSBs, and alcohol in 2018).

Table 3. Top sources of packaged food purchases (PFP) calories by store type in 2010 and 2018 [1] (percent of total calories (SE)).

	Grocery Store	Mass Merchandisers	Club Stores	Online Shopping	Dollar Stores	Convenience Stores	Other Stores	All Stores
Daily calories per capita (SE) 2010	802 (4.8)	356 (3.5)	257 (3.5)	112 (6.1)	55 (1.3)	51 (0.9)	72 (1.6)	1354 (5.7)
2018	686 (3.5)	358 (2.9)	243 (2.9)	73 (3.5)	60 (1.1)	36 (0.7)	60 (1.2)	1211 (4.5)
Top 5 Food Groups in 2010 (percent of total calories (SE))	Grains 18.1% (0.1%)	Grains 15.1% (0.1%)	Grains 12.3% (0.2%)	Grains 12.5% (0.4%)	Candy 24.5% (0.3%)	Candy 31.0% (0.3%)	Candy 15.4% (0.2%)	Grains 17.1% (0.1%)
	Desserts 8.3% (0.0%)	Candy 11.3% (0.1%)	Salty snacks 10.6% (0.2%)	Candy 12.4% (0.6%)	Desserts 15.6% (0.2%)	Salty snacks 9.0% (0.2%)	Grains 11.4% (0.2%)	Salty snacks 8.6% (0.0%)
	Salty snacks 7.9% (0.0%)	Salty snacks 10.3% (0.1%)	Mixed dishes 8.9% (0.1%)	Salty snacks 9.7% (0.4%)	Salty snacks 15.1% (0.2%)	Desserts 6.7% (0.1%)	Desserts 9.4% (0.2%)	Desserts 7.9% (0.0%)
	Mixed dishes 7.3% (0.0%)	Desserts 10.1% (0.1%)	Desserts 7.8% (0.1%)	Desserts 8.4% (0.4%)	Grains 8.4% (0.2%)	Grains 6.0% (0.1%)	Salty snacks 9.0% (0.2%)	Mixed dishes 7.3% (0.0%)
	Other dairy 6.8% (0.0%)	Mixed dishes 6.7% (0.1%)	Nuts 7.1% (0.1%)	Mixed dishes 6.1% (0.3%)	Mixed dishes 4.2% (0.1%)	Nuts 5.8% (0.1%)	Mixed dishes 3.2% (0.1%)	Fats and oils 6.6% (0.0%)
Top 5 Food Groups in 2018 (percent of total calories (SE))	Grains 16.1% (0.1%) **	Grains 14.3% (0.1%) *	Salty snacks 11.2% (0.1%) **	Grains 13.3% (0.4%)	Candy 27.5% (0.3%)	Candy 33.6% (0.3%)	Candy 16.5% (0.2%) **	Grains 15.3% (0.0%) **
	Salty snacks 8.6% (0.0%)	Candy 9.9% (0.1%) **	Grains 10.9% (0.1%) **	Salty snacks 10.2% (0.3%)	Desserts 15.0% (0.2%) **	Salty snacks 10.6% (0.2%) **	Salty snacks 10.6% (0.1%) **	Salty snacks 9.1% (0.0%) **
	Other dairy 7.8% (0.0%) **	Desserts 9.8% (0.1%)	Mixed dishes 10.2% (0.1%) **	Candy 9.0% (0.4%)	Salty snacks 11.9% (0.2%)	Desserts 6.4% (0.1%) *	Desserts 9.4% (0.2%)	Desserts 7.6% (0.0%) **
	Desserts 7.8% (0.0%) **	Salty snacks 9.6% (0.1%) **	Desserts 8.0% (0.1%)	Desserts 8.3% (0.3%)	Grains 8.2% (0.1%)	Nuts 5.2% (0.1%) **	Grains 8.2% (0.2%) **	Mixed dishes 7.5% (0.0%) **
	Mixed dishes 7.2% (0.0%) *	Mixed dishes 7.2% (0.1%) **	Nuts 7.0% (0.1%)	Mixed dishes 5.8% (0.3%)	Mixed dishes 4.8% (0.1%) **	Grains 4.8% (0.1%) **	Nuts 2.9% (0.1%)	Other dairy 7.3% (0.0%) **
Top 3 Beverage Groups in 2010 (percent of total calories (SE))	SSBs 5.1% (0.1%)	SSBs 6.5% (0.1%)	SSBs 4.0% (0.1%)	SSBs 6.5% (0.5%)	SSBs 7.3% (0.2%)	SSBs 11.1% (0.2%)	Alcohol 18.9% (0.3%)	SSBs 5.1% (0.0%)
	Milk 4.8% (0.0%)	Milk 3.4% (0.1%)	Milk 2.5% (0.1%)	Milk 3.9% (0.3%)	Milk 1.2% (0.1%)	Milk 7.7% (0.2%)	SSBs 6.3% (0.2%)	Milk 4.2% (0.0%)
	Juice 1.9% (0.0%)	Juice 1.7% (0.0%)	Juice 2.1% (0.1%)	Alcohol 2.4% (0.3%)	Juice 0.9% (0.1%)	Alcohol 5.1% (0.2%)	Milk 1.7% (0.1%)	Alcohol 2.1% (0.0%)
Top 3 Beverage Groups in 2018 (percent of total calories (SE))	SSBs 4.3% (0.0%) **	SSBs 4.5% (0.1%) **	SSBs 2.7% (0.1%) **	SSBs 5.4% (0.3%)	SSBs 7.7% (0.1%)	SSBs 11.6% (0.2%)	Alcohol 21.2% (0.3%) **	SSBs 4.1% (0.0%) **
	Milk 3.8% (0.0%) **	Milk 3.1% (0.0%) **	Alcohol 2.3% (0.1%) **	Milk 2.6% (0.2%) *	Milk 1.9% (0.1%) **	Alcohol 5.8% (0.1%) **	SSBs 5.8% (0.1%) *	Milk 3.5% (0.0%) **
	Alcohol 1.9% (0.0%) **	Alcohol 1.7% (0.0%) **	Milk 2.1% (0.1%) **	Alcohol 1.8% (0.2%)	Juice 0.9% (0.0%)	Milk 4.9% (0.1%) **	Milk 1.1% (0.0%) **	Alcohol 2.4% (0.0%) **

Table 3. Cont.

	Grocery Store	Mass Merchandisers	Club Stores	Online Shopping	Dollar Stores	Convenience Stores	Other Stores	All Stores
Other groups, 2010 (percent of total calories (SE))	Fruits 1.4% (0.0%)	Fruits 1.3% (0.0%)	Fruits 4.1% (0.1%)	Fruits 2.5% (0.2%)	Fruits 1.4% (0.1%)	Fruits 1.2% (0.1%)	Fruits 1.2% (0.0%)	Fruits 1.6% (0.0%)
	Vegetables 1.5% (0.0%)	Vegetables 0.8% (0.0%)	Vegetables 1.9% (0.1%)	Vegetables 1.3% (0.2%)	Vegetables 1.1% (0.1%)	Vegetables 0.4% (0.0%)	Vegetables 0.8% (0.0%)	Vegetables 1.2% (0.0%)
Other groups, 2018 (percent of total calories (SE))	Fruits 1.8% (0.0%) **	Fruits 1.7% (0.0%) **	Fruits 4.3% (0.1%) *	Fruits 2.3% (0.2%)	Fruits 1.1% (0.0%) **	Fruits 0.7% (0.0%) **	Fruits 1.4% (0.1%) *	Fruits 1.9% (0.0%) **
	Vegetables 1.9% (0.0%) **	Vegetables 1.3% (0.0%) **	Vegetables 2.1% (0.1%) *	Vegetables 1.7% (0.1%)	Vegetables 1.0% (0.1%)	Vegetables 0.4% (0.0%)	Vegetables 0.9% (0.0%)	Vegetables 1.6% (0.0%) **

[1] In 2010, the sample size across all store types was 61,105 household-year observations. In 2018, the sample size was 61,372 household-year observations. For each household-year observation, calories were summed for each food and beverage group as well as across all purchases to calculate a household's share of calories from each group for a given year. Results represent the average share of calories from each food/beverage group across households that purchased at least one PFP from a given store type in a given year. * 2010 vs. 2018 difference significant at $p < 0.05$ for share of calories purchased from food group within store type. ** 2010 vs. 2018 difference significant at $p < 0.001$ for share of calories purchased from food group within store type. SSB: Sugar-sweetened beverage. Nielsen disclaimer: Authors' calculations based in part on data reported by Nielsen through its Homescan Services for all food categories, including beverages and alcohol for the 2008–2018 periods across the U.S. market. The Nielsen Company, 2015. Nielsen is not responsible for and had no role in preparing the results reported herein.

3.2. Urban versus Rural Differences

There are statistically significant differences in the daily per capita calories from urban and rural households' PFPs from different store types, except for grocery stores and convenience/drug stores (Figure 1 and Table 4). Among households that shop at mass merchandisers, rural households purchase almost twice as many calories per person per day as urban households. Among households who shop at dollar stores, rural households also purchase slightly more calories compared to urban households. In comparison, urban households purchase more from club stores.

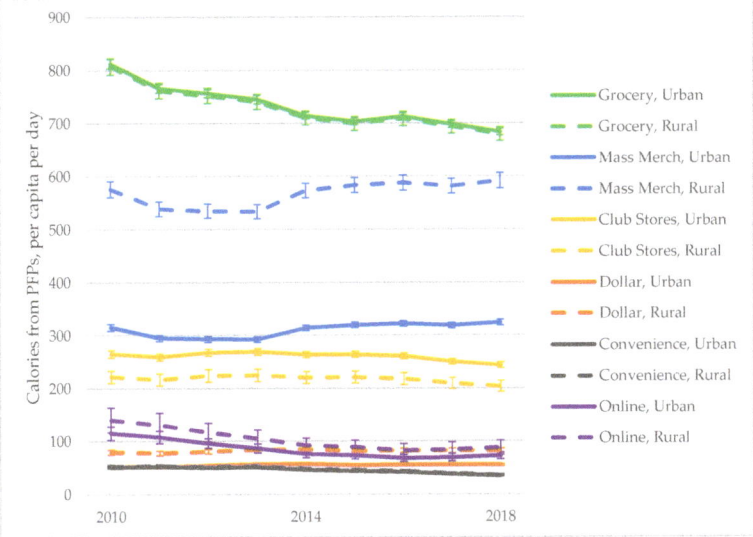

Figure 1. Trends in calories from PFPs by store type and urban/rural household residence. Trends reflect a "per consumer" analysis. Separate models were run for each store type where the analytic sample was limited to those households that purchased at least one packaged food or beverage from a given store type.

Table 4. Urban vs. rural nutritional quality of household packaged food purchases by store type, 2010–2018 [1] (predicted mean (SE)).

	Grocery Stores			Mass Merchandisers			Club Stores			Online Shopping			Dollar Stores			Convenience/Drug		
	Total	Rural	Urban	Total	Rural	Urban	Total	Rural	Urban	Total	Rural	Urban	Total	Rural	Urban	Total	Rural	Urban
Total calories, person/day [2]	730 (2)	728 (6)	731 (2)	349 (2)	565 (6) **	310 (2)	255 (2)	216 (5)	258 (2) **	85 (2)	100 (7)	82 (3)	59 (1)	81 (2) **	54 (1)	46 (1)	47 (1)	45 (1)
Fruits	10 (0)	9 (0)	11 (0) **	5 (0)	7 (0) **	4 (0)	10 (0)	7 (0)	10 (0) **	1 (0)	2 (0)	1 (0)	1 (0)	1 (0)	1 (0)	0 (0)	0 (0)	0 (0)
NS Vegetables	11 (0)	10 (0)	11 (0) **	4 (0)	6 (0) **	3 (0)	4 (0)	3 (0)	4 (0) **	1 (0)	1 (0)	1 (0)	0 (0)	0 (0)	0 (0)	0 (0)	0 (0)	0 (0)
Processed meats	33 (0)	39 (1) **	32 (0)	14 (0)	25 (0) **	12 (0)	10 (0)	9 (0)	10 (0) **	3 (0)	4 (1)	3 (0)	1 (0)	2 (0) **	1 (0)	0 (0)	1 (0)	0 (0)
Mixed dishes	53 (0)	49 (1)	54 (0) **	28 (0)	43 (1) **	25 (0)	21 (0)	15 (1)	22 (0) **	6 (0)	6 (1)	6 (0)	3 (0)	4 (0) **	3 (0)	1 (0)	1 (0)	1 (0)
Grains	124 (1)	119 (1)	125 (1) **	55 (0)	88 (1) **	49 (0)	33 (0)	26 (1)	34 (0) **	14 (1)	16 (1)	13 (1)	7 (0)	9 (0) **	6 (0)	3 (0)	4 (0)	3 (0)
SSBs	33 (0)	35 (1) **	33 (0)	17 (0)	28 (1) **	15 (0)	8 (0)	6 (0)	8 (0) **	4 (0)	4 (0)	4 (0)	4 (0)	7 (0) **	4 (0)	5 (0)	6 (0) **	4 (0)
Junk foods	170 (1)	173 (2)	169 (1)	103 (1)	167 (2) **	92 (1)	66 (1)	62 (2)	67 (1)	23 (1)	29 (2) **	22 (1)	28 (0)	38 (1) **	26 (0)	20 (0)	18 (1)	20 (0) **
Sugar g	45 (0)	45 (0)	45 (0)	23 (0)	37 (0) **	20 (0)	14 (0)	12 (0)	14 (0) **	5 (0)	6 (0) **	5 (0)	5 (0)	7 (0) **	4 (0)	4 (0)	4 (0)	4 (0)
Sugar, % Total calories	25% (0.0%)	25% (0.1%) **	24% (0.0%)	28% (0.0%)	28% (0.1%)	28% (0.0%) **	23% (0.1%)	24% (0.2%) **	23% (0.1%)	27% (0.2%)	28% (0.4%) **	27% (0.2%)	36% (0.1%)	37% (0.2%)	36% (0.1%)	39% (0.1%)	40% (0.2%) **	38% (0.1%)
Sat fat g	10 (0)	11 (0) **	10 (0)	5 (0)	8 (0) **	4 (0)	4 (0)	3 (0)	4 (0) **	1 (0)	1 (0)	1 (0)	1 (0)	1 (0) **	1 (0)	1 (0)	1 (0)	1 (0)
Sat fat, % Total calories	13% (0.0%)	13% (0.0%) **	13% (0.0%)	12% (0.0%)	12% (0.0%) **	12% (0.0%)	13% (0.0%)	12% (0.1%)	13% (0.0%)	11% (0.1%)	11% (0.2%)	11% (0.1%)	10% (0.0%)	10% (0.1%) **	10% (0.0%)	12% (0.0%)	12% (0.1%)	12% (0.0%) **
Sodium mg	1393 (5)	1412 (14)	1390 (5)	687 (4)	1123 (13) **	608 (4)	474 (5)	425 (11)	479 (5) **	172 (6)	204 (15)	167 (6)	148 (2)	184 (5) **	140 (2)	57 (1)	63 (2) **	57 (1)

[1] The estimates presented are based on a "per consumer" analysis, where the analytic sample for each store type was limited to households purchasing at least one item from a given store type in a year. In other words, an average of 733 calories per person per day are purchased from grocery stores among households who purchased at least one PFP from a grocery store. Estimates are generated using multivariate regression, controlling for household income, education, race/ethnicity, age composition, and year and are adjusted for Nielsen's survey design to be nationally representative. [2] Total calories and calories from specific food groups are expressed in units of calories per person per day. Grams of sugar and saturated fat are expressed in grams purchased per person per day. Percent purchased calories from sugar or saturated fat are calculated by dividing the calories attributable to sugar/saturated fat across all households by the total number of calories purchased from that store type across all households. Mixed dishes include foods such as frozen entrees and canned soups, and junk foods include salty snacks, grain-based desserts, candy, and sweeteners. Non-starchy (NS) vegetables include leafy greens but not potatoes, corn, etc. Examples of mixed dishes include frozen entrees and canned soups; examples of junk foods include candies and salty snacks. SSBs: sugar-sweetened beverages. ** Urban or rural value that is statistically higher at a significance value of $p < 0.01$. Nielsen disclaimer: Authors' calculations based in part on data reported by Nielsen through its Homescan Services for all food categories, including beverages and alcohol for the 2008–2018 periods across the U.S. market. The Nielsen Company, 2015. Nielsen is not responsible for and had no role in preparing the results reported herein.

Although online shopping makes up a small share of volume purchased among all households (<1% across all years), the number of calories purchased among households that did shop online exceeded calories purchased by dollar store shoppers. In 2010, online shoppers purchased an average of 112 calories per person per day while dollar store shoppers purchased 55 calories per person per day. In 2018, this difference narrowed: online shoppers purchased 73 calories per person per day while dollar store shoppers purchased 60 calories per person per day. In addition, rural households purchase more PFPs through online shopping compared to urban households.

To assess differences in quality, results for nutrients and food groups purchased at each store type are summarized in Table 4. Urban–rural differences in the calories purchased from specific foods groups follow the same patterns as total calories purchased. There is little difference in the quality of foods purchased by urban and rural households shopping at the same store type. However, there are differences in the average percent of calories from sugar and from saturated fat purchased by households across store types.

3.3. Interaction between Household Income and Urbanicity

Whether there is more variation in calories from PFPs by household income or by urban/rural residence depends on the store type (Figure 2). To assess differences in the nutritional quality of PFPs by income, and whether this further differs by urban/rural residence, results for nutrients and food groups are summarized in Table 5. Store types are condensed into four categories for ease of comparison: online purchases are included with their store type (i.e., purchases from Walmart.com are categorized as "mass merchandisers") and dollar stores are combined with convenience and drug stores (see Appendix A: Table A1 for all store types).

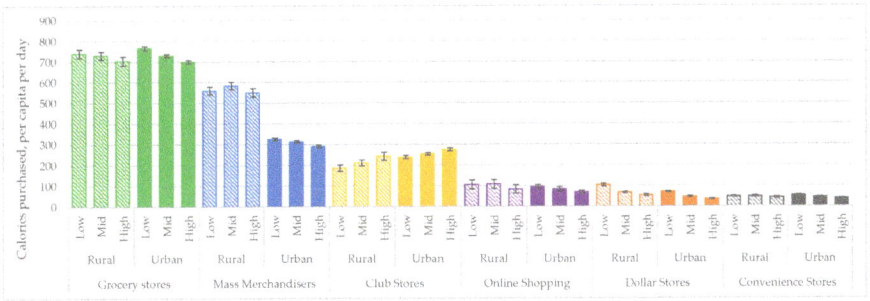

Figure 2. Calories (per person per day) from packaged food purchases, by store type, urban/rural household residence, and household income, 2010–2018.

Differences between high- and low-income households are similar for rural and urban households for all store types except for mass merchandisers. Among households who shop at grocery stores, low-income households purchase more calories from PFPs compared to high-income households. A similar pattern is found among dollar store shoppers. In comparison, among households who shop at club stores, high-income households purchase more calories than low-income households. Among households that shop at mass merchandisers, there is no difference between low-income and high-income rural households.

There are few rural–urban differences in the average calories per person per day purchased from each food group between low- and high-income households. Regardless of urbanicity or store type, high-income households purchase slightly more fruits and non-starchy vegetables. Where statistically significant difference-in-differences are found, the substantive differences are small. As in Table 4, the greatest contrasts can be found in the average percent of calories from sugar purchased by households at specific store types rather than between households categorized by income or urbanicity.

Table 5. Urban/Rural comparison of differences by income in the nutritional quality of household packaged food purchases by store type, 2010–2018 [1] (predicted margin (SE)).

Store Type	Grocery Stores				Mass Merchandisers				Club Stores				Convenience Stores			
County Type	Rural		Urban		Rural		Urban		Rural		Urban		Rural		Urban	
Income Tertile	Low	High	Low	High	Low	High	Low	High	Low	High	Low	High	Low	High	Low	High
Total calories, person/day [2]	740 (10.6) *	704 (10.9)	770 (4.6) **	702 (3.8)	564 (9.5)	555 (10.8)	329 (3.3) **	294 (3.2)	188 (7.6)	245 (10.0) **	242 (3.9)	281 (3.5) **	122 (3.4) **	74 (2.5)	94 (1.4) **	53 (0.9)
Fruits	9 (0.2)	10 (0.3) **	10 (0.1)	11 (0.1) **	6 (0.2)	8 (0.2) **	4 (0.1)	4 (0.1) *	5 (0.3)	8 (0.6) **	8 (0.2)	11 (0.2) **	1 (0.0) **	1 (0.1) **	1 (0.0)	1 (0.0)
NS Vegetables	9 (0.2)	11 (0.2) **	11 (0.1)	12 (0.1) **	5 (0.1)	6 (0.2) *	3 (0.0)	4 (0.1) **	2 (0.2)	4 (0.3) **	4 (0.1)	5 (0.1) **	0 (0.0) **	0 (0.0)	1 (0.0) **	0 (0.0)
Processed meats	41 (0.8) **	35 (0.9)	34 (0.3) **	30 (0.3)	25 (0.6) *	23 (0.6)	13 (0.2) **	11 (0.2)	8 (0.5)	10 (0.8) *	9 (0.2)	11 (0.2) **	2 (0.1) **	1 (0.1)	2 (0.1) **	1 (0.0)
Mixed dishes	53 (1.1) **	44 (1.0)	60 (0.6) **	48 (0.4)	46 (1.4) **	39 (1.2)	28 (0.4) **	22 (0.3)	13 (0.7)	17 (0.9) *	21 (0.4)	23 (0.4) *	6 (0.3) **	2 (0.2)	5 (0.1) **	2 (0.1)
Grains	121 (2.1) *	114 (2.0)	131 (1.0) **	120 (0.8)	87 (1.7)	85 (2.0)	52 (0.6) **	46 (0.5)	23 (1.2)	28 (1.8) *	32 (0.8)	34 (0.6)	13 (0.5) **	7 (0.3)	10 (0.2) **	5 (0.1)
SSBs	38 (1.1) **	30 (1.0)	39 (0.5) **	27 (0.4)	32 (1.0) **	24 (0.8)	17 (0.3) **	12 (0.2)	6 (0.4)	6 (0.6)	9 (0.3) *	8 (0.2)	13 (0.6) **	7 (0.4)	8 (0.2) **	4 (0.1)
Junk Foods	172 (2.6)	174 (1.4) **	166 (1.1)	169 (3.4)	162 (3.0)	95 (1.0) *	90 (1.0)	53 (2.3)	72 (3.4) **	61 (1.1)	74 (1.0) **	52 (1.4) **	34 (1.3)	42 (0.7) **	2.6 (0.5)
Sugar, g	47 (0.7) *	43 (0.8)	48 (0.3) **	42 (0.3)	38 (0.7) *	36 (0.7)	22 (0.2) **	19 (0.2)	11 (0.6)	14 (0.6) *	14 (0.3)	15 (0.2) **	11 (0.3) **	7 (0.2)	8 (0.1) **	5 (0.1)
Sugar, %	25%	25%	25%	24%	28%	28%	29%	28%	25%	23%	24%	23%	37%	37%	37%	37%
Total calories (0.1%) **	(0.1%)	(0.2%)	(0.1%)	(0.1%)	(0.2%) *	(0.2%)	(0.1%) **	(0.1%)	(0.5%) *	(0.3%)	(0.2%) **	(0.1%)	(0.3%)	(0.3%)	(0.1%)	(0.1%) *
Saturated fat, g	11 (0.2)	10 (0.2)	11 (0.1) **	10 (0.1)	8 (0.1)	8 (0.2)	5 (0.0) **	4 (0.0)	3 (0.1)	4 (0.2) **	4 (0.1)	4 (0.1) **	1 (0.0) **	1 (0.0)	1 (0.0) **	1 (0.0)
Saturated fat, % calories	13% (0.1%)	13% (0.1%) **	12% (0.0%)	13% (0.0%) *	12% (0.1%)	12% (0.1%)	12% (0.0%)	12% (0.0%)	12% (0.2%)	13% (0.1%)	13% (0.1%)	13% (0.1%)	11% (0.1%)	11% (0.1%) **	11% (0.0%)	12% (0.1%) **
Sodium, mg	1441 (21.9) *	1365 (23.4)	1468 (10.0) **	1346 (8.6)	1130 (20.6)	1089 (22.6)	652 (7.7) **	577 (7.7)	378 (15.3)	480 (19.0) **	472 (9.3)	512 (7.4) **	251 (8.4) **	131 (5.4)	182 (3.2) **	93 (2.1)

[1] The estimates presented are based on a "per consumer" analysis, where the analytic sample for each store type was limited to households purchasing at least one item from a given store type in a year. Estimates are generated using multivariate regression, controlling for household income, education, race/ethnicity, age composition, and year and are adjusted for Nielsen's survey design to be nationally representative. Store types are condensed into four categories for ease of comparison: online purchases are included with their store type (i.e., purchases from Walmart.com are categorized as "mass merchandisers") and dollar stores are combined with convenience and drug stores (see Table A1 in Appendix A for all store types). [2] Total calories and calories from specific food groups are expressed in units of calories per person per day. Grams of sugar and saturated fat are expressed in grams purchased per person per day. Percent purchased calories from sugar or saturated fat are calculated by dividing the calories attributable to sugar/saturated fat across all households by the total number of calories purchased from that store type across all households. Non-starchy (NS) vegetables include leafy greens but not potatoes, corn, etc. Mixed dishes include foods such as frozen entrees and canned soups, and junk foods include salty snacks, grain-based desserts, candy, and sweeteners. SSBs: sugar-sweetened beverages. * Indicates a statistically significant difference between low-income households and high-income households at $p < 0.05$. ** Indicates a statistically significant difference between low-income households and high-income households at $p < 0.001$. The shaded cells indicate that the income difference for rural (urban) households is significantly greater than for urban (rural) households—in other words, the difference-in-difference is significant, $p < 0.05$. Nielsen disclaimer: Authors' calculation based in part on data reported by Nielsen through its Homescan Services for all food categories, including beverages and alcohol for the 2008–2018 periods across the U.S. market. The Nielsen Company, 2015. Nielsen is not responsible for and had no role in preparing the results reported herein.

4. Discussion

Our study found differences in the nutritional quality of packaged foods and beverages purchased at different types of stores, although overall, quality has changed little from 2010 to 2018 and must be improved. In addition, we found that rural households purchased more calories per person per day from mass merchandisers and dollar stores compared to urban households, and that low-income households purchase more calories from convenience stores and fewer from club stores than high-income households. However, the nutritional quality of those purchases was similar across households shopping at the same store type.

While most packaged foods are obtained from grocery stores, the volume share of purchases has slowly declined, while the share of purchases from mass merchandisers, club stores, and dollar stores has increased. The relative share of volume purchases from 2010 to 2012 are consistent with results from prior research, and the trends we find represent a continuation of trends from 2000 to 2012. [2] Our findings also align with trends in an increasing number of dollar stores in recent years [44]. Our study adds that the share of purchases from other small convenience stores is decreasing. Dollar stores are likely to sustain their growth. If the economic impact of COVID-19 is similar to the Great Recession, dollar stores are likely to see an increase in sales as consumers look for less expensive products [45]. In comparison, while the volume share of purchases from online shopping remained quite low through 2018, COVID-19 has resulted in a rapid increase in online grocery shopping, which is likely to be sustained. This is because shoppers are likely to continue using online shopping once they try it, and companies are likely to accelerate their investment in the infrastructure needed for online shopping to meet demand [45,46]. In addition, by the end of October 2020, 45 states and D.C. had approved new pilot programs to allow online purchases using Supplemental Nutrition Assistance Program (SNAP) in response to COVID-19 [47]. After investing in the infrastructure for online SNAP purchases, these programs are likely to continue.

Top packaged foods and beverages as a share of total calories have not changed meaningfully since 2000. [2] The top food and beverage groups across store types in 2010–2012 were consistent with findings from prior research [2]. Across all years, top groups include a few examples of healthy foods or beverages, apart from unsweetened milk. One exception is that juice has been replaced by alcohol as a top beverage, which is consistent with other findings that juice consumption is declining [48]. Grains are a top contributor of calories and include a mix of healthy and unhealthy grain-based foods. This is notable because it suggests that our unhealthy food groups provide a conservative estimate of low-quality purchases. One recent study compared the nutrient densities of foods to thresholds used by the Chilean government in assigning foods unhealthy warning labels and found that 66% of calories from breads and 100% of calories from ready-to-eat cereals qualified as junk foods by these standards [49]. Therefore, since all breads and cereals were included under grains in our study and grains were the top contributor of calories, our categorization of foods based on Nielsen groupings likely understates the proportion of calories from unhealthy junk foods.

However, while there was little difference in which groups were the top contributors of calories between store types, the relative proportion of calories from these groups differed between stores. The largest difference is in candies, which are not a top contributor of calories from grocery stores or club stores but comprise 10% of calories from mass merchandisers and 28% and 34% of calories from dollar stores and convenience stores, respectively. While the nutritional quality of PFPs is low among all store types, our findings indicate there are important differences between stores. PFPs from dollar stores and convenience stores are particularly high in sugar as a percent of total calories (36% and 39% respectively), and PFPs from mass merchandisers and online shopping (28% and 27%) are slightly higher in sugar than PFPs from grocery stores and club stores (25% and 23%). As a point of reference, the *Dietary Guidelines for Americans* recommend that added sugar not exceed 10% of total caloric intake [50]. While added sugars are a component of our study measure of total sugars, dollar stores and convenience stores are a negligible source of packaged fruits and vegetables with naturally occurring sugars. Relative differences in the percent of calories from sugar in these store types is likely to drive the high numbers of calories from junk foods. Our findings using nutrient outcomes align with previous research using expenditures from Nielsen 2004–2010 to calculate a single healthfulness score of purchases, which found supermarket purchases to be the healthiest, followed by club stores, supercenters (e.g., Walmart), convenience stores, and dollar stores [44]. Store stocking requirements [51] are a potential policy lever to increase the ratio of healthful to unhealthful foods (e.g., eligibility criteria for stores to accept SNAP or local ordinances). However, a recent evaluation of the Minneapolis Staple Food Ordinance found that corporate-owned stores made greater gains in complying with healthy stocking requirements compared to independently owned stores [52]. Therefore, such requirements should be coupled with financing initiatives [53,54] to help independently owned stores stock healthy foods (e.g., refrigerated storage) and community engagement to increase demand for healthy foods to support the commercial viability of such efforts [55].

We find few differences between urban and rural households in the nutritional quality of foods purchased among shoppers at a given store type. However, since meaningful differences do exist in the quality of purchases between stores, the mix of stores that households shop at matters. In particular, rural households tend to shop slightly more at dollar stores and substantially more at mass merchandisers. Therefore, interventions in these store types should be prioritized to reduce urban vs. rural diet-related disparities. Rural households may shop at these stores more frequently due to the lack of grocery stores and/or the convenience of shopping in bulk for food and non-food items at mass merchandisers to save on transportation costs [56,57]. While aspects of food marketing, including the product selection, pricing, point-of-sale promotion, and product placement, influence the healthfulness of purchases (the 4 Ps) [58], further research is needed to understand how these strategies differ between mass merchandisers, dollar stores, grocery stores, and club stores. Since both dollar stores and mass merchandisers consist of only a few large national chains, corporate engagement may be a potential strategy to shift marketing strategies in these stores to improve the quality of PFPs. Advantages of working with national chains include that decisions to shift to healthier products affect many store locations, chains have reliable supplier distribution networks, and chains can negotiate lower prices through buying in bulk [59]. For example, Dollar General aims to equip 5000 of its roughly 15,000 stores with the ability to sell fresh produce, and the Natural Resources Defense Council has secured commitments from Dollar General to prioritize locally sourced produce [60] (product selection). However, evidence suggests that voluntary initiatives by large food retail chains to encourage healthier purchases, through strategies such as reformulation (product selection), reducing prices on healthy foods, and healthy front-of-package labels (promotion) [61], may not be successful by themselves [62] and that corporate stores are more likely to sell and market more unhealthy foods compared to independently owned stores [63]. More research is needed to identify effective healthy retail strategies that are scalable across these large chains and how retailers can be held accountable to voluntary pledges.

We found few differences in the nutritional quality of purchases by the intersection of household income and urban or rural residence. Some patterns in overall shopping emerged. Low-income households purchase more calories from supermarkets, while higher income households purchase more calories from club stores, which is likely due to the membership fees required for these stores. Among households who shop at mass merchandisers, we find in urban counties that low-income households purchase more than high-income households, which is consistent with previous findings [64,65]. However, we find no income difference in purchases from mass merchandisers among rural households. This may be because most barriers faced by rural households, such as the lack of local food stores and long travel time to retailers [66], affect households of all income levels. These findings have implications for the types of retail interventions mass merchandisers should prioritize to promote equity. For example, since rural households purchase far more calories from mass merchandisers compared to urban households but there is no difference in calories purchased by low- vs. high-income rural households, it is important to improve the selection, promotion, and placement of healthy products for all consumers in rural locations. In comparison, mass merchandiser stores located in urban counties should prioritize making healthier PFPs more affordable, since low-income households purchase more than high-income households from these stores.

The use of household purchase data has several limitations. First, the participant burden of scanning each purchase is high, resulting in underreporting, especially for small purchases. However, the degree of measurement error found in Nielsen Homescan is no different than in other household panel datasets [67]. Second, packaged foods are an incomplete picture of household food purchases. Without the inclusion of unpackaged, random-weight purchases (e.g., deli meats, loose produce, bakery goods), we are unable to examine the overall healthfulness of purchases. However, packaged foods make up the majority of foods purchased from stores [19]. Lastly, purchases do not equal consumption. Not all food purchased at the store is consumed, and we are unable to account for food waste. However, the nutritional profile of purchases is correlated with diet quality as measured by 24-h recalls and therefore a good representation of overall intake [68]. Lastly, since Nielsen predominantly samples urban counties, the rural sample is much smaller than our urban sample, and rural households are more likely to be sampled from counties closer to major markets. Therefore, they may not be fully reflective of all rural areas/households.

However, our study has several important strengths. Compared to food retail sales data, household purchase data are directly tied to the sociodemographic characteristics of the household. This allows us to understand how purchasing patterns in urban and rural areas differ among high and low SES households. In comparison, retail sales data can only be linked to area-level measures of socioeconomic characteristics, precluding epidemiological analysis to understand the behavior of different consumer groups. Compared to dietary 24-h recalls, panel data are collected over a longer period of time, which better captures usual intake and avoids bias from seasonality in purchases [30]. In addition, our research group annually updates links between food items and brand-specific Nutrition Facts Panel data, capturing product reformulation and the entry/exit of products to better reflect the nutritional quality of products in a rapidly changing food market. Importantly, our access to data as recent as 2018 allows us to understand how sociodemographic factors are related to the healthfulness of purchasing patterns today.

5. Conclusions

While the quality of PFPs must be improved across all store types, we find the quality of PFPs from dollar stores and convenience stores to be worse compared to club stores and supermarkets. Although we find few differences in the quality of foods purchased by urbanicity or household income among shoppers at the same store type, there are significant differences in the types of stores frequented by rural and urban shoppers. Rural shoppers tend to purchase more calories from mass merchandisers and dollar stores with less healthful PFPs. Therefore, interventions should focus on engaging with these chains to offer healthier packaged foods.

Author Contributions: Conceptualization, A.L., S.W.N. and B.P.; methodology, A.L. and S.W.N.; software, A.L.; formal analysis, A.L.; investigation, A.L.; writing—original draft preparation, A.L.; writing—reviewing and editing, A.L., S.W.N. and B.P.; visualization, A.L.; funding acquisition, A.L., S.W.N. All authors have read and agreed to the published version of the manuscript.

Funding: This research received primary financial support from Healthy Eating Research, a national program of the Robert Wood Johnson Foundation. We would also like to acknowledge support from Arnold Ventures, NIH's Population Research Infrastructure Program (P2C HD050924) and the Population Research Training grant (T32 HD007168) at The University of North Carolina at Chapel Hill by the Eunice Kennedy Shriver National Institute of Child Health and Human Development.

Acknowledgments: Donna Miles for exceptional assistance with the data management and Emily Yoon for administrative assistance.

Conflicts of Interest: The authors declare no conflict of interest. The funders had no role in the design of the study; in the collection, analyses, or interpretation of data; in the writing of the manuscript, or in the decision to publish the results.

Appendix A. All Store Types

Table A1. Urban/Rural comparison of differences by income in the nutritional quality of household packaged food purchases by store type, 2010-2018 [1] (predicted margin (SE)).

Store Type	Grocery Stores						Mass Merchandisers						Club Stores						Online Shopping						Dollar Stores						Convenience Stores					
County Type	Rural			Urban			Rural			Urban			Rural			Urban			Rural			Urban			Rural			Urban			Rural			Urban		
Income Tertile	Low		High	Low		High	Low		High	Low		High	Low		High	Low		High	Low		High	Low		High	Low		High	Low		High	Low		High	Low		High
Total calories, person/day [2]	740 (10.6)*		704 (10.9)	766 (4.6)**		700 (3.8)	559 (9.5)		549 (10.7)	324 (3.3)		291 (3.2)	186 (7.8)		242 (10.0)**	238 (3.9)		275 (3.5)	105 (10.9)		84 (10.2)	95 (4.4)**		69 (3.2)	103 (3.4)**		53 (2.4)	70 (1.3)**		35 (1.0)	48 (1.8)*		42 (1.9)	53 (1.0)**		38 (0.7)
Fruits	9 (0.2)		10 (0.3)**	10 (0.1)		11 (0.1)**	6 (0.2)		8 (0.2)**	4 (0.1)		4 (0.1)*	5 (0.3)		8 (0.6)**	8 (0.2)		11 (0.2)**	2 (0.2)		2 (0.2)	1 (0.1)		1 (0.1)	1 (0.1)**		1 (0.1)	1 (0.0)**		0 (0.0)	0 (0.0)		0 (0.0)	0 (0.0)**		0 (0.0)
NS Vegetables	9 (0.2)		11 (0.2)**	11 (0.1)		12 (0.1)**	5 (0.1)		6 (0.2)*	3 (0.0)		3 (0.1)**	2 (0.1)		4 (0.3)**	3 (0.1)		5 (0.1)**	1 (0.1)		1 (0.1)	1 (0.1)		1 (0.1)	0 (0.0)**		0 (0.0)	1 (0.0)**		0 (0.0)	0 (0.0)		0 (0.0)	0 (0.0)*		0 (0.0)
Processed meats	41 (0.8)**		35 (0.9)	34 (0.3)**		30 (0.3)	25 (0.6)*		23 (0.6)	13 (0.2)**		11 (0.2)**	8 (0.5)		10 (0.8)*	9 (0.2)		11 (0.2)**	4 (0.6)		4 (0.9)	3 (0.3)*		3 (0.2)	2 (0.2)**		1 (0.1)	2 (0.1)**		1 (0.0)	1 (0.1)*		1 (0.1)	2 (0.1)**		1 (0.0)
Mixed dishes	53 (1.1)**		44 (1.0)	60 (0.6)**		48 (0.4)	46 (1.5)**		38 (1.2)	28 (0.4)**		22 (0.3)	13 (0.7)		16 (0.9)**	21 (0.4)		22 (0.4)*	7 (1.0)*		4 (0.6)	7 (0.5)**		5 (0.3)	5 (0.3)**		2 (0.1)	5 (0.1)**		2 (0.1)	1 (0.1)		3 (0.3)	4 (0.1)**		3 (0.1)
Grains	121 (2.1)*		114 (2.0)	131 (1.0)**		119 (0.8)	51 (1.7)		84 (2.0)	46 (0.6)**		46 (0.5)	23 (1.2)		28 (1.8)	32 (0.8)		34 (0.6)	17 (2.5)		14 (2.0)	15 (0.8)**		11 (0.6)	12 (0.5)**		6 (0.3)	9 (0.2)**		4 (0.2)	3 (0.2)		3 (0.3)	4 (0.1)**		3 (0.1)
SSBs	38 (1.1)**		30 (1.0)	39 (0.5)**		27 (0.4)	31 (1.0)**		24 (0.8)	17 (0.3)**		12 (0.2)	6 (0.4)		6 (0.6)	9 (0.3)*		7 (0.2)	3 (0.3)		3 (0.3)	5 (0.3)**		2 (0.2)	10 (0.6)**		4 (0.3)	5 (0.2)**		2 (0.1)	6 (0.4)**		5 (0.3)	6 (0.1)**		3 (0.1)
Junk foods	172 (2.7)		172 (3.2)	174 (1.4)*		165 (1.1)	161 (3.0)		167 (3.4)	93 (1.0)*		89 (1.0)	52 (2.3)		71 (3.4)**	59 (1.2)		72 (1.0)**	29 (2.8)		26 (2.9)	25 (1.1)		19 (0.9)	47 (1.4)**		26 (1.1)	33 (0.6)**		18 (0.5)	17 (0.6)		18 (1.1)	23 (0.5)**		18 (0.4)
Sugar, g	46 (0.7)*		43 (0.8)	48 (0.3)**		42 (0.3)	38 (0.7)*		36 (0.7)	22 (0.2)**		19 (0.2)	11 (0.6)		13 (0.6)*	14 (0.3)		15 (0.3)*	7 (0.7)		5 (0.6)	6 (0.3)**		4 (0.2)	9 (0.1)**		5 (0.2)	6 (0.1)**		3 (0.1)	4 (0.2)		3 (0.1)	5 (0.1)**		3 (0.1)
Sugar, % total calories	25%** (0.1%)		25% (0.2%)	25%** (0.1%)		24% (0.1%)	28%* (0.2%)		26% (0.2%)	29%** (0.1%)		28% (0.1%)	25%** (0.9%)		23% (0.3%)	24%** (0.1%)		22% (0.1%)	30%* (0.7%)		27% (0.7%)	29%** (0.3%)		26% (0.3%)	36% (0.3%)		37% (0.4%)	39% (0.1%)		37% (0.2%)	41%** (0.4%)		39% (0.4%)	39%** (0.2%)		38% (0.2%)
Saturated fat, g	11 (0.2)		10 (0.2)	11 (0.1)**		10 (0.1)*	8 (0.1)		8 (0.2)	4 (0.0)**		4 (0.0)	3 (0.1)		4 (0.2)**	3 (0.1)		4 (0.1)**	1 (0.2)		1 (0.2)	1 (0.1)**		1 (0.0)	1 (0.0)**		1 (0.0)	1 (0.0)**		1 (0.0)	1 (0.0)		1 (0.0)	1 (0.0)**		1 (0.0)
Saturated fat, % calories	13% (0.1%)*		13% (0.1%)**	12% (0.0%)*		13% (0.0%)**	12% (0.1%)		12% (0.1%)*	12% (0.0%)		12% (0.0%)	12% (0.2%)		13% (0.1%)	13% (0.1%)		13% (0.0%)	11% (0.3%)		11% (0.3%)	11% (0.1%)		11% (0.1%)	10% (0.1%)		11% (0.1%)*	10% (0.0%)		10% (0.1%)	11% (0.1%)		12%* (0.2%)	12% (0.1%)		12%** (0.1%)
Sodium, mg	1440 (21.9)*		1366 (23.4)	1460 (9.9)**		1341 (8.6)	1120 (20.5)		1077 (22.4)	642 (7.7)**		570 (7.7)	367 (15.3)		470 (19.1)**	459 (9.3)		497 (7.4)*	224 (25.3)		168 (23.8)	198 (12.7)**		137 (7.3)	242 (9.2)**		117 (5.8)	181 (3.7)**		95 (2.9)	65 (3.5)*		53 (2.9)	67 (1.7)**		47 (1.4)

[1] The estimates presented are based on a "per consumer" analysis, where the analytic sample for each store type was limited to households purchasing at least one item from a given store type in a year. Estimates are generated using multivariate regression, controlling for household income, education, race/ethnicity, age composition, and year and are adjusted for Nielsen's survey design to be nationally representative. [2] Total calories and calories from specific food groups are expressed in units of calories per person per day. Grams of sugar and saturated fat are expressed in grams purchased per person per day. Percent purchased calories from sugar or saturated fat are calculated by dividing the calories attributable to sugar/saturated fat across all households by the total number of calories purchased from that store type across all households. Non-starchy (NS) vegetables include leafy greens but not potatoes, corn, etc. Examples of mixed dishes include frozen entrees and canned soups; examples of junk foods include candies and salty snacks. SSBs: sugar-sweetened beverages. * Indicates a statistically significant difference between low-income households and high-income households at $p < 0.05$. ** Indicates a statistically significant difference between low-income households and high-income households at $p < 0.001$. Shaded cells indicate that the income difference for rural (urban) households is significantly greater than for urban (rural) households—in other words, the difference-in-difference is significant, $p < 0.05$. Nielsen disclaimer: University of North Carolina calculation based in part on data reported by Nielsen through its Homescan Services for all food categories, including beverages and alcohol for the 2008–2018 periods across the U.S. market. The Nielsen Company, 2015. Nielsen is not responsible for and had no role in preparing the results reported herein.

References

1. Langellier, B.A.; Garza, J.R.; Prelip, M.L.; Glik, D.; Brookmeyer, R.; Ortega, A.N. Corner Store Inventories, Purchases, and Strategies for Intervention: A Review of the Literature. *Calif. J. Health Promot.* **2013**, *11*, 1–13. [CrossRef] [PubMed]
2. Stern, D.; Ng, S.W.; Popkin, B.M. The Nutrient Content of U.S. Household Food Purchases by Store Type. *Am. J. Prev. Med.* **2016**, *50*, 180–190. [CrossRef] [PubMed]
3. Walker, R.E.; Keane, C.R.; Burke, J.G. Disparities and access to healthy food in the United States: A review of food deserts literature. *Health Place* **2010**, *16*, 876–884. [CrossRef] [PubMed]
4. Liese, A.D.; Weis, K.E.; Pluto, D.; Smith, E.; Lawson, A. Food Store Types, Availability, and Cost of Foods in a Rural Environment. *J. Am. Diet. Assoc.* **2007**, *107*, 1916–1923. [CrossRef] [PubMed]
5. Findholt, N.E.; Izumi, B.T.; Nguyen, T.; Pickus, H.; Chen, Z. Availability of healthy snack foods and beverages in stores near high-income urban, low-income urban, and rural elementary and middle schools in Oregon. *Child. Obes.* **2014**, *10*, 342–348. [CrossRef]
6. Hardin-Fanning, F.; Rayens, M.K. Food Cost Disparities in Rural Communities. *Health Promot. Pract.* **2014**, *16*, 383–391. [CrossRef] [PubMed]
7. Dean, W.R.; Sharkey, J.R. Rural and Urban Differences in the Associations between Characteristics of the Community Food Environment and Fruit and Vegetable Intake. *J. Nutr. Educ. Behav.* **2011**, *43*, 426–433. [CrossRef]
8. Smith, C.; Morton, L.W. Rural Food Deserts: Low-income Perspectives on Food Access in Minnesota and Iowa. *J. Nutr. Educ. Behav.* **2009**, *41*, 176–187. [CrossRef] [PubMed]
9. Pinard, C.A.; Byker Shanks, C.; Harden, S.M.; Yaroch, A.L. An integrative literature review of small food store research across urban and rural communities in the U.S. *Prev. Med. Rep.* **2016**, *3*, 324–332. [CrossRef]
10. Nelson, M.C.; Gordon-Larsen, P.; Song, Y.; Popkin, B.M. Built and social environments associations with adolescent overweight and activity. *Am. J. Prev. Med.* **2006**, *31*, 109–117. [CrossRef]
11. NCD Risk Factor Collaboration. Rising rural body-mass index is the main driver of the global obesity epidemic in adults. *Nature* **2019**, *569*, 260–264. [CrossRef] [PubMed]
12. Donahue, M. *The Impact of Dollar Stores and How Communities Can Fight Back*; Institute for Local Self-Reliance: Washington, DC, USA, 2018.
13. Romell, R. Dollar General's aggressive expansion into small Wisconsin towns has hurt locally owned grocery stores. *Milwaukee Journal Sentinel*, 23 May 2019.
14. Misra, T. The Dollar Store Backlash Has Begun. *City Lab*, 20 December 2018.
15. Dockter, M. As Dollar General rapidly expands in rural Siouxland, small-town grocers report losses. *Sioux City Journal*, 11 August 2019.
16. McGreal, C. Where even Walmart won't go: How Dollar General took over rural America. *The Guardian*, 13 August 2018.
17. Meyersohn, N. Dollar stores are everywhere. That's a problem for poor Americans. *CNN Business*, 19 July 2019.
18. Pantries Padded With Produce as North Americans Prepare for the COVID-19 Long Haul. *Nielsen Insights: CPG, FMCG & Retail*, 17 April 2020.
19. Slining, M.M.; Ng, S.W.; Popkin, B.M. Food Companies' Calorie-Reduction Pledges to Improve U.S. Diet. *Am. J. Prev. Med.* **2013**, *44*, 174–184. [CrossRef]
20. Poti, J.M.; Yoon, E.; Hollingsworth, B.; Ostrowski, J.; Wandell, J.; Miles, D.R.; Popkin, B.M. Development of a food composition database to monitor changes in packaged foods and beverages. *J. Food Compos. Anal.* **2017**, *64*, 18–26. [CrossRef] [PubMed]
21. Poti, J.M.; Mendez, M.A.; Ng, S.W.; Popkin, B.M. Is the degree of food processing and convenience linked with the nutritional quality of foods purchased by US households? *Am. J. Clin. Nutr.* **2015**, *101*, 1251–1262. [CrossRef] [PubMed]
22. Moubarac, J.-C.; Batal, M.; Louzada, M.L.; Martinez Steele, E.; Monteiro, C.A. Consumption of ultra-processed foods predicts diet quality in Canada. *Appetite* **2017**, *108*, 512–520. [CrossRef]
23. Hall, K.D. Ultra-processed diets cause excess calorie intake and weight gain: A one-month inpatient randomized controlled trial of ad libitum food intake. *Cell Matabolism* **2019**, *30*, 1–10. [CrossRef]
24. Company, T.N. (Ed.) *Nielsen Homescan Consumer Panel. Authors' Calculations Based in Part on Data Reported by Nielsen through Its Homescan Services for All Food Categories, Including Beverages and Alcohol for the 2010–2018 Periods Across the U.S. Market*; The Nielsen Company: New York, NY, USA, 2015.

25. Einav, L.; Leibtag, E.; Nevo, A. *On the Accuracy of Nielsen Homescan Data*; USDA, Economic Research Service: Washington, DC, USA, 2008.
26. Parker, T. *Rural-Urban Continuum Codes*; USDA, Economic Research Service: Washington, DC, USA, 2013.
27. Cromartie, J.; Parker, T. What is Rural? 20 August 2019. Available online: https://www.ers.usda.gov/topics/rural-economy-population/rural-classifications/what-is-rural/ (accessed on 15 October 2019).
28. Bureau of Economic Analysis. Regional Price Parities by State and Metro Area. 16 May 2019. Available online: https://www.bea.gov/data/prices-inflation/regional-price-parities-state-and-metro-area (accessed on 10 May 2019).
29. U.S. Department of Health and Human Services. Poverty Guidelines. 2020. Available online: https://aspe.hhs.gov/poverty-guidelines (accessed on 10 May 2019).
30. Ng, S.W.; Popkin, B.M. Monitoring foods and nutrients sold and consumed in the United States: Dynamics and challenges. *J. Acad. Nutr. Diet.* **2012**, *112*, 41–45.e44. [CrossRef] [PubMed]
31. Ng, S.W.; Slining, M.M.; Popkin, B.M. Use of Caloric and Noncaloric Sweeteners in US Consumer Packaged Foods, 2005–2009. *J. Acad. Nutr. Diet.* **2012**, *112*, 1828–1834.e6. [CrossRef] [PubMed]
32. Krebs-Smith, S.M.; Pannucci, T.E.; Subar, A.F.; Kirkpatrick, S.I.; Lerman, J.L.; Tooze, J.A.; Wilson, M.M.; Reedy, J. Update of the Healthy Eating Index: HEI-2015. *J. Acad. Nutr. Diet.* **2018**, *118*, 1591–1602. [CrossRef] [PubMed]
33. Brewster, P.J.; Guenther, P.M.; Jordan, K.C.; Hurdle, J.F. The Grocery Purchase Quality Index-2016: An innovative approach to assessing grocery food purchases. *J. Food Compos. Anal.* **2017**, *64*, 119–126. [CrossRef]
34. McGuire, S. Scientific Report of the 2015 Dietary Guidelines Advisory Committee. Washington, DC: US Departments of Agriculture and Health and Human Services, 2015. *Adv. Nutr.* **2016**, *7*, 202–204. [CrossRef]
35. Norat, T.; Scoccianti, C.; Boutron-Ruault, M.-C.; Anderson, A.; Berrino, F.; Cecchini, M.; Espina, C.; Key, T.; Leitzmann, M.; Powers, H.; et al. European Code against Cancer 4th Edition: Diet and cancer. *Cancer Epidemiol.* **2015**, *39*, S56–S66. [CrossRef] [PubMed]
36. Forouhi, N.G.; Krauss, R.M.; Taubes, G.; Willett, W. Dietary fat and cardiometabolic health: Evidence, controversies, and consensus for guidance. *BMJ* **2018**, *361*, k2139. [CrossRef] [PubMed]
37. He, F.J.; MacGregor, G.A. Reducing Population Salt Intake Worldwide: From Evidence to Implementation. *Prog. Cardiovasc. Dis.* **2010**, *52*, 363–382. [CrossRef]
38. He, F.; Nowson, C.; Lucas, M.; MacGregor, G. Increased consumption of fruit and vegetables is related to a reduced risk of coronary heart disease: Meta-analysis of cohort studies. *J. Human Hypertens.* **2007**, *21*, 717. [CrossRef]
39. Bouvard, V.; Loomis, D.; Guyton, K.Z.; Grosse, Y.; Ghissassi, F.E.; Benbrahim-Tallaa, L.; Guha, N.; Mattock, H.; Straif, K. Carcinogenicity of consumption of red and processed meat. *Lancet Oncol.* **2015**, *16*, 1599–1600. [CrossRef]
40. Wilde, P.; Pomeranz, J.L.; Lizewski, L.J.; Ruan, M.; Mozaffarian, D.; Zhang, F.F. Legal Feasibility of US Government Policies to Reduce Cancer Risk by Reducing Intake of Processed Meat. *Milbank Q.* **2019**, *97*, 420–448. [CrossRef] [PubMed]
41. Malik, V.S.; Popkin, B.M.; Bray, G.A.; Després, J.-P.; Hu, F.B. Sugar-Sweetened Beverages, Obesity, Type 2 Diabetes Mellitus, and Cardiovascular Disease Risk. *Circulation* **2010**, *121*, 1356–1364. [CrossRef] [PubMed]
42. *Stata Statistical Software: Release 15*; StataCorp LP: College Station, TX, USA, 2017.
43. Heeringa, S.G.; West, B.T.; Berglund, P.A. *Applied Survey Data Analysis*, 2nd ed.; CRC Press: Boca Raton, FL, USA, 2017.
44. Volpe, R.; Jaenicke, E.C.; Chenarides, L. Store formats, market structure, and consumers' food shopping decisions. *Appl. Econ. Perspect. Policy* **2018**, *40*, 672–694. [CrossRef]
45. The fight to remain relevant if the U.S. enters a recession. *Nielsen Insights: CPG, FMCG & Retail*, 9 April 2020.
46. Tracking the unprecedented impact of covid-19 on U.S. CPG shopping behavior. *Nielsen Insights: CPG, FMCG & Retail*, 30 March 2020.
47. SNAP: FNS Launches the Online Purchasing Pilot. Food and Nutrition Services, United States Department of Agriculture. Available online: https://www.fns.usda.gov/snap/online-purchasing-pilot (accessed on 20 April 2020).
48. Miller, G.; Merlo, C.; Demissie, Z.; Sliwa, S.; Park, S. Trends in beverage consumption among high school students—United States, 2007–2015. *MMWR. Morb. Mortal. Wkly. Rep.* **2017**, *66*, 112. [CrossRef]
49. Dunford, E.K.; Popkin, B.M.; Ng, S.W. Recent Trends in Junk Food Intake in U.S. Children and Adolescents, 2003–2016. *Am. J. Prev. Med.* **2020**, *59*, 49–58. [CrossRef] [PubMed]

50. U.S. Department of Health and Human Services and U.S. Department of Agriculture. *2015–2020 Dietary Guidelines for Americans*, 8th ed.; December 2015. Available online: http://health.gov/dietaryguidelines/2015/guidelines/ (accessed on 1 December 2019).
51. Laska, M.; Pelletier, J. *Minimum Stocking Levels and Marketing Strategies of Healthful Foods for Small Retail Food Stores*; Healthy Eating Research: Durham, NC, USA, 2016.
52. Caspi, C.E.; Winkler, M.R.; Lenk, K.M.; Harnack, L.J.; Erickson, D.J.; Laska, M.N. Store and neighborhood differences in retailer compliance with a local staple foods ordinance. *BMC Public Health* **2020**, *20*, 172. [CrossRef] [PubMed]
53. Fleischhacker, S.E.; Flournoy, R.; Moore, L.V. Meaningful, measurable, and manageable approaches to evaluating healthy food financing initiatives: An overview of resources and approaches. *J. Public Health Manag. Pract.* **2013**, *19*, 541–549. [CrossRef] [PubMed]
54. Harries, C.; Koprak, J.; Young, C.; Weiss, S.; Parker, K.M.; Karpyn, A. Moving from policy to implementation: A methodology and lessons learned to determine eligibility for healthy food financing projects. *J. Public Health Manag. Pract. JPHMP* **2014**, *20*, 498–505. [CrossRef] [PubMed]
55. Middel, C.N.; Schuitmaker-Warnaar, T.J.; Mackenbach, J.D.; Broerse, J.E. Systematic review: A systems innovation perspective on barriers and facilitators for the implementation of healthy food-store interventions. *Int. J. Behav. Nutr. Phys. Act.* **2019**, *16*, 108. [CrossRef]
56. Harnack, L.; Valluri, S.; French, S.A. Importance of the Supplemental Nutrition Assistance Program in Rural America. *Am. J. Public Health* **2019**, *109*, 1641–1645. [CrossRef]
57. Andress, L.; Fitch, C. Juggling the five dimensions of food access: Perceptions of rural low income residents. *Appetite* **2016**, *105*, 151–155. [CrossRef]
58. Glanz, K.; Bader, M.D.M.; Iyer, S. Retail Grocery Store Marketing Strategies and Obesity: An Integrative Review. *Am. J. Prev. Med.* **2012**, *42*, 503–512. [CrossRef]
59. Houghtaling, B.; Serrano, E.L.; Kraak, V.I.; Harden, S.M.; Davis, G.C.; Misyak, S.A. A systematic review of factors that influence food store owner and manager decision making and ability or willingness to use choice architecture and marketing mix strategies to encourage healthy consumer purchases in the United States, 2005–2017. *Int. J. Behav. Nutr. Phys. Act.* **2019**, *16*, 5. [CrossRef]
60. Karst, T. Produce expectations for Dollar General rise too quickly. *The Packer*, 13 June 2019.
61. Wal-Mart Stores Inc. Making Healthier Food a Reality for All. 2013. Available online: https://corporate.walmart.com/global-responsibility/hunger-nutrition/our-commitments (accessed on 10 October 2020).
62. Taillie, L.S.; Ng, S.W.; Popkin, B.M. Gains made by Walmart's healthier food initiative mirror preexisting trends. *Health Aff.* **2015**, *34*, 1869–1876. [CrossRef]
63. Winkler, M.R.; Lenk, K.M.; Caspi, C.E.; Erickson, D.J.; Harnack, L.; Laska, M.N. Variation in the food environment of small and non-traditional stores across racial segregation and corporate status. *Public Health Nutr.* **2019**, *22*, 1624–1634. [CrossRef]
64. Hausman, J.; Leibtag, E. Consumer benefits from increased competition in shopping outlets: Measuring the effect of Wal-Mart. *J. Appl. Econom.* **2007**, *22*, 1157–1177. [CrossRef]
65. Carpenter, J.M.; Moore, M. Consumer demographics, store attributes, and retail format choice in the US grocery market. *Int. J. Retail Distrib. Manag.* **2006**, *34*, 434–452. [CrossRef]
66. Sharkey, J.R. Measuring Potential Access to Food Stores and Food-Service Places in Rural Areas in the U.S. *Am. J. Prev. Med.* **2009**, *36*, S151–S155. [CrossRef]
67. Zhen, C.; Taylor, J.L.; Muth, M.K.; Leibtag, E. Understanding Differences in Self-Reported Expenditures between Household Scanner Data and Diary Survey Data: A Comparison of Homescan and Consumer Expenditure Survey. *Appl. Econ. Perspect. Policy* **2009**, *31*, 470–492. [CrossRef]
68. Basu, S.; Meghani, A.; Siddiqi, A. Evaluating the health impact of large-scale public policy changes: Classical and novel approaches. *Annu. Rev. Public Health* **2017**, *38*, 351–370. [CrossRef] [PubMed]

Publisher's Note: MDPI stays neutral with regard to jurisdictional claims in published maps and institutional affiliations.

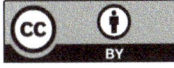

© 2020 by the authors. Licensee MDPI, Basel, Switzerland. This article is an open access article distributed under the terms and conditions of the Creative Commons Attribution (CC BY) license (http://creativecommons.org/licenses/by/4.0/).

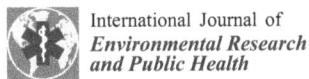

Article

A Model Depicting the Retail Food Environment and Customer Interactions: Components, Outcomes, and Future Directions

Megan R. Winkler [1], Shannon N. Zenk [2], Barbara Baquero [3], Elizabeth Anderson Steeves [4], Sheila E. Fleischhacker [5], Joel Gittelsohn [6], Lucia A Leone [7] and Elizabeth F. Racine [8,*]

1. Division of Epidemiology and Community Health, University of Minnesota School of Public Health, Minneapolis, MN 55455, USA; mwinkler@umn.edu
2. Department of Population Health Nursing Science, University of Illinois Chicago, Chicago, IL 60612, USA; szenk@uic.edu
3. Department of Health Services, University of Washington School of Public Health, Seattle, WA 98198, USA; Bbaquero@uw.edu
4. Department of Nutrition, University of Tennessee, Knoxville, TN 37996, USA; Eander24@utk.edu
5. Law Center, Georgetown University, Washington, DC 20001, USA; sef80@georgetown.edu
6. Center for Human Nutrition, Johns Hopkins Bloomberg School of Public Health, Baltimore, MD 21205, USA; jgittel1@jhu.edu
7. Department of Community Health and Health Behavior, School of Public Health and Health Professions, University at Buffalo, Buffalo, NY 14214, USA; lucialeo@buffalo.edu
8. Department of Public Health Sciences, University of North Carolina, Charlotte, NC 28223, USA
* Correspondence: efracine@uncc.edu; Tel.: +1-704-687-8979

Received: 7 September 2020; Accepted: 16 October 2020; Published: 19 October 2020

Abstract: The retail food environment (RFE) has important implications for dietary intake and health, and dramatic changes in RFEs have been observed over the past few decades and years. Prior conceptual models of the RFE and its relationships with health and behavior have played an important role in guiding research; yet, the convergence of RFE changes and scientific advances in the field suggest the time is ripe to revisit this conceptualization. In this paper, we propose the Retail Food Environment and Customer Interaction Model to convey the evolving variety of factors and relationships that convene to influence food choice at the point of purchase. The model details specific components of the RFE, including business approaches, actors, sources, and the customer retail experience; describes individual, interpersonal, and household characteristics that affect customer purchasing; highlights the macro-level contexts (e.g., communities and nations) in which the RFE and customers behave; and addresses the wide-ranging outcomes produced by RFEs and customers, including: population health, food security, food justice, environmental sustainability, and business sustainability. We believe the proposed conceptualization helps to (1) provide broad implications for future research and (2) further highlight the need for transdisciplinary collaborations to ultimately improve a range of critical population outcomes.

Keywords: grocery store; restaurant; environment; retail; food purchasing behavior; dietary intake

1. Introduction

Dramatic changes in the retail food environment (RFE) are evident over the past few decades, and even the past few years [1,2]. The number of traditional supermarkets are declining, while alternative grocery formats such as discount and convenience focused grocers are proliferating [1]. Food is increasingly found everywhere, across stores and businesses that are not traditionally considered "food" outlets [3,4]. Exponential growth in the number of dollar stores, pharmacies, and their grocery offerings exemplifies both of these trends [1,2,5]. Due in part to technological advances, online grocery shopping with delivery or curbside pick-up may be the wave of the future, further accelerated by consumer and federal responses (e.g., expanding online shopping options for US Department of Agriculture Supplemental Nutrition Assistance Program (SNAP) participants) to the coronavirus pandemic [6]. Still, prior to the pandemic, the majority of the American food dollar went to food prepared away from home [7]. Prepared food delivery has surged, with digital ordering and third-party delivery services helping to fuel its rise [8,9]. These changes partially reflect a growing consumer demand for convenience due to time scarcity [10–12], but also the decisions of a variety of other food actors including outlet owners, suppliers, and manufacturers to compete for customers through facilitating convenience. The RFE—including these recent trends—has implications for health, but also for other outcomes such as community and economic development.

Over the past 15 years, conceptual models of the RFE have played an important role in guiding research and intervention efforts, and thus have advanced the field. In 2005, the Model of Community Nutrition Environments by Glanz and colleagues identified several key components of the RFE, such as the "consumer" and "community" nutrition environments, which facilitated communication in the field [13]. The ecological framework depicting multilevel, interacting influences on what people eat by Story and colleagues positioned retail food sources as a key aspect of the physical environment [14]. In her book, Morland expanded on the pathways by which the RFE affects obesity and personal factors that moderate these relationships [15]. Yet, the recent convergence of changes in the RFE and advances in the field suggest the time is ripe to revisit how we conceptualize the RFE. Previous models tend to miss important components of the current and emerging environment, such as the wide varieties of retail food sources, involved actors, and business models, focus solely on diet and/or health as the outcomes of interest, and underemphasize the broader context that influences and interacts with the RFE to affect a diverse range of population outcomes.

The proposed model in this paper was prepared by The Healthy Food Retail Working Group leadership team. The Healthy Food Retail Working Group is a US collaboration of over 150 researchers and stakeholders jointly supported by Healthy Eating Research, a national program of the Robert Wood Johnson Foundation, and the Nutrition and Obesity Policy Research and Evaluation Network (NOPREN), which is supported by a cooperative agreement from the Centers for Disease Control and Prevention's Division of Nutrition, Physical Activity, and Obesity. The Healthy Food Retail Working Group holds bimonthly webinars on retail food topics and convenes smaller sub-groups to explore topics in further depth and develop collaborative research, practice, or policy projects.

In March 2019, the working group leadership met at the annual NOPREN meeting and strategized on research needs and future directions including a conceptual model to guide research. This process began as a brainstorming activity and a review of the previously published RFE conceptual models. We agreed that there were elements of the RFE missing from previous conceptualizations. To address this, we began meeting throughout the next year, and with feedback from the wider membership, developed a conceptual model to reflect RFE evolutions and its complexity, as well as what has been learned about the RFE over the past 20 years of public health research. Our focus was on developing a model that captured the chronic, ongoing processes, and outcomes of the RFE, and much of our efforts preceded the recent COVID-19 pandemic and historic protests against police brutality across the U.S. While we believe some model components and outcomes are highlighted by the COVID-19 pandemic and the movement for racial justice, there are others we do not address (e.g., state-mandated restaurant closures). As a compliment, Leone and colleagues (see Special Issue "Retail Strategies to Support Healthy Eating" https://www.mdpi.com/1660-4601/17/20/7397) offer ways that the proposed model could be used to inform research directions during significant disruptions, such as pandemics.

The aim of this paper is to propose an updated conceptual model of the RFE and its relationships with customer behavior that produce a host of significant population outcomes. Below, we present an overview of the conceptual model and our underlying assumptions and motivations. We then describe and justify each of the model components. Last, we discuss how the model can be used to direct broad future directions in observational, intervention, and policy research to understand and modify the interactions between customers and the RFE with the intention of improving societal outcomes.

2. Overview and Motivation for the Retail Food Environment and Customer Interaction Model

As an overview, the Retail Food Environment and Customer Interaction Model (Figure 1) breaks the RFE down into business models, actors, and sources and their influence on the customer retail experience (e.g., food availability, promotion, quality). Our model depicts reciprocal relationships and influence between the RFE and customers, including their individual, interpersonal, and household characteristics that affect sales/purchases. The model highlights the multilevel context in which the RFE and customers operate and expands the population outcomes produced by RFEs and customers that should be considered moving forward: health, food security, food justice, environmental sustainability, and business sustainability. See Table 1 for component definitions.

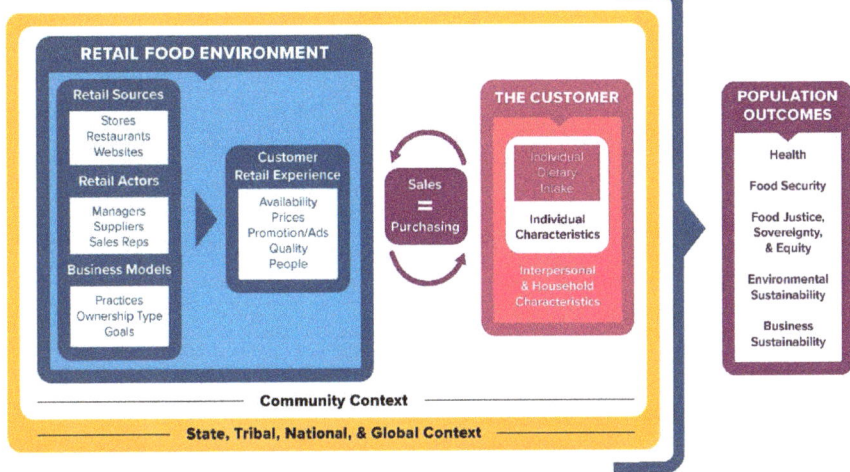

Figure 1. Retail Food Environment and Customer Interaction Model. The retail food environment consists of retail sources, retail actors, and business models that influence the customer retail experience. Customers involve individual, interpersonal, and household characteristics that affect customer purchasing and thus the retail sales of foods and beverages. Both the retail food environment and customers and their households are embedded in macro-level contexts (e.g., communities and nations), and as a result of the interactions and dynamics among these multiple model components, a host of population outcomes are produced: health, food security, food justice, environmental sustainability, and business sustainability. Definitions for model components are provided in Table 1.

Several underlying assumptions motivated the proposed model components and relationships. First, we took a highly-inclusive posture to address the multifactorial nature of the RFE in the US and its wide-ranging, discipline-crossing implications for society. However, we recognize as predominantly public health scholars that our focus remains on health and thus describe much of the model from that evidence base. We also conceptualized the model's diverse and multidimensional components as a complex dynamic system. This is represented not only in the reciprocal relationship between RFEs and customers, but also by the inclusion of multilevel contexts that can affect RFEs, customers, and their interactions. Finally, we speculated that an important driver of the RFE evolution has been the supply and demand for convenience and highlighted this in several model components. Time scarcity [10–12], growing mental fatigue and stress [16], and changing social norms [17] around daily food preparation may all contribute to customers' increasing demand for highly-accessible, limited-preparation products [18]. This demand has often been met by RFEs providing an abundance of ultra-processed, highly palatable, calorically-dense products through an ever-growing accessibility [19–21]. Yet, these patterns are juxtaposed by others that suggest that large swaths of the US are devoid of a variety of convenient foods and sources [22–24]. Thus, even an important driver, such as convenience, must be considered in a larger system of relationships and factors in order to understand why diverse outcomes can be produced.

Table 1. Definitions for key model components.

Retail Food Environment	
Sources	• The settings (e.g., stores, restaurants, online websites/apps) where people can purchase and obtain food/beverage products
Actors	• The people who interact, make decisions, and behave in various ways that create and support the current food environment, such as: store managers, owners, distributors, wholesalers, and sales representatives
Business Models	• The business design (e.g., targeted customer base, product/service selection), practices, goals, and ownership types (e.g., independent, publicly-traded, franchise) that characterize retail food businesses
Customer Retail Experience	• The features (e.g., price, availability) that customers encounter when they obtain and purchase food/beverage products
The Customer	
Individual Dietary Intake	• The specific foods and beverages consumed
Individual Characteristics	• Factors at an intrapersonal level that contribute and influence individual dietary intake and/or purchasing behavior
Interpersonal and Household Characteristics	• Factors at the interpersonal and household levels that contribute to an individual's behavior and characteristics
Sales and Purchasing	• The point of a transaction where a product is sold by the retailer and equivalently purchased by the customer
Community Context	• Macro-level factors from neighborhoods and city/local jurisdictions that influence the retail food environment, customers, and their relationships.
State, Tribal, National, and Global Context	• Macro-level factors from state, tribal, national, and global contexts that can influence the community context, retail food environment, customers, and their relationships.

3. Retail Food Environment

A key focus of our efforts to advance prior conceptualizations was to more comprehensively identify specific components of the RFE. We define the RFE as the environment where all food and beverages are purchased by consumers, including foodservice operations such as restaurants. We also recognize that the RFE is part of a larger food system, including agriculture, farming, and food production. However, in our model, we focus on the retail components most immediate to where food is sourced and purchased by customers, including: Retail Food Sources, Retail Food Actors, Retail Food Business Models, and the Retail Food Customer Experience. While differentiating the various components of the food environment is helpful, we acknowledge that overlap can and does exist among these components.

3.1. Retail Food Sources

Retail food sources (e.g., stores, restaurants, websites) are settings where people can purchase food and beverages, and are a well-known, well-studied concept in food environment research. Most investigations have studied these sources by examining the geographic-related aspects, such as number of, proximity to, and density of food outlets (i.e., the physical locations whose primary business is to sell food, such as restaurants and stores) [13]. Using these measures, research has aimed to characterize community food environments and examine their associations with community residents' diet and health related outcomes [25–28]. For example, prior evidence suggests positive relationships between convenience store availability and obesity among children [25] and between relative availability of unhealthy (e.g., fast food, convenience stores) to healthy (e.g., supermarkets, farmers' markets) sources with adult obesity [28].

Yet, such conceptualizations of retail food sources have insufficiently addressed the full and evolving range of settings and modalities where food and beverages can be purchased.

Business responses to address customer convenience (i.e., reduce customer time and effort in food preparation and acquisition) have likely driven a growth in retail food sources in the US [29] and contributed to an ever-increasing ubiquity of ready-to-eat foods and beverages available for purchase. Thus, our conceptualization (Figure 2) aims to capture a more complete range of retail food sources that have evolved and classifies them across two dimensions of customer convenience: food preparation and accessibility.

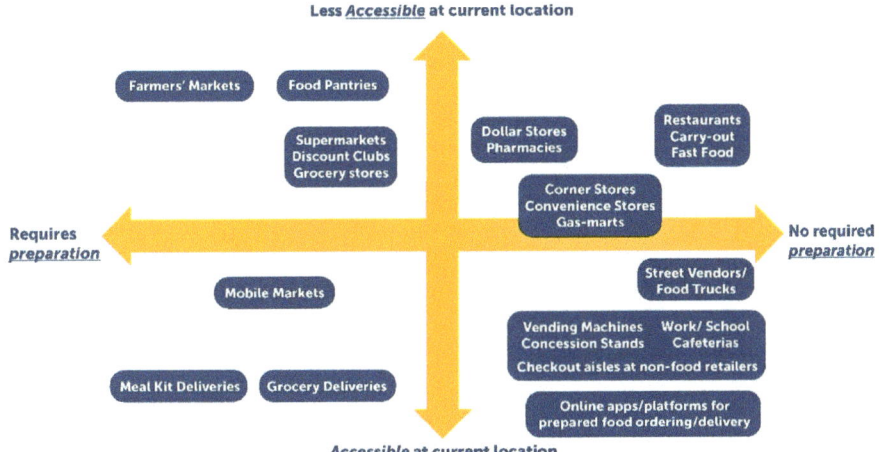

Figure 2. Common and Emerging Retail Food Sources across Two Dimensions of Customer Convenience: Accessibility and Degree of Required Preparation. Accessibility involves the ability for customers to obtain food products from a retail source from their immediate location (e.g., food can be delivered to their location or customers are required to travel to source). Degree of required preparation captures the typical proportion of products offered by the source that is prepared: ready-to-eat versus unprepared.

The first convenience dimension—food preparation—demonstrates the variation across sources in the typical proportion of products offered that are prepared: ready-to-eat versus unprepared. As shown in Figure 2, there is an apparent imbalance in the types of sources that primarily offer products that eliminate at-home food preparation versus those that offer unprepared versions. Some sources, such as fast food, restaurants, and food trucks, only offer ready-to-eat products. However, ready-to-eat foods are also staples in gas-marts and convenience stores through offerings of pre-packaged foods and increasingly grab-and-go delis and hot prepared food [30]. Even grocery stores and supermarkets are part of this prepared food trend [7,31], though continue to offer a greater percentage of products that require some (e.g., frozen pizza) or complete (e.g., eggs) at-home preparation. These offerings stand in contrast to other sources, such as farmer's markets and meal kit deliveries, which continue to sell a majority of products that require some degree of preparation (e.g., cut, chop, and sauté fresh vegetables).

Sources have also evolved to address customer convenience through the dimension of accessibility. We view accessibility as the ability of customers to purchase products from their immediate location (e.g., home, work, school). Changes in accessibility were first observed through the staggering spread of brick-and-mortar food sources that narrowed customers' travel distances to venues. For instance, evidence suggests that the density of fast food chains and restaurants near US homes and workplaces significantly increased between 1971 and 2008—in some cases doubling [32]. While these changes contributed to today's approximately 200,000 fast food venues [33] and 153,000 convenience stores/gas-marts [34], accessibility has also recently evolved to no longer require people to travel to and visit brick-and-mortar locations. Such immediate accessibility has in some respects been around for decades through vending machines, worksite cafeterias, and pizza delivery. However, accessibility in recent years seems to be exponentially expanding. Ready-to-eat packaged foods (e.g., candy) are offered in non-food outlets and checkout aisles (e.g., barber shops, home improvement stores, clothing stores) [3,4]; sit-down and fast food restaurants regularly offer options for delivery, often via third-party online applications and platforms [9]; and even sources that primarily sell products requiring preparation are now delivering (e.g., meal kit deliveries, online grocery delivery). Moving forward, we need a better understanding of the impacts of these increasing forms of accessibility and prepared food products offered by retail sources. Future research can investigate how some modalities might be used to improve the ubiquity of healthier ready-to-eat options as well as disentangle for whom these convenience dimensions are more or less available.

3.2. Retail Food Actors

Retail food actors are the people that work in the RFE whom, at various steps in the process typically towards the middle and ends of the food supply chain, determine the foods and beverages available at a source (e.g., managers/owners, suppliers/distributors, merchandising managers, and sales representatives). The retail food actors interact to determine which items are feasible to sell, store, and transport while maintaining quality and minimizing waste. For instance, when source managers or restaurant owners plan to sell a new item, they identify potential suppliers and understand the space, cost, and shelf life requirements necessary to sell the product in a safe and profitable way. Food manufacturer sales representatives are another example, who work with store managers to promote products and marketing strategies, such as in-store displays [35].

Each actor has their own specialty and focus. A sales representative's focus is often to develop relationships with retail outlets that will provide environments for food products to reach consumers and cultivate demand. A distributor's focus may be to develop a supply chain that efficiently moves food from warehouses to stores and restaurants. Alternatively, a store manager or restaurant owner's focus may be to provide an array of items that customers demand in an efficient and pleasant environment [36,37]. The varying foci and goals of these actors have often resulted in an efficient system that provides an abundance of convenient, non-perishable, manufactured food and beverage items, as these are often more logistically and financially appealing to manage [38–40].

Relative to other RFE components in the model, very little literature in public health nutrition has investigated the impact of these actors on the RFE, though there is a growing base of research examining the role of store managers [36,41–43]. Such research is important as these actors develop reciprocal and deterministic processes that influence the current RFE (e.g., informal and formal product contract agreements [44,45], managers requesting products from distributors based on customer demand and what they can maintain due to resources and infrastructure) [46,47]. A better understanding of how the retail food source is influenced by the goals, foci, and decisions of these actors may be necessary to develop more effective policies and sustainable interventions to improve population outcomes.

3.3. Retail Food Business Models

Another RFE component that requires additional research is the business models used across each retail food source. Business models direct a source's operations, financing, target customer base, and mission. Understanding the business model of a source, particularly products sold and services provided, helps to understand their priorities. For example, sources offering culturally-tailored products might be demonstrating a priority to address the needs and preferences of a specific ethnic community [48–50], while sources offering products with specific values, such as locally-sourced, or dietary requirements, such as gluten-free [51], may be targeting and prioritizing other customer groups. Services provided (e.g., fast food versus "dining experience") can also indicate a source's targeted customer base (e.g., income/class, available time, cooking abilities/preferences). Products sold might also reflect a source's priorities to generate additional revenue streams, such as stores that participate in federal assistance nutrition programs [52] to expand their customer base, as well as how much local demand is valued over operational convenience (e.g., product variation versus the same products at all locations) [53].

Business outcomes, including revenue and profits, are often the ultimate goal for many sources. Such goals are at times a necessity, given that some source types (e.g., grocery wholesalers and stores) struggle with low profit margins [54]. Yet, some sources may have additional goals beyond profit. For example, institutional foodservice companies might be profit driven, but they contract with community-based institutions, such as colleges, workplaces, prisons, or hospitals [55]. This partnership creates a mix of profit motive and community benefit where the institution's goals, such as for healthy eating and/or locally-sourced products, influences the foods that the foodservice company provides.

Ownership is another indicator of the business model, and a range of ownership types with diverse goals exist across the RFE. The majority of foods and beverages purchased in US are sold by publicly-traded corporations [56–58], such as Walmart, Kroger, McDonalds, Sysco, and Starbucks. However, there are a number of large-chain food retailers that are privately-owned such as Chick-fil-A, Publix, Meijer, and Subway. Such privately-owned chains, while not always held to produce profits for shareholders, continue to dominate RFE spaces (in terms of profits, reach, etc.) over the private and independently-owned source with only one or two locations. Other examples of ownership models include food cooperatives (co-ops) and community-owned businesses. Co-ops involve groups of people that use membership fees to collectively operate a food retailer. Some co-ops are not-for-profit companies, allowing more flexibility to operate the co-op in a manner aligning with the co-op's mission or changing member needs. Community-owned business food retailers are often for-profit businesses that are financed, owned [59], and operated collectively by community members (e.g., Baldwin Market in Florida), and differing from co-ops often raise more capital and investments to allow "capital-intensive enterprises to start at scale [59]".

The past several decades have brought an important RFE transformation from small independent ownership to large chain often corporate/franchise ownership [60–62]. In some cases, entire groups of sources may be corporately-owned, such as fast food. In other cases, ownership at sources, such as grocery stores and supermarkets, remains relatively diverse; though, these also show growing declines in the presence (number and market share) of independent ownership [60]. With these shifts in centralizing ownership to fewer hands, much remains to be investigated and understood about how these different ownership types and business models contribute to the RFE [63,64].

3.4. Customer Retail Experience

Together, retail actors, business models, and retail sources combine and lead to the final component of the RFE: the customer retail experience. This component consists of the characteristics of food and beverage products for sale and the broader environment that people encounter when making their purchases. Referred to by Glanz and colleagues as the "consumer nutrition environment" [13], these features were mainly conceptualized as occurring within a physical location. Yet, given increasing shifts to online purchasing, customers are now also experiencing retail food spaces through webpages and mobile applications.

The traditional marketing mix of product, price, place, promotion, and people remains a helpful way to classify the customer retail experience [65]. In comparison to research on retail food sources, fewer studies in the field have examined how features of the customer retail experience within those sources relate to purchasing, consumption, or health outcomes [26,27]. This work is important as studies examining links with sources often rely on classifying entire source types as either healthy (e.g., supermarkets) or unhealthy (e.g., fast food); yet, this can neglect the variation in product mixes (e.g., supermarkets offer plenty of unhealthy products), placement, and other marketing features within a source that influence customer purchasing [66–68].

Of the limited evidence examining features of the customer retail experience, many have studied food product availability or prices. Both the absolute and relative availability and prices of healthful and unhealthy foods, as well as availability of culturally-appropriate products [49,50], may be relevant for consumers' purchasing decisions [69–71]. Often, unhealthy products are more available [72–75] and less expensive than healthful products [76]. Product quality and variety (i.e., number of options), such as for produce or milk options, also influence purchasing decisions [77–81] and can vary across source type and neighborhood [82–84].

Other features, including placement and promotion, have been less studied, although industry practices provide indirect evidence that these, too, are important for creating a customer retail experience that translates into sales. For instance, food/beverage manufacturers spend an estimated USD 50 billion per year, or 70% of their marketing budget, on in-store trade-promotion fees [35]. Such fees can guarantee certain product placement (e.g., checkout aisles) and/or promotion through cooperative advertising (e.g., store circulars) and discount campaigns (e.g., "2 for 1"). These practices also occur in online shopping spaces, such as pop-up advertisements, notifications, and cart "reminders" [85]. Promotion also occurs at the packaging level, as significant efforts have been made by manufacturers to attract customers (e.g., children's cereal boxes [86]) and by public health to inform customers of a product's nutritional composition and quality (e.g., nutrition label reform [87], front-of-package, and traffic-light labeling [88–90]). Even newer features of shelf promotion, such as undershelf lighting in the candy aisle, signals that these features will continue to evolve as the competition for customer attention and thus sales endure among companies and product categories [91].

The final feature—people—also affects customers' decisions on where to shop and the food and beverage products to which they have access. Despite limited literature, studies indicate that negative social interactions influence people's shopping locations and can range from inefficient, unenthusiastic service to forms of discrimination and stigma [92–95]. For instance, Black Americans have described employees watching, following, or treating them with less respect and experienced this behavior while shopping in predominantly White neighborhoods or in stores owned by individuals of a race/ethnicity different than their own [94,96–99]. Research also highlights that some customers frequent sources that they trust and especially those with which they have a built relationship [100,101].

4. Retail Sales and Customer Purchasing

The conceptual model involves two sides—an RFE side that presents key components that are most immediate to where food is sourced and purchased by customers and a customer side that presents the many aspects relevant to individual variation in customer purchasing and dietary intake (see Section 5). The two sides connect at the point of a transaction or where a product is sold by the retailer and equivalently purchased by the customer (Figure 1). In comparison to prior models, we view the relationship between the two sides as reciprocal: actions of RFEs influence customer behaviors and customer behaviors influence RFE actions. Moreover, aspects of both the RFE and individual customers can interact to lead to a customer purchase.

5. The Customer: Individual Dietary Intake, Individual Characteristics, and Household Characteristics

The right-side of the model (Figure 1) represents the customer and the multidimensional characteristics that influence decisions about personal dietary intake and food and beverage purchasing. The relationship between dietary intake and purchasing is bidirectional, and we propose that a wide range of individual, interpersonal, and household characteristics influence individual purchasing and ultimately dietary intake (Table 2) [14]. At the individual level are the intrapersonal factors that influence dietary intake and purchasing behaviors. Previous models and a large body of evidence indicate that factors such as attitudes, knowledge, food preferences, socio-demographic characteristics, lifestyle behaviors (e.g., smoking), stress, and cultural norms influence these behaviors. For example, individuals who have less education and/or poor employment consistently report lower dietary quality [102,103], which may be due to limited time or financial resources. Individuals' food knowledge and attitudes are also important, as greater nutrition knowledge has been associated with better dietary quality and may reflect a better nutrition label literacy and ability to overcome food marketing tactics to make healthier purchases [104].

Table 2. Examples of individual, interpersonal, and household characteristics relevant to food and beverage purchasing and dietary intake behavior.

Domain	Individual Characteristics	Interpersonal and Household Characteristics
Examples	<ul><li>Eating behaviors</li><li>Food cooking skills and behaviors</li><li>Taste/food preference/meal selection</li><li>Cognitions (attitudes, knowledge, preferences)</li><li>Time availability and pressure</li><li>Perceived stress and physiologic stress responses</li><li>Lifestyle/other health behaviors</li><li>Weight status</li><li>Eating disorders and chronic health conditions</li><li>Biological (age, genes)</li><li>Demographics (education, race/ethnicity, employment)</li><li>Immigration status</li><li>Cultural values</li><li>Prior experiences/memories with food</li></ul>	<ul><li>Household membership</li><li>Food preparation equipment, tools, and space</li><li>Household member with food preparation skills</li><li>Work schedules</li><li>Transportation</li><li>US Department of Agriculture Supplemental Nutrition Assistance Program (SNAP) status</li><li>Time of month (food benefit cycle)</li><li>Household preferences for food/drinks available</li><li>Social influences (role modeling, support, norms)</li><li>Food purchase frequency</li><li>Time of the day</li><li>Access to and placement of foods in the home</li><li>Food choice incentives</li><li>Rules and norms about eating (family eats together)</li></ul>

Individuals are embedded in households and other interpersonal contexts, and much evidence suggests that characteristics from these contexts, such as SNAP status, income, social support, social norms, shopping behaviors, and food preparation skills and decision-making, are also related to dietary intake and purchasing. For example, sources and timing of food benefits (e.g., SNAP benefit schedule) shape the number of food shopping trips and their food baskets, as diets tend to be healthier around the weeks that SNAP household benefits are redeemed versus other times of the month [105,106]. Household income is also consistently related to purchases with higher household incomes purchasing healthier foods and beverages and having greater access (e.g., fruits and vegetables) compared to lower income households [107]. In households of immigrant families, the level of acculturation of the head of household influences what food is purchased [108,109]. Additionally, household members' work schedules and transportation options are related to shopping trip frequency and foods purchased and may contribute to customers' increasing need for convenience [110].

6. Community, State, Tribal, National, and Global Contexts

As shown in Figure 1, the RFE, as well as customers do not operate in a vacuum. Instead, macro-level factors, including economic, social, media, built environment, policy, and others, influence the RFE, customers, and their relationships. A growing body of evidence examines factors at this macro-level, and we group these factors under two contextual levels: community context, including neighborhoods and city/local jurisdictions, and the broader state, tribal, national, and global context. Table 3 provides examples of relevant factors in each context. These factors may directly affect the RFE and customers, as well as modify RFE–dietary intake relationships.

Table 3. Macro-level contexts with example factors that influence the retail food environment; customer purchasing, dietary intake, and individual and household characteristics; and their relationships.

	Retail Food Environment	Customer: Diets and Individual and Household Characteristics	Community Context
Community Context	<ul><li>Licensing fees</li><li>Taxes (e.g., sweetened beverage taxes)</li><li>Local subsidies</li><li>Income level and purchasing power</li><li>Cost of living</li><li>Local ordinances (e.g., default beverage in restaurant child meals, staple foods)</li><li>Food industry contracts with schools, hospitals, and other institutions</li><li>Zoning codes</li></ul>	<ul><li>Economic development</li><li>Employment opportunities</li><li>Safety</li><li>Retailer-community relations</li><li>Social and cultural norms</li><li>Stressors (e.g., disorder, violence)</li><li>Educational system</li><li>Transportation systems</li><li>Walkability</li><li>Public health campaigns</li><li>Food industry sponsorship of community activities (e.g., child sports/summer camps)</li></ul>	
State, Tribal, National, and Global Context	<ul><li>Food assistance programs-retailer requirements (e.g., SNAP, WIC)</li><li>Banking and lending practices</li><li>Societal values and ideologies</li><li>Broadband internet infrastructure</li><li>School, daycare, worksite policies</li><li>Regional planning</li><li>Food safety standards</li><li>Food labeling laws</li><li>Food production</li><li>Product development</li><li>Food processing/manufacturing</li><li>Marketing (e.g., trade promotion fees)</li><li>Agriculture policies and subsidies</li><li>International trade agreements</li></ul>	<ul><li>Federal nutrition assistance programs-benefits and food packages (e.g., SNAP, WIC)</li><li>Minimum wage laws</li><li>Regulations for media advertising to children</li><li>Advertising (e.g., commercials, social media, sponsorships)</li></ul>	<ul><li>Funding for education</li><li>Transportation funding</li><li>Preemption laws</li></ul>

Note. SNAP, US Department of Agriculture Supplemental Nutrition Assistance Program; WIC, US Department of Agriculture Special Supplemental Nutrition Program for Women, Infants, and Children.

Under the community context, zoning codes and commercial real estate professionals can directly influence where food sources are located; transportation systems can affect the food sources that consumers can reach; local social norms might ultimately influence the food options available; and tax policies such as municipal sugar-sweetened beverage taxes affect the prices that consumers face [111]. Under the broader contexts, numerous factors from the state, tribal, and federal levels influence food retail and customer behavior such as the following examples. First, stocking requirements for participating retailers in SNAP and the Special Supplemental Nutrition Program for Women, Infants, and Children (WIC) affect the products they carry, and these are particularly impactful in smaller sources, such as dollar stores, that may not otherwise carry as many healthier items [43,112]. Second, minimum wage laws affect the financial resources that consumers have to purchase foods. Third, industry advertising of food products may affect food choices and thus dietary intake. Finally, healthy food purchasing incentive programs and nutrition education programs (e.g., within SNAP) increase financial access and education about healthy foods and beverages. As suggested by the embedding of the community context within the broader context in Figure 1, factors at the state, tribal, national, and global levels can influence the community context as well. For example, preemptive laws can prevent state and local governments from enacting policies that influence the RFE, such as taxes and labeling [113].

Moreover, community and broader contexts may modify effects of the RFE on sales/purchasing and in turn individual dietary intake. For instance, the effect of retail food outlet availability on where people purchase foods may depend on safety of the surrounding community environment, as shoppers have reported avoiding stores or certain shopping times due to unsafe neighborhood conditions, including drug sales, violence, and harassment [93,94]. Because consumption of high-fat, sugary foods and beverages can alleviate stress, exposure to such community stressors may also increase the effect of household availability of these food types on individual consumption choices. With regard to the broader state, tribal, national, or federal context, for example, the impact of in-store food/beverage marketing to children on purchasing may vary depending on regulations for television food advertising to children. That is, it is possible that being exposed to both in-store marketing and television food advertising will have a stronger impact on purchasing than when one is only exposed to one or the other. Thus, our model recognizes a wide variety of factors that may influence the RFEs, customers, and their sales/purchasing interface as well as alter these relationships.

7. Population Outcomes

We posit that the dynamics and interactions between RFEs, individuals and households, and their larger contexts can produce a host of population outcomes. Scholars have previously articulated the importance of examining the multiple outcomes produced by national and global food systems [114,115]. In this conceptualization, we offer five for consideration: health; food security; environmental sustainability; business sustainability; and food sovereignty, equity, and justice.

Population health is the outcome most familiar to RFE researchers from the discipline of public health. It aims to uncover the ways this system contributes to diet-related non-communicable diseases, such as obesity, type 2 diabetes, and cardiovascular disease [13,14]. Those interested in improving this outcome often offer RFE modifications that help "make the healthy choice, the easy choice," such as offering and widely promoting products consistent with national dietary guidelines [116].

Food insecurity is another outcome, and one that at the time of this writing has dramatically risen as a result of the economic implications from executive orders required to curb the spread of COVID19 (e.g., miles of cars waiting at food pantries [117]) as well as damage to RFE locations that accompanied peaceful protests for racial justice [118]. In usual times, food insecurity is likely to occur when federal nutrition assistance is not accepted at all sources, price structures lead high-fat and high-sugar products to be most affordable (i.e., lowest-cost dietary option), and fresh and healthier options are not equally available across communities. As such, healthy food and beverages are not affordable or accessible to all groups, and this most often impacts the economically and socially disadvantaged [14,116].

Outcomes of the system not only relate to people but to the environment. Food waste is one example, as more than 400 pounds of approximate waste per person was observed at the US retailer and consumer levels in 2010 [119]. Other examples relate to the agriculture and transportation practices required for the types of products sold and purchased. Many suggest that the majority of available products are produced and commonly transported in a way that leads to environmental degradation, as they require methods that can diminish soil fertility, emit greenhouse gases, deplete freshwater resources, and/or neglect biodiversity [114,115].

The system also contributes to business and economic outcomes, which reflect the "health" of the source's business performance in the US market economy [120]. Here, goals of generating sales, profits, and competitiveness are key and for some businesses may be the primary motivators for decision-making [120–123]. Food retailers and companies often aim to achieve such goals by interrogating consumer "choice" and the predictors of which retailers will be shopped and which products purchased (e.g., price strategies, product mix, store layout) [122,124]. Of the outcomes identified, this outcome has arguably been the best performing in recent decades, as US supermarket and fast food industries experienced an estimated annual revenue in 2019 of USD 682 billion and 293 billion [125,126], respectively. However, the COVID-19 pandemic is likely to change this success for some industries, such as restaurants, which observed a 51% drop in food-away-from-home monthly expenditures in March 2020 compared to March 2019 [127].

Finally, there are also significant outcomes of the system characterized through the lens of food sovereignty, equity, and justice. In this perspective, inequalities in power are central, and the rights of individuals and communities to define, produce, and sell their own food are emphasized [116,128]. To achieve such outcomes requires addressing the socio-structural barriers (e.g., economic inequality, racism, sexism) that have historically-marginalized, inequitably targeted, and resource-deprived certain groups and populations [129]. It also demands the development of sustained opportunities for communities to create the RFE that best serves their needs and interests (e.g., supporting tribal food sovereignty and Black-owned businesses).

Articulating these five outcomes is necessary to not only highlight the multiple outcomes produced and that need to be considered in future research but the challenges and opportunities that also lie ahead. For instance, when we focus on a single RFE goal and ignore that other outcomes are produced, we create solutions that may address our goal but simultaneously produce harm in other areas. Such consequences may be unintentional or well-known (e.g., promotion of unhealthy, processed foods which increase profits, but are associated with non-communicable disease [130–132]). Yet, moving forward it may be important to reframe these varying outcomes from inevitable systemic trade-offs to sites of opportunity. Diverse groups working to improve the RFE could identify ways to work at cross-purposes, achieve goals for multiple outcome areas, and potentially do so with greater efficiency and less duplication and resources. Working together will also push discipline-centric change agents to consider the feasibility and sustainability of their proposed solutions and may help spur the creation of more worthwhile and effective transformations. While collaboration and attention to multiple outcomes will be easy for some, other groups may require support or even accountability measures to help cultivate "common ground" (e.g., reframing from businesses profitability to sustainability), and many have already been calling for and provided specific strategies to do so [115,129,131,133].

8. Future Directions

The Retail Food Environment and Customer Interaction Model attempts to capture key RFE and customer components in the US that converge to shape food and beverage purchases with diverse societal outcomes. Expanding upon previous frameworks [13–15], we believe this updated model highlights: (1) the multifactorial nature of the RFE; (2) the wide-ranging and discipline-crossing outcomes produced for society; (3) the reciprocal and dynamic relationships between RFEs and customers as well as with factors from multilevel contexts creating a complex system; and (4) the importance supply and demand for convenience has and continues to play in shaping the US RFE. As such, the model adds important information that can guide future research on the broader RFE context for dietary intake and help to inform public health interventions and policies aimed at improving RFE settings.

The encompassing nature of our model has broad implications for future research and can guide numerous research questions. However, here for the sake of brevity, we focus our comments on three important gaps that we identified throughout model development. First, additional research is necessary to investigate the role and influence of certain understudied RFE components: retail actors, business models, and the customer retail experience. A better understanding of these components is required to develop effective interventions and partnerships that are more likely to improve outcomes. Second, there is a need, especially in public health, to broaden our awareness of outcomes beyond health in an attempt to anticipate the wide array outcomes that a single change to the RFE and customer interaction can generate. Finally, while literature examining why convenience is an important driver of behavior exists in the disciplines of psychology, behavioral economics, and cognitive science, there remain relatively less investigation and understanding of nutrition and public health. Uncovering what convenience means to customers and how best to capitalize on it to improve health and other population outcomes are important directions moving forward.

Given the complexity, dynamics, and reciprocal processes of the Retail Food Environment and Customer Interaction Model, we also suggest a need for more sophisticated research methods and transdisciplinary partnerships. Two recommended research approaches are systems science and multilevel, multicomponent (MLMC) interventions [134–136]. Systems science involves methodological approaches, often computational models, that aim to understand the impacts produced from complex interrelated mechanisms and relationships among multiple factors [134,135]. Except for a few exceptions [137–140], relatively little work has studied the RFE using such methods, and incorporating these approaches could help to not only identify solutions that improve multiple outcomes but identify those to avoid to circumvent unexpected consequences. MLMC interventions are large, complex, multidimensional interventions that often require significant coordination, stakeholder buy-in, and resources; yet, their utility also lies in identifying which individual and/or set of components most effectively improves outcomes [141,142]. Both the model's complexity and these research approaches suggest that transdisciplinary, collaborative leadership will be required. Bringing together stakeholders from many disciplines, such as agriculture, business, public policy, regional/urban planning, nutrition, social sciences, and public health, could help to build more and stronger transdisciplinary projects that are better positioned to effectively improve the RFE for a variety of societal outcomes.

9. Conclusions

This paper provides a model depicting the interactions of the RFE and consumer behavior while also highlighting some of the outcomes of this system as witnessed in the US. We view the Retail Food Environment and Customer Interaction Model as a "living" conceptualization and hope that it inspires many additional, more refined versions. We encourage research utilizing this model to help us better understand why food sources operate in certain locations, how food sources decide which foods to carry, and why customers choose to purchase certain foods. Then using this insight, transdisciplinary efforts should work to develop solutions that modify the RFE-customer relationship in ways that ultimately improve a range of population outcomes.

Author Contributions: Conceptualization, M.R.W., S.N.Z., B.B., E.A.S., S.E.F., J.G., L.A.L., and E.F.R.; methodology, B.B., E.F.R., M.R.W., and S.N.Z.; writing—original draft preparation and writing, B.B., E.F.R., M.R.W., and S.N.Z.; review and editing, E.A.S., S.E.F., J.G., and L.A.L. All authors have read and agreed to the published version of the manuscript and contributed substantially to the work reported.

Funding: All of the authors are on the leadership team of the Healthy Food Retail Working Group, jointly supported by Healthy Eating Research (HER), a national program of the Robert Wood Johnson Foundation (RWJF), and the Nutrition and Obesity Policy Research and Evaluation Network (NOPREN). NOPREN is supported by Cooperative Agreement No. 5U48DP00498–05 from the Centers for Disease Control and Prevention (CDC), Prevention Research Centers Program. All authors receive a stipend from HER for their leadership role with the working group. Support for MRW's effort was provided by the National Heart, Lung, and Blood Institute (NHLBI), grant number K99HL144824 (Principal Investigator: MRW). Publication fees were supported by Healthy Eating Research, a national program of the Robert Wood Johnson Foundation. The content is solely the responsibility of the authors and does not necessarily represent the official views of the HER, RWJF, NOPREN, CDC, or NHLBI.

Conflicts of Interest: The authors declare no conflict of interest. The funders had no role in the design of the study; in the collection, analyses, or interpretation of data; in the writing of the manuscript, or in the decision to publish the results.

References

1. Kuijpers, D.; Simmons, V.; van Wamelen, J. Reviving Grocery Retail: Six Imperatives. Available online: https://www.mckinsey.com/industries/retail/our-insights/reviving-grocery-retail-six-imperatives# (accessed on 22 August 2020).
2. Redman, R. Tradional Supermarkets Lose Share as Playing Field Shifts. Available online: https://www.supermarketnews.com/retail-financial/traditional-supermarkets-lose-share-playing-field-shifts (accessed on 22 August 2020).

3. Lucan, S.C.; Maroko, A.R.; Patel, A.N.; Gjonbalaj, I.; Elbel, B.; Schechter, C.B. Healthful and less-healthful foods and drinks from storefront and non-storefront businesses: Implications for 'food deserts', 'food swamps' and food-source disparities. *Public Health Nutr.* **2020**, *23*, 1428–1439. [CrossRef] [PubMed]
4. Farley, T.A.; Baker, E.T.; Futrell, L.; Rice, J.C. The ubiquity of energy-dense snack foods: A national multicity study. *Am. J. Public Health* **2010**, *100*, 306–311. [CrossRef] [PubMed]
5. Discount & Dollar Retailers. Available online: https://www.gordonbrothers.com/insights/industry-insights/retail-dollar-stores (accessed on 14 June 2020).
6. Berthiaume, D. Survey: COVID-19 Drives Online Grocery Sales to New High. Available online: https://chainstoreage.com/survey-covid-19-drives-online-grocery-sales-new-high (accessed on 22 August 2020).
7. Saksena, M.J.; Okrent, A.M.; Anekwe, T.D.; Cho, C.; Dicken, C.; Effland, A.; Elitzak, H.; Guthrie, J.; Hamrick, K.S.; Hyman, J.; et al. America's Eating Habits: Food Away from Home. Available online: https://www.ers.usda.gov/webdocs/publications/90228/eib-196.pdf (accessed on 22 August 2020).
8. The NPD Group. Foodservice Delivery in U.S. Posts Double-Digit Gains Over Last Five Years With Room to Grow. Available online: https://www.npd.com/wps/portal/npd/us/news/press-releases/2018/foodservice-delivery-in-us-posts-double-digit-gains-over-last-five-years-with-room-to-grow/ (accessed on 22 August 2020).
9. Poelman, M.P.; Thornton, L.; Zenk, S.N. A cross-sectional comparison of meal delivery options in three international cities. *Eur. J. Clin. Nutr.* **2020**. [CrossRef] [PubMed]
10. Celnik, D.; Gillespie, L.; Lean, M.E.J. Time-scarcity, ready-meals, ill-health and the obesity epidemic. *Trends Food Sci. Technol.* **2012**, *27*, 4–11. [CrossRef]
11. Strazdins, L.; Griffin, A.L.; Broom, D.H.; Banwell, C.; Korda, R.J.; Dixon, J.; Paolucci, F.; Glover, J. Time Scarcity: Another Health Inequality? *Environ. Plan. A. Space* **2011**, *43*, 545–559. [CrossRef]
12. Jabs, J.; Devine, C.M. Time scarcity and food choices: An overview. *Appetite* **2006**, *47*, 196–204. [CrossRef]
13. Glanz, K.; Sallis, J.F.; Saelens, B.E.; Frank, L.D. Healthy Nutrition Environments: Concepts and Measures. *Am. J. Heal. Promot.* **2005**, *19*, 330–333. [CrossRef]
14. Story, M.; Kaphingst, K.M.; Robinson-O'Brien, R.; Glanz, K. Creating Healthy Food and Eating Environments: Policy and Environmental Approaches. *Annu. Rev. Public Health* **2008**, *29*, 253–272. [CrossRef]
15. Morland, K. *Local Food Environments: Food Access in America*; CRC Press: Boca Raton, FL, USA, 2015.
16. Pew Research Center. Raising Kids and Running a Household: How Working Parents Share the Load. Available online: https://www.pewsocialtrends.org/2015/11/04/raising-kids-and-running-a-household-how-working-parents-share-the-load/ (accessed on 12 July 2020).
17. Share Our Strength's Cooking Matters, APCO Insight. It's Dinnertime: A Report on Low-Income Families' Efforts on Plan, Shop for and Cook Healthy Meals. 2012, pp. 1–54. Available online: http://cookingmatters.org/sites/default/files/pdf/ITSDINNERTIME-report.pdf (accessed on 2 August 2020).
18. Yang, Y.; Davis, G.C.; Muth, M.K. Beyond the sticker price: Including and excluding time in comparing food prices. *Am. J. Clin. Nutr.* **2015**, *102*, 165–171. [CrossRef]
19. Singleton, C.R.; Li, Y.; Duran, A.C.; Zenk, S.N.; Odoms-Young, A.; Powell, L.M. Food and beverage availability in small food stores located in healthy food financing initiative eligible communities. *Int. J. Environ. Res. Public Health* **2017**, *14*, 1242. [CrossRef]
20. Vandevijvere, S.; Waterlander, W.; Molloy, J.; Nattrass, H.; Swinburn, B. Towards healthier supermarkets: A national study of in-store food availability, prominence and promotions in New Zealand. *Eur. J. Clin. Nutr.* **2018**, *72*, 971–978. [CrossRef] [PubMed]
21. Caspi, C.E.; Pelletier, J.E.; Harnack, L.; Erickson, D.J.; Laska, M.N. Differences in healthy food supply and stocking practices between small grocery stores, gas-marts, pharmacies and dollar stores. *Public Health Nutr.* **2016**, *19*, 540–547. [CrossRef]
22. Racine, E.F.; Delmelle, E.; Major, E.; Solomon, C.A. Accessibility landscapes of supplemental nutrition assistance program-authorized stores. *J. Acad. Nutr. Diet.* **2018**, *118*, 836–848. [CrossRef]
23. Bitto, E.A.; Morton, L.W.; Oakland, M.J.; Sand, M. Grocery store acess patterns in rural food deserts. *J. Study Food Soc.* **2003**, *6*, 35–48. [CrossRef]
24. Morton, L.W.; Blanchard, T.C. Starved for Access: Life in Rural America's Food Deserts. Available online: https://www.ruralsociology.org/assets/docs/rural-realities/rural-realities-1-4.pdf (accessed on 22 August 2020).

25. Cobb, L.K.; Appel, L.J.; Franco, M.; Jones-Smith, J.C.; Nur, A.; Anderson, C.A. The relationship of the local food environment with obesity: A systematic review of methods, study quality, and results. *Obesity (Silver Spring)* **2015**, *23*, 1331–1344. [CrossRef]
26. Caspi, C.E.; Sorensen, G.; Subramanian, S.V.; Kawachi, I. The local food environment and diet: A systematic review. *Health Place* **2012**, *18*, 1172–1187. [CrossRef] [PubMed]
27. Zenk, S.N.; Thatcher, E.; Reina, M.; Odoms-Young, A. Local Food Environments and Diet-Related Health Outcomes: A Systematic Review of Local Food Environments, Body Weight, and Other Diet-Related Health Outcomes. In *Local Food Environments: Food Access in America*; Morland, K., Ed.; CRC Press: Boca Raton, FL, USA, 2015; pp. 167–204.
28. Cooksey-Stowers, K.; Schwartz, M.B.; Brownell, K.D. Food swamps predict obesity rates better than food deserts in the United States. *Int. J. Environ Res. Public Health* **2017**, *14*, 1366. [CrossRef]
29. Sarasin, L.G. How Everything We Know about Consumers Is Being Flipped and What That Means for Leadership. Available online: https://www.fmi.org/blog/view/fmi-blog/2018/05/16/how-everything-we-know-about-consumers-is-being-flipped-and-what-that-means-for-leadership (accessed on 15 June 2020).
30. National Association of Convenience Stores. State of the Industry Report: 2018 Data: Strong Sales for Convenience Stores. 2019. Available online: https://mma.prnewswire.com/media/846231/NACS_Sales_Report_2018.pdf (accessed on 4 June 2020).
31. Zenk, S.N.; Powell, L.M.; Isgor, Z.; Rimkus, L.; Barker, D.C.; Chaloupka, F.J. Prepared food availability in U.S. food stores: A national study. *Am. J. Prev. Med.* **2015**, *49*, 553–562. [CrossRef] [PubMed]
32. James, P.; Seward, M.W.; James O'Malley, A.; Subramanian, S.V.; Block, J.P. Changes in the food environment over time: Examining 40 years of data in the Framingham Heart Study. *Int. J. Behav. Nutr. Phys. Act.* **2017**, *14*, 84. [CrossRef] [PubMed]
33. IBISWorld. Fast Food Restaurants in the US: Number of Businesses 2001–2026. Available online: https://www.ibisworld.com/industry-statistics/number-of-businesses/fast-food-restaurants-united-states/) (accessed on 14 June 2020).
34. National Association of Convenience Stores. U.S. Convenience Store Count. Available online: https://www.convenience.org/Research/FactSheets/ScopeofIndustry/IndustryStoreCount (accessed on 14 June 2020).
35. Rivlin, G. *Rigged: Supermarket Shelves for Sale*; Center for Science in the Public Interest: Washington, DC, USA, 2016.
36. Houghtaling, B.; Serrano, E.L.; Kraak, V.I.; Harden, S.M.; Davis, G.C.; Misyak, S.A. A systematic review of factors that influence food store owner and manager decision making and ability or willingness to use choice architecture and marketing mix strategies to encourage healthy consumer purchases in the United States, 2005–2017. *Int. J. Behav. Nutr. Phys. Act.* **2019**, *16*, 5. [CrossRef]
37. Hansen, T.H.; Skytte, H. Retailer buying behaviour: A review. *Int. Rev. Retail. Distrib. Consum. Res.* **1998**, *8*, 277–301. [CrossRef]
38. Rong, A.; Akkerman, R.; Grunow, M. An optimization approach for managing fresh food quality throughout the supply chain. *Int. J. Prod. Econ.* **2011**, *131*, 421–429. [CrossRef]
39. Turi, A.; Goncalves, G.; Mocan, M. Challenges and competitiveness indicators for the sustainable development of the supply chain in food industry. *Procedia Soc. Behav. Sci.* **2014**, *124*, 133–141. [CrossRef]
40. Gokarn, S.; Kuthambalayan, T.S. Analysis of challenges inhibiting the reduction of waste in food supply chain. *J. Clean. Prod.* **2017**, *168*, 595–604. [CrossRef]
41. Ayala, G.X.; Laska, M.N.; Zenk, S.N.; Tester, J.; Rose, D.; Odoms-Young, A.; McCoy, T.; Gittelsohn, J.; Foster, G.D.; Andreyeva, T. Stocking characteristics and perceived increases in sales among small food store managers/owners associated with the introduction of new food products approved by the Special Supplemental Nutrition Program for Women, Infants, and Children. *Public Health Nutr.* **2012**, *15*, 1771–1779. [CrossRef]
42. Gittelsohn, J.; Laska, M.N.; Karpyn, A.; Klingler, K.; Ayala, G.X. Lessons learned from small store programs to increase healthy food access. *Am. J. Health Behav.* **2014**, *38*, 307–315. [CrossRef]
43. Wallace, L.A.; Morris, V.G.; Hudak, K.M.; Racine, E.F. Increasing access to WIC through discount variety stores: Findings from qualitative research. *J. Acad. Nutr. Diet* **2020**. [CrossRef]

44. Gittelsohn, J.; Ayala, G.X.; D'Angelo, H.; Kharmats, A.; Ribisl, K.M.; Sindberg, L.S.; Liverman, S.P.; Laska, M.N. Formal and informal agreements between small food stores and food and beverage suppliers: Store owner perspectives from four cities. *J. Hunger. Env. Nutr.* **2018**, *13*, 517–530. [CrossRef]
45. Laska, M.N.; Sindberg, L.S.; Ayala, G.X.; D'Angelo, H.; Horton, L.A.; Ribisl, K.M.; Kharmats, A.; Olson, C.; Gittelsohn, J. Agreements between small food store retailers and their suppliers: Incentivizing unhealthy foods and beverages in four urban settings. *Food Policy* **2018**, *79*, 324–330. [CrossRef]
46. Kim, M.; Budd, N.; Batorsky, B.; Krubiner, C.; Manchikanti, S.; Waldrop, G.; Trude, A.; Gittelsohn, J. Barriers to and facilitators of stocking healthy food options: Viewpoints of Baltimore City small storeowners. *Ecol. Food Nutr.* **2017**, *56*, 17–30. [CrossRef]
47. O'Malley, K.; Gustat, J.; Rice, J.; Johnson, C.C. Feasibility of increasing access to healthy foods in neighborhood corner stores. *J. Community Health* **2013**, *38*, 741–749. [CrossRef] [PubMed]
48. Song, H.J.; Gittelsohn, J.; Kim, M.; Suratkar, S.; Sharma, S.; Anliker, J. Korean American storeowners' perceived barriers and motivators for implementing a corner store-based program. *Health Promot. Pract.* **2011**, *12*, 472–482. [CrossRef]
49. Khojasteh, M.; Raja, S. Agents of change: How immigrant-run ethnic food retailers improve food environments. *J. Hunger Environ. Nutr.* **2017**, *12*, 299–327. [CrossRef]
50. Grigsby-Toussaint, D.S.; Zenk, S.N.; Odoms-Young, A.; Ruggiero, L.; Moise, I. Availability of commonly consumed and culturally specific fruits and vegetables in African-American and Latino neighborhoods. *J. Acad. Nutr. Diet* **2010**, *110*, 746–752. [CrossRef] [PubMed]
51. Inmarket Insights Report. Where Vegetarian-Leaning Consumers Grub & Grocery Shop. 2019. Available online: https://medium.com/inmarket-insights/where-vegetarian-leaning-consumers-grub-grocery-shop-1406f5684416 (accessed on 2 August 2020).
52. Hudak, K.M.; Paul, R.; Gholizadeh, S.; Zadrozny, W.; Racine, E.F. Special Supplemental Nutrition Program for Women, Infants, and Children (WIC) authorization of discount variety stores: Leveraging the private sector to modestly increase availability of healthy foods. *Am. J. Clin. Nutr.* **2020**, *111*, 1278–1285. [CrossRef]
53. Hübner, A.H.; Kuhn, H.; Sternbeck, M.G. Demand and supply chain planning in grocery retail: An operations planning framework. *Int. J. Retail Distrib.* **2013**. [CrossRef]
54. Biery, M.E. The 15 Least Profitable Industries in the U.S. Available online: https://www.forbes.com/sites/sageworks/2016/10/03/the-15-least-profitable-industries-in-the-u-s/#6635c5c618ab (accessed on 22 August 2020).
55. Egan, B. Introduction to Food Production and Service. Licensed under Creative Commons Attributes 4.0. Available online: https://psu.pb.unizin.org/hmd329/ (accessed on 2 August 2020).
56. U.S. Department of Agriculture; Economic Research Service. Retail Trends. Available online: https://www.ers.usda.gov/topics/food-markets-prices/retailing-wholesaling/retail-trends.aspx (accessed on 22 August 2020).
57. Palmer, B. The World's 10 Biggest Restaurant Companies. Available online: https://www.investopedia.com/articles/markets/012516/worlds-top-10-restaurant-companies-mcdsbux.asp (accessed on 22 August 2020).
58. Dun & Bradstreet. Food Service Contractors Companies in United States of America. Available online: https://www.dnb.com/business-directory/company-information.food-service-contractors.us.html?page=1 (accessed on 22 August 2020).
59. American Independant Business Alliance. Community Ownership: Helping People Fill Local Needs Through Shared Vision, Investment. Available online: https://www.amiba.net/resources/community-ownership/ (accessed on 31 July 2020).
60. Cho, C.; Volpe, R. Independent Grocery Stores in the Changing Landscape of the U.S. Food Retail Industry. Available online: https://www.ers.usda.gov/webdocs/publications/85783/err-240.pdf?v=0 (accessed on 22 August 2020).
61. Food & Water Watch. Consolidation and Buyer Power in the Grocery Industry. Available online: https://www.foodandwaterwatch.org/sites/default/files/consolidation_buyer_power_grocery_fs_dec_2010.pdf (accessed on 31 July 2020).
62. Loria, K. What Is Fueling Grocery Consolidation? Available online: https://www.grocerydive.com/news/why-grocery-consolidation/535608/ (accessed on 31 July 2020).

63. Winkler, M.R.; Lenk, K.M.; Caspi, C.E.; Erickson, D.J.; Harnack, L.; Laska, M.N. Variation in the food environment of small and non-traditional stores across racial segregation and corporate status. *Public Health Nutr.* **2019**, *22*, 1624–1634. [CrossRef]
64. Caspi, C.E.; Winkler, M.R.; Lenk, K.M.; Harnack, L.J.; Erickson, D.J.; Laska, M.N. Store and neighborhood differences in retailer compliance with a local staple foods ordinance. *BMC Public Health* **2020**, *20*, 172. [CrossRef]
65. Armstrong, G.; Adam, S.; Denize, S.; Kotler, P. *Principles of Marketing*; Pearson Australia: Melbourne, Australia, 2015.
66. Lucan, S.C. Concerning limitations of food-environment research: A narrative review and commentary framed around obesity and diet-related diseases in youth. *J. Acad. Nutr. Diet* **2015**, *115*, 205–212. [CrossRef]
67. Thornton, L.E.; Cameron, A.J.; McNaughton, S.A.; Waterlander, W.E.; Sodergren, M.; Svastisalee, C.; Blanchard, L.; Liese, A.D.; Battersby, S.; Carter, M.A.; et al. Does the availability of snack foods in supermarkets vary internationally? *Int. J. Behav. Nutr. Phys. Act.* **2013**, *10*, 56. [CrossRef] [PubMed]
68. Cameron, A.J.; Thornton, L.E.; McNaughton, S.A.; Crawford, D. Variation in supermarket exposure to energy-dense snack foods by socio-economic position. *Public Health Nutr.* **2013**, *16*, 1178–1185. [CrossRef] [PubMed]
69. Caspi, C.E.; Lenk, K.; Pelletier, J.E.; Barnes, T.L.; Harnack, L.; Erickson, D.J.; Laska, M.N. Association between store food environment and customer purchases in small grocery stores, gas-marts, pharmacies and dollar stores. *Int. J. Behav. Nutr. Phys. Act.* **2017**, *14*, 76. [CrossRef] [PubMed]
70. Lin, B.-H.; Ver Ploeg, M.; Kasteridis, P.; Yen, S.T. The roles of food prices and food access in determining food purchases of low-income households. *J. Policy Model.* **2014**, *36*, 938–952. [CrossRef]
71. Webber, C.B.; Sobal, J.; Dollahite, J.S. Shopping for fruits and vegetables. Food and retail qualities of importance to low-income households at the grocery store. *Appetite* **2010**, *54*, 297–303. [CrossRef] [PubMed]
72. Kelly, B.; Flood, V.M.; Bicego, C.; Yeatman, H. Derailing healthy choices: An audit of vending machines at train stations in NSW. *Health Promot. J. Austr.* **2012**, *23*, 73–75. [CrossRef]
73. Ko, L.K.; Enzler, C.; Perry, C.K.; Rodriguez, E.; Mariscal, N.; Linde, S.; Duggan, C. Food availability and food access in rural agricultural communities: Use of mixed methods. *BMC Public Health* **2018**, *18*, 634. [CrossRef]
74. Zenk, S.N.; Powell, L.M.; Rimkus, L.; Isgor, Z.; Barker, D.C.; Ohri-Vachaspati, P.; Chaloupka, F. Relative and absolute availability of healthier food and beverage alternatives across communities in the United States. *Am. J. Public Health* **2014**, *104*, 2170–2178. [CrossRef]
75. Farley, T.A.; Rice, J.; Bodor, J.N.; Cohen, D.A.; Bluthenthal, R.N.; Rose, D. Measuring the food environment: Shelf space of fruits, vegetables, and snack foods in stores. *J. Urban Health* **2009**, *86*, 672–682. [CrossRef]
76. Drewnowski, A.; Darmon, N. The economics of obesity: Dietary energy density and energy cost. *Am. J. Clin. Nutr.* **2005**, *82*, 265S–273S. [CrossRef]
77. Haynes-Maslow, L.; Parsons, S.E.; Wheeler, S.B.; Leone, L.A. A qualitative study of perceived barriers to fruit and vegetable consumption among low-income populations, North Carolina, 2011. *Prev. Chronic. Dis.* **2013**, *10*, E34. [CrossRef]
78. Anzman-Frasca, S.; Mueller, M.P.; Sliwa, S.; Dolan, P.R.; Harelick, L.; Roberts, S.B.; Washburn, K.; Economos, C.D. Changes in children's meal orders following healthy menu modifications at a regional US restaurant chain. *Obesity* **2015**, *23*, 1055–1062. [CrossRef] [PubMed]
79. Zenk, S.N.; Schulz, A.J.; Hollis-Neely, T.; Campbell, R.T.; Holmes, N.; Watkins, G.; Nwankwo, R.; Odoms-Young, A. Fruit and vegetable intake in African Americans income and store characteristics. *Am. J. Prev. Med.* **2005**, *29*, 1–9. [CrossRef] [PubMed]
80. Sharkey, J.R.; Johnson, C.M.; Dean, W.R. Food access and perceptions of the community and household food environment as correlates of fruit and vegetable intake among rural seniors. *BMC Geriatr.* **2010**, *10*, 32. [CrossRef]
81. Caldwell, E.M.; Miller Kobayashi, M.; DuBow, W.M.; Wytinck, S.M. Perceived access to fruits and vegetables associated with increased consumption. *Public Health Nutr.* **2009**, *12*, 1743–1750. [CrossRef]
82. Zenk, S.N.; Schulz, A.J.; Israel, B.A.; James, S.A.; Bao, S.; Wilson, M.L. Fruit and vegetable access differs by community racial composition and socioeconomic position in Detroit, Michigan. *Ethn. Dis.* **2006**, *16*, 275–280. [CrossRef]

83. Andreyeva, T.; Blumenthal, D.M.; Schwartz, M.B.; Long, M.W.; Brownell, K.D. Availability and prices of foods across stores and neighborhoods: The case of New Haven, Connecticut. *Health Aff.* **2008**, *27*, 1381–1388. [CrossRef]
84. Gosliner, W.; Brown, D.M.; Sun, B.C.; Woodward-Lopez, G.; Crawford, P.B. Availability, quality and price of produce in low-income neighbourhood food stores in California raise equity issues. *Public Health Nutr* **2018**, *21*, 1639–1648. [CrossRef]
85. Chester, J.; Kopp, K.; Montgomery, K.C. Does Buying Groceries Online Put SNAP Participants at Risk? Available online: https://www.democraticmedia.org/sites/default/files/field/public-files/2020/cdd_snap_report_ff_0.pdf (accessed on 31 July 2020).
86. Page, R.; Montgomery, K.; Ponder, A.; Richard, A. Targeting children in the cereal aisle. *Am. J. Health Educ.* **2008**, *39*, 272–282. [CrossRef]
87. Malik, V.S.; Willett, W.C.; Hu, F.B. The revised nutrition facts label: A step forward and more room for improvement. *JAMA* **2016**, *316*, 583–584. [CrossRef]
88. Goodman, S.; Vanderlee, L.; Acton, R.; Mahamad, S.; Hammond, D. The impact of front-of-package label design on consumer understanding of nutrient amounts. *Nutrients* **2018**, *10*, 1624. [CrossRef]
89. Roseman, M.G.; Joung, H.W.; Littlejohn, E.I. Attitude and behavior factors associated with front-of-package label use with label users making accurate product nutrition assessments. *J. Acad. Nutr. Diet* **2018**, *118*, 904–912. [CrossRef]
90. Emrich, T.E.; Qi, Y.; Lou, W.Y.; L'Abbe, M.R. Traffic-light labels could reduce population intakes of calories, total fat, saturated fat, and sodium. *PLoS ONE* **2017**, *12*, e0171188. [CrossRef]
91. Almy, J.; Wootan, M.G. The Food Industry's Sneaky Strategy for Selling More. Available online: https://cspinet.org/temptation-checkout (accessed on 22 August 2020).
92. Chauvenet, C.; De Marco, M.; Barnes, C.; Ammerman, A.S. WIC recipients in the retail environment: A qualitative study assessing customer experience and satisfaction. *J. Acad. Nutr. Diet* **2019**, *119*, 416–424. [CrossRef]
93. Cannuscio, C.C.; Hillier, A.; Karpyn, A.; Glanz, K. The social dynamics of healthy food shopping and store choice in an urban environment. *Soc. Sci. Med.* **2014**, *122*, 13–20. [CrossRef] [PubMed]
94. Zenk, S.N.; Odoms-Young, A.M.; Dallas, C.; Hardy, E.; Watkins, A.; Hoskins-Wroten, J.; Holland, L. "You have to hunt for the fruits, the vegetables": Environmental barriers and adaptive strategies to acquire food in a low-income African American neighborhood. *Health Educ. Behav.* **2011**, *38*, 282–292. [CrossRef] [PubMed]
95. Odoms-Young, A.M.; Zenk, S.; Mason, M. Measuring food availability and access in African-American communities: Implications for intervention and policy. *Am. J. Prev. Med.* **2009**, *36*, S145–S150. [CrossRef]
96. Zenk, S.N.; Schulz, A.J.; Israel, B.A.; Mentz, G.; Miranda, P.Y.; Opperman, A.; Odoms-Young, A.M. Food shopping behaviours and exposure to discrimination. *Public Health Nutr.* **2014**, *17*, 1167–1176. [CrossRef]
97. Brewster, Z.W.; Rusche, S.N. Quantitative evidence of the continuing significance of race: Tableside racism in full-service restaurants. *J. Black Stud.* **2012**, *43*, 359–384. [CrossRef] [PubMed]
98. Rusche, S.E.; Brewster, Z.W. 'Because they tip for shit!': The social psychology of everyday racism in restaurants. *Sociol. Compass* **2008**, *2*, 2008–2029. [CrossRef]
99. Lee, J. The salience of race in everyday life: Black customers' shopping experiences in Black and White neighborhoods. *Work Occup.* **2000**, *27*, 353–376. [CrossRef]
100. Haynes-Maslow, L.; Auvergne, L.; Mark, B.; Ammerman, A.; Weiner, B.J. Low-income individuals' perceptions about fruit and vegetable access programs: A qualitative study. *J. Nutr. Educ. Behav.* **2015**, *47*, 317–324.e311. [CrossRef] [PubMed]
101. Emond, J.A.; Madanat, H.N.; Ayala, G.X. Do Latino and non-Latino grocery stores differ in the availability and affordability of healthy food items in a low-income, metropolitan region? *Public Health Nutr.* **2012**, *15*, 360–369. [CrossRef] [PubMed]
102. Darmon, N.; Drewnowski, A. Contribution of food prices and diet cost to socioeconomic disparities in diet quality and health: A systematic review and analysis. *Nutr. Rev.* **2015**, *73*, 643–660. [CrossRef] [PubMed]

103. Rehm, C.D.; Penalvo, J.L.; Afshin, A.; Mozaffarian, D. Dietary intake among US adults, 1999–2012. *JAMA* **2016**, *315*, 2542–2553. [CrossRef] [PubMed]
104. Spronk, I.; Kullen, C.; Burdon, C.; O'Connor, H. Relationship between nutrition knowledge and dietary intake. *Br. J. Nutr.* **2014**, *111*, 1713–1726. [CrossRef]
105. Schwartz, G.; Grindal, T.; Wilde, P.; Klerman, J.; Bartlett, S. Supermarket shopping and the food retail environment among SNAP participants. *J. Hunger. Environ. Nutr.* **2018**, *13*, 154–179. [CrossRef]
106. Kinsey, E.W.; Oberle, M.; Dupuis, R.; Cannuscio, C.C.; Hillier, A. Food and financial coping strategies during the monthly Supplemental Nutrition Assistance Program cycle. *SSM Popul. Health* **2019**, *7*, 100393. [CrossRef]
107. French, S.A.; Tangney, C.C.; Crane, M.M.; Wang, Y.; Appelhans, B.M. Nutrition quality of food purchases varies by household income: The SHoPPER study. *BMC Public Health* **2019**, *19*, 231. [CrossRef]
108. Arandia, G.; Sotres-Alvarez, D.; Siega-Riz, A.M.; Arredondo, E.M.; Carnethon, M.R.; Delamater, A.M.; Gallo, L.C.; Isasi, C.R.; Marchante, A.N.; Pritchard, D.; et al. Associations between acculturation, ethnic identity, and diet quality among U.S. Hispanic/Latino Youth: Findings from the HCHS/SOL Youth Study. *Appetite* **2018**, *129*, 25–36. [CrossRef]
109. Ayala, G.X.; Mueller, K.; Lopez-Madurga, E.; Campbell, N.R.; Elder, J.P. Restaurant and food shopping selections among Latino women in Southern California. *J. Am. Diet Assoc.* **2005**, *105*, 38–45. [CrossRef]
110. Nilsson, E.; Garling, T.; Marell, A.; Nordvall, A. Who shops groceries where and how?-the relationship between choice of store format and type of grocery shopping. *Int. Rev. Retail. Distrib. Consum. Res.* **2014**, *25*, 1–19. [CrossRef]
111. Change Lab Solutions. A Legal and Practical Guide for Designing Sugary Drink Taxes. 2018. Available online: https://www.changelabsolutions.org/sites/default/files/Sugary_Drinks-TAX-GUIDE_FINAL_20190114.pdf (accessed on 2 August 2020).
112. Zenk, S.N.; Odoms-Young, A.; Powell, L.M.; Campbell, R.T.; Block, D.; Chavez, N.; Krauss, R.C.; Strode, S.; Armbruster, J. Fruit and vegetable availability and selection: Federal food package revisions, 2009. *Am. J. Prev. Med.* **2012**, *43*, 423–428. [CrossRef]
113. Pomeranz, J.L.; Zellers, L.; Bare, M.; Pertschuk, M. State preemption of food and nutrition policies and litigation: Undermining government's role in public health. *Am. J. Prev. Med.* **2019**, *56*, 47–57. [CrossRef] [PubMed]
114. Willett, W.; Rockstrom, J.; Loken, B.; Springmann, M.; Lang, T.; Vermeulen, S.; Garnett, T.; Tilman, D.; DeClerck, F.; Wood, A.; et al. Food in the anthropocene: The EAT-Lancet Commission on healthy diets from sustainable food systems. *Lancet* **2019**, *393*, 447–492. [CrossRef]
115. Swinburn, B.A.; Kraak, V.I.; Allender, S.; Atkins, V.J.; Baker, P.I.; Bogard, J.R.; Brinsden, H.; Calvillo, A.; De Schutter, O.; Devarajan, R.; et al. The Global Syndemic of Obesity, Undernutrition, and Climate Change: The Lancet Commission report. *Lancet* **2019**, *393*, 791–846. [CrossRef]
116. Swinburn, B.; Sacks, G.; Vandevijvere, S.; Kumanyika, S.; Lobstein, T.; Neal, B.; Barquera, S.; Friel, S.; Hawkes, C.; Kelly, B.; et al. INFORMAS (International Network for Food and Obesity/non-communicable diseases Research, Monitoring and Action Support): Overview and key principles. *Obes. Rev.* **2013**, *14*, 1–12. [CrossRef]
117. Kulish, N. 'Never Seen Anything Like It': Cars Line Up for Miles at Food Banks; New York Times. 2020. Available online: https://www.nytimes.com/2020/04/08/business/economy/coronavirus-food-banks.html (accessed on 2 June 2020).
118. Bleich, S.N.; Fleiechhacker, S.; Laska, M.N. Protecting Hungry Children during the Fight for Racial Justice. Available online: https://thehill.com/opinion/civil-rights/500656-protecting-hungry-children-during-the-fight-for-racial-justice (accessed on 14 June 2020).
119. U.S. Department of Agriculture. How much food waste is there in the United States? Available online: https://www.usda.gov/foodwaste/faqs (accessed on 22 August 2020).
120. Blake, M.R.; Backholer, K.; Lancsar, E.; Boelsen-Robinson, T.; Mah, C.; Brimblecombe, J.; Zorbas, C.; Billich, N.; Peeters, A. Investigating business outcomes of healthy food retail strategies: A systematic scoping review. *Obes. Rev.* **2019**, *20*, 1384–1399. [CrossRef]

121. Gittelsohn, J.; Mhs, M.C.F.; Ba, I.R.R.; Ries, A.V.; Ho, L.S.; Pavlovich, W.; Santos, V.T.; Ms, S.M.J.; Frick, K.D. Understanding the Food Environment in a Low-Income Urban Setting: Implications for Food Store Interventions. *J. Hunger. Environ. Nutr.* **2008**, *2*, 33–50. [CrossRef]
122. Carpenter, J.M.; Moore, M. Consumer demographics, store attributes, and retail format choice in the US grocery market. *Int. J. Retail. Distrib.* **2006**, *34*, 434–452. [CrossRef]
123. Gravlee, C.C.; Boston, P.Q.; Mitchell, M.M.; Schultz, A.F.; Betterley, C. Food store owners' and managers' perspectives on the food environment: An exploratory mixed-methods study. *BMC Public Health* **2014**, *14*, 1031. [CrossRef] [PubMed]
124. Dong, D.; Stewart, H. Modeling a household's choice among food store types. *Am. J. Agric. Econ.* **2012**, *94*, 702–717. [CrossRef]
125. The Food Industry Association. Supermarket Facts. Available online: https://www.fmi.org/our-research/supermarket-facts (accessed on 14 June 2020).
126. IBISWorld. Fast Food Restaurants Industry in the US-Market Research Report. Available online: https://www.ibisworld.com/united-states/market-research-reports/fast-food-restaurants-industry/ (accessed on 14 June 2020).
127. U.S. Department of Agriculture; Economic Research Service. Eating-out Expenditures in March 2020 Were 28 Percent Below March 2019 Expenditures. Available online: https://www.ers.usda.gov/data-products/chart-gallery/gallery/chart-detail/?chartId=98556 (accessed on 31 July 2020).
128. Patel, R. Food sovereignty. *J. Peasant. Stud.* **2009**, *36*, 663–706. [CrossRef]
129. Anderson, M.D. Food and Farming Research for the Public Good. For Whom? Questioning the Food and Farming Research Agenda; A Special Edition Magazine from the Food Ethics Council. 2018, pp. 28–29. Available online: https://www.foodethicscouncil.org/app/uploads/For%20whom%20-%20questioning%20the%20food%20and%20farming%20research%20agenda_FINAL.pdf (accessed on 24 May 2019).
130. Monteiro, C.A.; Moubarac, J.C.; Cannon, G.; Ng, S.W.; Popkin, B. Ultra-processed products are becoming dominant in the global food system. *Obes. Rev.* **2013**, *14*, 21–28. [CrossRef] [PubMed]
131. White, M.; Aguirre, E.; Finegood, D.T.; Holmes, C.; Sacks, G.; Smith, R. What role should the commercial food system play in promoting health through better diet? *BMJ* **2020**, *368*, m545. [CrossRef]
132. Ludwig, D.S.; Nestle, M. Can the food industry play a constructive role in the obesity epidemic? *JAMA* **2008**, *300*, 1808–1811. [CrossRef] [PubMed]
133. Smith Taillie, L.; Jaacks, L.M. Toward a just, nutritious, and sustainable food system: The false dichotomy of localism versus supercenterism. *J. Nutr.* **2015**, *145*, 1380–1385. [CrossRef] [PubMed]
134. Gittelsohn, J.; Mui, Y.; Adam, A.; Lin, S.; Kharmats, A.; Igusa, T.; Lee, B.Y. Incorporating systems science principles into the development of obesity prevention interventions: Principles, benefits, and challenges. *Curr. Obes. Rep.* **2015**, *4*, 174–181. [CrossRef]
135. Barnhill, A.; Palmer, A.; Weston, C.M.; Brownell, K.D.; Clancy, K.; Economos, C.D.; Gittelsohn, J.; Hammond, R.A.; Kumanyika, S.; Bennett, W.L. Grappling with complex food systems to reduce obesity: A US public health challenge. *Public Health Rep.* **2018**, *133*, 44S–53S. [CrossRef]
136. Ewart-Pierce, E.; Ruiz, M.J.M.; Gittelsohn, J. "Whole-of-Community" obesity prevention: A review of challenges and opportunities in multilevel, multicomponent interventions. *Curr. Obes. Rep.* **2016**, *5*, 361–374. [CrossRef]
137. Auchincloss, A.H.; Riolo, R.L.; Brown, D.G.; Cook, J.; Diez Roux, A.V. An agent-based model of income inequalities in diet in the context of residential segregation. *Am. J. Prev. Med.* **2011**, *40*, 303–311. [CrossRef]
138. Mui, Y.; Lee, B.Y.; Adam, A.; Kharmats, A.Y.; Budd, N.; Nau, C.; Gittelsohn, J. Healthy versus unhealthy suppliers in food desert neighborhoods: A network analysis of corner stores' food supplier networks. *Int. J. Environ. Res. Public Health* **2015**, *12*, 15058–15074. [CrossRef] [PubMed]
139. Orr, M.G.; Kaplan, G.A.; Galea, S. Neighbourhood food, physical activity, and educational environments and black/white disparities in obesity: A complex systems simulation analysis. *J. Epidemiol. Commun. Health* **2016**, *70*, 862. [CrossRef]
140. Wong, M.S.; Nau, C.; Kharmats, A.Y.; Vedovato, G.M.; Cheskin, L.J.; Gittelsohn, J.; Lee, B.Y. Using a computational model to quantify the potential impact of changing the placement of healthy beverages in stores as an intervention to "Nudge" adolescent behavior choice. *BMC Public Health* **2015**, *15*, 1284. [CrossRef] [PubMed]

141. Trude, A.C.B.; Surkan, P.J.; Cheskin, L.J.; Gittelsohn, J. A multilevel, multicomponent childhood obesity prevention group-randomized controlled trial improves healthier food purchasing and reduces sweet-snack consumption among low-income African-American youth. *Nutr. J.* **2018**, *17*, 96. [CrossRef]
142. Redmond, L.C.; Jock, B.; Gadhoke, P.; Chiu, D.T.; Christiansen, K.; Pardilla, M.; Swartz, J.; Platero, H.; Caulfield, L.E.; Gittelsohn, J. OPREVENT (Obesity Prevention and Evaluation of InterVention Effectiveness in NaTive North Americans): Design of a Multilevel, Multicomponent Obesity Intervention for Native American Adults and Households. *Curr. Dev. Nutr.* **2019**, *3*, 81–93. [CrossRef] [PubMed]

Publisher's Note: MDPI stays neutral with regard to jurisdictional claims in published maps and institutional affiliations.

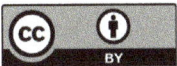

© 2020 by the authors. Licensee MDPI, Basel, Switzerland. This article is an open access article distributed under the terms and conditions of the Creative Commons Attribution (CC BY) license (http://creativecommons.org/licenses/by/4.0/).

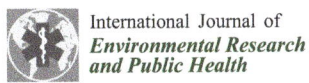

International Journal of
Environmental Research and Public Health

Communication

Healthy Food Retail during the COVID-19 Pandemic: Challenges and Future Directions

Lucia A. Leone [1,*], Sheila Fleischhacker [2], Betsy Anderson-Steeves [3], Kaitlyn Harper [4], Megan Winkler [5], Elizabeth Racine [6], Barbara Baquero [7] and Joel Gittelsohn [4]

1 School of Public Health and Health Professions, University at Buffalo, Buffalo, NY 14213, USA
2 Law Center, Georgetown University, Washington, DC 20001, USA; sef80@georgetown.edu
3 Department of Nutrition, University of Tennessee, Knoxville, TN 37996, USA; Eander24@utk.edu
4 Bloomberg School of Public Health, Johns Hopkins University, Baltimore, MD 21205, USA; kharpe14@jhu.edu (K.H.); jgittel1@jhu.edu (J.G.)
5 School of Public Health, University of Minnesota, Minneapolis, MN 55455, USA; mwinkler@umn.edu
6 Department of Public Health Sciences, College of Health and Human Services University of North Carolina at Charlotte, Charlotte, NC 28223, USA; efracine@uncc.edu
7 Department of Health Services School of Public Health, University of Washington Seattle, WA 98195, USA; bbaquero@uw.edu
* Correspondence: lucialeo@buffalo.edu; Tel.: +1-716-829-6953

Received: 7 September 2020; Accepted: 8 October 2020; Published: 11 October 2020

Abstract: Disparities in dietary behaviors have been directly linked to the food environment, including access to retail food outlets. The Coronavirus Disease of 2019 (COVID-19) pandemic has led to major changes in the distribution, sale, purchase, preparation, and consumption of food in the United States (US). This paper reflects on those changes and provides recommendations for research to understand the impact of the pandemic on the retail food environment (RFE) and consumer behavior. Using the Retail Food Environment and Customer Interaction Model, we describe the impact of COVID-19 in four key areas: (1) community, state, tribal, and federal policy; (2) retail actors, business models, and sources; (3) customer experiences; and (4) dietary intake. We discuss how previously existing vulnerabilities and inequalities based on race, ethnicity, class, and geographic location were worsened by the pandemic. We recommend approaches for building a more just and equitable RFE, including understanding the impacts of changing shopping behaviors and adaptations to federal nutrition assistance as well as how small food business can be made more sustainable. By better understanding the RFE adaptations that have characterized the COVID-19 pandemic, we hope to gain greater insight into how our food system can become more resilient in the future.

Keywords: retail food environment; food purchasing; federal nutrition assistance; COVID-19; grocery stores; restaurants; dietary intake

1. Introduction

In the United States (US), substantial socioeconomic and racial disparities exist in dietary behaviors [1]. Limited access to fresh food, coupled with a greater prevalence of fast food outlets in lower-income and minority neighborhoods, is partially responsible for sub-optimal eating patterns among residents [2]. The Coronavirus Disease of 2019 (COVID-19) pandemic has placed unprecedented strain on the US food system and changed the way food is distributed, sold, obtained, prepared, and consumed [3,4]. In the early weeks of the pandemic, grocery retailers saw overwhelming demand paired with panic buying resulting in empty shelves [5]. Restaurants have been temporarily closed in many communities and some have even permanently closed as they were unable to weather the financial burden of the temporary closures and/or the required additional pandemic safeguards [6].

To reduce risk of exposure, many consumers shifted to online food shopping and opted for curbside pickup or home delivery over entering retail stores [7]. Changes in consumer purchasing, coupled with government-mandated business closures, also negatively impacted food growers and producers. Due to the lack of demand from restaurants, there were reports of farmers who found it more economical to plow under crops and cull their herds [8–12].

The virus has disproportionality impacted food access for groups that already had higher rates of food insecurity (see Table 1) [13]. COVID-19 has also further exacerbated existing disparities as coping strategies (e.g., bulk purchasing, online ordering, food delivery) are largely unavailable to those with already limited food access [11,14]. Food insecurity disproportionately affects communities who have been historically oppressed, most notably communities of color, due to policies and structures obstructing access to affordable foods [15]. Individuals in these communities often do not have equal access to resources and are more likely to have lost jobs during the COVID-19 crisis, leading to a further increased risk of food insecurity [16]. Before the pandemic, 21% of Non-Hispanic Black households experienced food insecurity [17]; currently, that proportion is estimated at 38% and will likely continue to rise the longer the pandemic persists and during the resulting economic recovery [18]. Many communities have also been impacted by uprisings against police brutality and structural racism that may have damaged, disrupted, or destroyed food retail outlets and other infrastructure, creating even more food access issues [19].

Table 1. Food insecurity rates before and during COVID-19 for select population groups.

Population Group	Food Insecurity Rate	
	Before COVID	During COVID
All US households [17]	11%	23%
Households with children (<18 years) [20,21]	15%	35%
Mothers with children 12 years and under [20]	15%	41%
Non-Hispanic Black households [18]	21%	38%

Factors contributing to food insecurity during COVID-19:
- Structural inequities regarding race and class
- Job loss
- Holding a low-wage job(s)
- Limited savings/access to credit

Despite the many possible effects of the pandemic on components of the retail food environment (RFE), no literature exists that explores these effects in a systematic manner, and then uses these findings to suggest and prioritize next steps. To address this gap, we used the Retail Food Environment and Customer Interaction Model developed by Winkler and colleagues (also in this issue) to describe the impact of COVID-19 on the US RFE in four key areas outlined by the model: (1) community, state, tribal, and federal policy; (2) retail actors, business models, and retail sources; (3) customer experiences in retail setting; and (4) customer dietary intakes. This new model is the first attempt to describe the role of RFE on diet, and the unprecedented change in RFE due to the pandemic allowed an opportunity to both test the new model and to systematically structure our paper. For the purposes of the model and this paper, the RFE includes food stores (grocery, supermarket), food service (restaurants, institutional food), and emergency food (food pantries, food banks). In an effort to build a stronger, more sustainable food system for the future, we also identified research priorities and strategic programmatic directions related to the RFE in the pandemic context.

2. Community, State, Tribal, and Federal Policy Affecting the Retail Food Environment

During the pandemic, a variety of macrolevel factors at the community, state, tribal, federal, and global levels have influenced the RFE and customers' behaviors. Table 2 lists a range of COVID-19-relevant US federal government responses, including policies, programs, and operational guidelines related to food distribution and donations, household food handling and eating out, federal nutrition assistance, and federal nutrition education and promotion. The key US government departments and agencies charged with RFE-related pandemic responses include the Department of Agriculture (USDA), the Department of Commerce, the Department of Health and Human Services, Centers for Disease Control and Prevention (CDC), the Food and Drug Administration (FDA), and the Department of Homeland Security, specifically the Federal Emergency Management Agency (FEMA). Policies targeting retailers included new guidance from the CDC related to safe operations, a Paycheck Protection Program (PPP) which provided forgivable business loans, and rapid dissemination and utilization of existing laws such as those that protect organizations donating food [22]. On the consumer side, the CDC published guidelines on food safety and running essential errands including food shopping. The USDA provided relief to many people struggling to afford food through the Farmers to Families Food Box Program [23]. For this program, the USDA contracted with food distributers and other retail actors to distribute excess farm products (which normally would have gone to restaurants) through emergency food channels. A variety of existing federal nutrition education and promotion materials have been disseminated, modified, or created during the pandemic, particularly around food safety [24–26]. The USDA denied waivers from several states to use SNAP Education (SNAP-Ed) funding to pay for staff to perform work for other federal programs such as school meal distribution [27]. SNAP-Ed is an evidence-based program that works to promote healthy eating at the community, state, and tribal levels by using policies, systems, and environmental supports, providing direct nutrition education, and supporting social marketing campaigns [28].

Table 2. Selected US federal government COVID-19 initiatives targeting the retail food environment and customers *.

Food Distribution and Donations
Retail Food Establishments
• CDC released guiding principles for restaurants and bars to keep in mind to reduce the risk of COVID-19 spread
• FDA released the Best Practices for Retail Food Stores, Restaurants, and Food Pick-Up/Delivery Services During the COVID-19 Pandemic and also Best Practices for Re-Opening Retail Food Establishments During the COVID-19 Pandemic—Food Safety Checklist, among other fact sheets and guidance documents
• Stimulus relief packages included support for retail food establishments (i.e., Paycheck Protection Program, which is a small business loan that helps businesses keep their workforce employed during the COVID-19 pandemic)
• USDA supported Gus Schumacher Nutrition Incentive Program, which supports projects to increase the purchase of fruits and vegetables among low-income consumers participating in SNAP by providing incentives at the point of purchase, allowed for operational flexibilities during the pandemic, including awarding mini-grants to enable operational changes at farmers' markets and grocery stores to expand affordable access to fruits and vegetables during this time of need
Charitable Food Network
• FEMA Emergency Food and Shelter National Board Program FY 2019 appropriations, which helps provide supplemental funding allocations to local jurisdictions across the country to help support local service organizations that provide critical resources to people with economic emergencies, which include our hungry and homeless populations
• FEMA public assistance grants, which could be utilized to support emergency food distribution during this pandemic
• Stimulus relief packages provided increased appropriations and allowed for certain operational flexibilities for The Emergency Food Assistance Program (TEFAP), which helps supplement the food needs of income-eligible Americans by providing emergency food assistance at no cost by providing American-grown USDA Foods and administrative funds to states to operate the program
• USDA announced the Farmers to Families Food Box initiative, which uses congressional authority to purchase and distribute up to USD 4 billion in agricultural products to food banks and other eligible vendors to distribute to individuals and families in need

Table 2. *Cont.*

Home Delivery
• USDA announced partnership with PepsiCo and the Baylor Collaborative on Hunger and Poverty to provide boxes with 5 days of healthy, shelf-stable, individually packaged foods
• Older American Act, which aims to provide comprehensive funding for critical disease prevention and health promotion services, among other supports such as elder nutrition meal provision, was reauthorized in March 2020 and allowed for flexibilities during this pandemic for drive-through, take-out, or home-delivered meals, providing for grocery delivery, etc.
Export Services
• US Department of Commerce announced temporary reductions in or eliminations of costs of several of their export services, which provides relief to US businesses and economic development organizations during this pandemic and encourages the promotion of foreign direct investment and the export of "Made in the USA" foods and beverages around the world during this economic depression
State, Tribal, and Local Governments
• FEMA public assistance grants, which could be utilized to support emergency food distribution during this pandemic
Household Food Handling and Eating Out
• CDC released Running Essential Errands, including grocery shopping and take-out
• CDC released Food and Coronavirus Disease 2019
• FDA released and compiled a variety of food safety and COVID-19 resources, including FAQs related to COVID-19 in general and specific to the temporary policy on food labeling
Federal Nutrition Assistance—Local Access and Purchasing
• Stimulus relief packages provided increased appropriations to help with anticipated increased enrollments in the WIC, which provides federal grants to states for supplemental foods, health care referrals, and nutrition education for income-eligible pregnant, breastfeeding, and non-breastfeeding postpartum women, and to infants and children up to age five who are found to be at nutritional risk, and SNAP, which provides nutrition benefits to supplement the food budget of income-eligible families so they can purchase healthy foods and beverages
• USDA used congressional authority to expand the SNAP Online Purchasing Pilot, with 45 states and the District of Columbia currently participating in the pilot program
• USDA issued guidance regarding congressionally authorized increased flexibilities during the COVID-19 pandemic such as online enrollment for federal nutrition assistance (i.e., WIC and SNAP, among other programs in the suite of 15 federal nutrition assistance programs)
• USDA used congressional authority to approve state plans for temporary emergency standards of eligibility and levels of benefits for school children (and now during the extension of this program for school year 2020–2021 to children in childcare) during school and childcare closures, known as P-EBT
• USDA used congressional authority to provide additional foods for families in the Food Distribution Program on Indian Reservations (FDPIR), which provides USDA Foods to eligible households living on Indian reservations and to American Indian households residing in approved areas near reservations and in Oklahoma
Federal Nutrition Education and Promotion
• USDA developed, modified, or created a variety of federal nutrition education and promotion materials during the pandemic, particularly around food safety and eating on a budget

Note: CDC = Centers for Disease Control and Prevention; USDA = United States Department of Agriculture; FEMA = Federal Emergency Management Agency; FDA = Food and Drug Administration; WIC = Special Supplemental Nutrition Assistance Program for Women, Infants and Children; P-EBT = Pandemic Electronic Benefits Transfer. * Additional tribal, state, and local laws, along with retailer policies and practices, impacted the retail food environment during this pandemic and several other national and international responses impacted the broader food system.

Early in the pandemic, Congress made unprecedented short- and long-term changes to federal nutrition assistance [29]. A key change for the USDA Supplemental Nutrition Assistance Program (SNAP), which provides funding to supplement the food budgets of income-eligible individuals and families, was the expansion of online purchasing, which is now available in 45 states and the District of Columbia, impacting more than 90% of SNAP participants [30,31]. More work remains to expand the SNAP-authorized retailers beyond Walmart and Amazon and to ensure proper protections against predatory exposures to unhealthy food marketing [32–35]. Despite increasing access to online shopping, SNAP benefits have not yet been increased [32]. However, states could request waivers from the USDA to provide additional SNAP benefits through emergency allotments (up to USD 646 for a family of four) through Pandemic Electronic Benefits Transfer (P-EBT) for households with children who would normally receive free or reduced-price school meals (estimated USD 114 per child per month) [36]. The Special Supplemental Nutrition Program for Women, Infants, and Children (WIC) regularly provides supplemental foods, health care referrals, and nutrition education for income-eligible pregnant, breastfeeding, and non-breastfeeding postpartum women, and to infants and children up to age five who are found to be at nutritional risk. Online food payment is not currently possible with WIC benefits, though workarounds are available to order online with curbside payment and pickup [37,38]. A recent brief detailed key COVID-19 provisions to help optimize program impacts, including modernizing and streamlining WIC enrollment, extending eligibility for mothers and children, enhancing and expanding outreach, examining WIC food package flexibilities, scaling up nationwide best practices, and evaluating changes in breastfeeding practices during the pandemic [39].

Tribes, states, and local governments have played significant roles in shaping the RFE including creating food retail capacity and opening restrictions aimed at reducing the transmission of COVID-19. They have also increased technical assistance and communication regarding enrollment in new and existing federal nutrition assistance programs (e.g., P-EBT and Grab-n-Go meals), funding to support emergency feeding programs, and policies and resource allocations that support home delivery to vulnerable populations (e.g., state agencies covering delivery fees for SNAP online purchases) [40–42]. To offer Grab-n-Go meals to children during school closures, the USDA granted schools and other community sites flexibility to serve meals that do not meet the National School Lunch and School Breakfast programs' nutrition standards [43].

3. Retail Sources

COVID-19 has had multiple impacts on access to the places and the means by which people obtain food. Perhaps the most notable effects have come from restaurant closures. As about half of America's food dollars and a third of the food products produced in this country go to food service (food prepared away from home), including both restaurants and institutional food service (e.g., schools, hospital cafeterias), the closing of many of these venues significantly shifted both where Americans get their food and where food supplies are sent (or not sent). March 2020 spending on food away from home was 51% percent lower than it was in March of 2019 [44]. More cooking and eating at home has meant that other sources, like grocery stores and fresh food delivery services, have seen a surge in demand.

Since dollar stores and larger retailers like Target and Walmart sell groceries, they have been able to stay open when other retail outlets have been forced to close and may have seen increased sales as a result. Even as food sales have shifted from prepared food sources to retail food stores, shopping access has been limited by shorter store hours that allowed staff more time for cleaning or by designated shopping times for vulnerable community members (e.g., seniors, immunocompromised) [45]. Grocery workers protesting poor working conditions have also threatened to limit grocery store access [46].

During the initial onset of the pandemic, online ordering and sales, which allow for no or low-contact purchasing, surged with as many as 78.7% of consumers reporting having shopped online (compared with 39% pre-pandemic) [7]. However, regular online shopping rates have remained modest, with 33% of people reporting shopping online at least once a week compared to 27% in 2019 [47,48]. Prior to COVID-19, online grocery shopping rates were highest in the 30–44 age group with 28.3% reporting shopping for groceries online in 2019. This trend, mainly driven by families with children who desire convenience, has continued during COVID-19 [49]. Younger shoppers in general are more likely to embrace the technology needed to shop online than their older counterparts [50]; only 10% of baby boomers report that they will continue shopping for food online after the pandemic is over compared with 35–40% of younger shoppers [51].

Online shopping may also be disproportionately observed among wealthier, urban consumers as opposed to people who have limited income or live in rural communities, who may lack credit cards or reliable internet [52,53]. Federal nutrition assistance benefits are not accepted online at all (in the case of WIC) or only by select retailers (in the case of SNAP). On the business side, the switch to online sales may have left some small businesses behind. Larger supermarkets with existing online ordering capability have more easily adapted to the online order environment, while smaller stores without dedicated e-commerce platforms have been left scrambling to complete phone orders or create homespun website solutions [54].

For restaurants, many delivery services (e.g., Grubhub, Skip the Dishes) are expensive and can cut into already reduced margins [55]. Consumers may assume that restaurants that do not use these services are closed or they may merely overlook them. Local food purveyors such as farmers and mobile markets that directly sell produce and other foods to consumers have also struggled to adapt to online sales and home delivery as they may have limited staff for deliveries or are unable to take orders from customers with limited internet access [56,57]. Regardless of the food source (restaurant, grocery delivery, mobile market), delivery options may be limited, or totally unavailable to many rural consumers due to the extensive distances needed to travel to provide delivery in those areas, further exacerbating disparities in accessing food in rural communities [47].

Finally, food banks and food pantries have seen a huge surge as consumers who lost their jobs have turned to food aid. Emergency food is also an important source for those not eligible for federal nutrition assistance or those who fear the chilling effect of the Public Charge Rule, which threatens the legal status of immigrants who accept certain forms of government assistance [58,59]. At the same time, food banks and pantries were impacted by disruptions in the food supply as well as decreases in donations and volunteers, who tend to be older and more vulnerable to COVID-19.

4. Retail Actors

Important retail actors affected by the pandemic include the owners and managers of food retail and food distribution businesses that control what food is available where. The most notable pandemic challenges for food distributors has been that supply chains and products developed for food service and restaurants need to be adjusted to get food to grocery stores and other retail outlets (i.e., packaging sizes are different for stores vs. restaurants) [3]. For many distributors, switching from food service to food retail sales requires flexible packing lines and transportation channels as well as diverse distribution relationships which most of them do not currently have [3]. Without the ability to quickly readjust distribution channels, the shift in demand has led to temporary decreases in availability of many foods at retail outlets (see additional detail in Customer Retail Experience below). However, some smaller producers and distributors were able to transition to selling food directly to the public. In addition to shifting supply, there has been a redirection in the workforce as grocery stores have had to hire more employees and restaurants in turn have laid off workers. The pandemic has also precipitated an increase in "gig" economy positions including food delivery for popular restaurant and grocery delivery apps like Instacart and Grubhub [60]. Despite being labeled as essential workers, many food retail and delivery jobs have limited benefits such as hazard pay or sick leave and may leave these workers vulnerable to food insecurity themselves [61].

5. Business Models

Many retail food businesses have been forced to change and adapt their business models to both serve the needs of their communities and ensure their survival. In addition to the rapid expansion of online shopping and delivery services observed in grocery stores and restaurants, many retail food businesses have transitioned their products or target markets. For example, some restaurants have transitioned to mission-driven work (e.g., providing food for hospital workers or laid-off restaurant workers) and are relying on donations from customers to keep their businesses afloat [42]. Others have pivoted by creating prepare-at-home food or by opening a farm stand or mobile grocery store which has allowed them both to sell-off excess stock and take some of the burden off of over-crowded grocery stores [62]. Many restaurants have enhanced outdoor seating thanks to parking lots and sidewalks that were turned into make-shift patios.

While the large majority of grocery stores remained open with adjustments, some non-traditional retailers (mobile markets, farmers' markets, community-supported agriculture) initially shut down over fears of not being able to safely serve their customers, especially those who served primarily senior populations [44]. This has resulted in increased sales for grocery stores while 74% of farmers' markets say that they have lost income [63]. Other farmers and small markets have found ways to stay open by converting to pre-packaged foods (i.e., bundle or box models) that eliminate having customers touch the food or spend extra time making selections. Many small stores (corner stores, bodegas, etc.) in urban settings were already outfitted with plexiglass partitions and had existing practices that limited the number of clients entering the store; therefore, these small stores were paradoxically better prepared for the pandemic in some ways compared to larger food stores [64,65]. There has also been a rise in direct sales by producers including food manufacturers' bulk shipping of canned goods, snacks, and other shelf-stable items directly to customers [66]. Notably, in May 2020, PepsiCo launched Snacks.com and PantryShop.com to sell its products directly to consumers. On a smaller scale, farmers and fishermen started community-supported farm or fishery programs [62].

6. Customer Retail Experience

COVID-19 has had an unprecedented impact on all aspects of the customer retail experience, most notably availability and prices. Customers have reported having to visit multiple retailers to find desired foods and beverages or say they are not able to find the types of foods and beverages their families prefer [67]. These reductions in food availability disproportionately impact communities that already had reduced access to retail food sources like rural communities and communities of color [68]. Supply chain issues limited the availability of many foods and beverages, including infant formula, but empty grocery store shelves were more a result of consumer behavior [69]. Many consumers started stocking up on food, either because they were afraid they would not be able to find the items or wanted to limit the number of times they had to leave their home [70]. These customer behaviors inadvertently deepened inequities in food access. People with limited income do not generally have enough disposable income to make bulk purchases and may be limited in how much they can buy if they rely on public transit. Limited stock may force them to make multiple trips or rely on more expensive small stores closer to home. Although flexibilities were available in some states due to the pandemic, WIC participants are limited to shopping in WIC-approved stores, are generally limited to specific sizes and brands, and cannot substitute when a WIC-approved brand is sold out, essentially making them unable to redeem much-needed benefits.

The shift to more grocery shopping and at-home preparation has led to some price increases (Table 3). In April 2020, the cereal and bakery index saw the largest monthly price increase ever recorded by the Bureau of Labor Statistics (3.1%) [71]. In May 2020, consumer prices for meats and eggs rose 10% which was the largest 12-month percentage increase since 2004; these increases were partially due to changes in meat supply due to COVID outbreak-related closures in meat processing facilities [71]. In addition to higher prices, consumers have seen fewer promotions and advertisements during the pandemic as stores are already dealing with increased demand and want to decrease traffic. Some food companies even pledged not to offer any promotions for at least the initial pandemic months [72]. However, marketing may have shifted to different venues; Kraft Heinz, Kellogg's, and McDonald's were forced to temporarily cease advertising on online learning platforms after advocacy groups raised concerns over ads for unhealthy foods being advertised to children [73].

Table 3. Twelve-month percent change in the US Consumer Price Index for food at home Jan–May 2020.

Month	All Items	Food at Home	Cereals and Bakery Products	Meats, Poultry, Fish, and Eggs	Fruits and Vegetables	Dairy and Related Products	Nonalcoholic Beverages and Beverage Materials
Jan 2020	2.5	0.7	0.3	1.9	−1.0	2.7	0.6
Feb 2020	2.3	0.8	0.2	1.9	−1.6	3.6	0.4
Mar 2020	1.5	1.1	0.1	2.3	−1.9	3.7	1.4
Apr 2020	0.3	4.1	3.1	6.8	0.4	5.2	5.0
May 2020	0.1	4.8	2.6	10.0	1.5	5.7	4.1

Note: U S Bureau of Labor Statistics data for urban consumers [74].

7. The Customer and Individual Dietary Intake

The RFE changes described here have likely had profound and lasting effects on the shopping behavior and diets of customers. Customers have reduced in-person shopping frequency; only 20% of customers reported multiple shopping trips each week (down from 28% in 2019) [44]. Preliminary data collected during the pandemic indicates increases in cooking at home, following a diet, snacking, and eating plant-based foods [47]. Importantly, these effects appear to be differentially felt depending on the individual, interpersonal, and household level characteristics of each customer. Individuals or households who live in communities with greater access to a variety of food sources, and who have sufficient resources, steady employment, and credit are more able to adapt to the pandemic food environment. In addition to financial savings, the positive benefits of transitioning to fewer prepared foods may include consumption of more locally produced foods (especially local produce) and decreased reliance on ultraprocessed foods [75,76].

Changes in food intake are likely very different among the economically and nutritionally vulnerable members of our society. Individuals experiencing food insecurity are more likely to buy less expensive and less healthy foods and beverages, such as packaged and ultraprocessed items. A study of the early effects of COVID-19 indicated that 41% of food-insecure individuals reported buying fewer fresh items (i.e., milk, meat, fruits and vegetables) compared to 21% of food-secure individuals [77]. Food-insecure individuals are also more likely to need to access other components of the food system, including food pantries and free meal distribution sites, such as school meal distribution. Lower diet quality associated with food insecurity could potentially exacerbate already higher rates of diet-related diseases that resulted in part from historic structural barriers in food access [15,78]. This is especially problematic as diet-related diseases, such as hypertension, obesity, and diabetes, are associated with COVID-19 hospitalizations and higher mortality [79,80].

8. Future Directions

The COVID-19 pandemic has put unexpected strains on our nation's food system, upending many traditional food supply and access strategies employed by retailers and customers, and establishing new ones. It will not only be important to study the direct impact of changes to the RFE during the pandemic, but to look at the implications for building more resilient food systems following the pandemic. This work in particular should focus on our most under-resourced community members, including low-income communities and communities of color, whose access to healthy foods was already limited. Recommendations for further research at the consumer, retail, community, and policy levels are outlined.

Little is yet known about the effects of the pandemic on consumer behavior, including shopping frequency and the types of foods purchased. Fewer shopping trips due to pandemic exposure concerns may have led to less purchasing of fresh foods, such as fruits and vegetables [81]. It is likely that far greater quantities of ultraprocessed and long-term storage foods were purchased, but the longer-term impacts of these food system shifts on the diet of households and individuals are not known. Future research is needed to understand how changes in shopping patterns due to the pandemic have affected what people buy and eat. The pandemic accelerated an existing trend towards online ordering of both groceries and prepared foods. Research on online food purchasing behaviors is still nascent and there is an urgent need to better understand who is buying online and from what types of sellers (i.e., retailers, manufactures). We also need to better understand the role of marketing and other behavioral economic factors, especially given the reports of increased surveillance and marketing of unhealthy foods to SNAP participants shopping online [32,33]. It is also critical that accessibility needs for underserved populations, including rural customers and SNAP and WIC recipients, be better understood and addressed.

The movement of food retail towards alternative (and in some instances, more community-minded) models combined with the closure of many restaurants underscores a need for research looking at business sustainability, especially in lower-income and minority communities. Food retail already operates on very slim margins and the US has some of the cheapest food in the world in relation to income with low costs coming at the expense of small farmers, food workers, and our environment. Research to understand what it will take to change this exploitive relationship is needed. This is particularly relevant as business interest expands outside profit to include public health, supporting local producers and economies, and simultaneously being able to advance equity through affordable pricing and paying a living wage. Outlining how private companies can meet these goals will help retail food actors move past the purely profit-driven model which has contributed to current health disparities. More diversity within business models and retail actors (e.g., minority and immigrant-owned businesses) who live and support the communities they serve may be one step towards this goal. Research is needed to understand how the effectiveness of existing policies and community programs (e.g., business incubators, healthy food financing, public procurement) can support business diversity at the local level. We also need more community-engaged research to understand the impact of food policy councils and other forms of community representation, particularly among Indigenous peoples and communities of color.

At the federal level, we need to advance our understanding of the impacts on families and retailers, among others, of the quick and large-scale expansion of federal nutrition assistance. While there has been an increase in SNAP enrollment and some SNAP benefits, current benefit levels are inadequate and legislative attention is needed to define, calculate, and provide adequate SNAP benefits, especially since increasing benefits has been shown to help stabilize the economy [32]. Understanding how flexibilities made to programs like WIC and SNAP in certain states affected program effectiveness can help with creating future resilience and understanding which adaptations should remain during "normal times" [13,82]. We also need to understand the impact of the USDA Farmers to Families Food Box program on both food security and the broader RFE. It is still unclear how this large influx of free food affected small retailers and distributors in lower-income communities.

In thinking about how we can build resilience in our food system and be better prepared for future crises, one possible food system adaptation may be referred to as "smaller is better." This would include enhancing and supporting local production and shorter supply chains [83]. Although more research is required, smaller enterprises may respond to market disruptions more effectively as they have more ability to shift to new markets and products as they gain insights from an engaged customer base (e.g., the Scale paradox) [84]. We see that when food supply chains are developed to only serve one type of food business (e.g., restaurants), it has ripple effects that head back to the source and negatively affect farmers and producers. Efforts to improve local food control and sovereignty have the potential to enhance food system resilience, but the format and impact of these efforts are just beginning to be explored [85].

9. Conclusions

The RFE and Customer Interaction Model provided a useful framework for outlining adaptations and research needs related to the US RFE during the COVID-19 pandemic. Using this model helped highlight vulnerabilities in our food system and future research needs. However, we emphasize that many of the challenges that COVID-19 has brought to the forefront are not new, but instead are the result of a deepening of previously existing inequities, notably in communities of color. Using the model, we were able to identify potential strategies that could help build a more equitable RFE, which may not only benefit our country during normal times but could help build resilience against future pandemics or similar crises.

Author Contributions: Conceptualization, J.G., L.A.L., S.F. and B.A.-S.; investigation, J.G., L.A.L., S.F., B.A.-S. and K.H.; resources, B.B., M.W. E.R.; writing—original draft preparation, L.A.L., K.H., S.F., B.A.-S. and J.G.; writing—review and editing, all authors. All authors have read and agreed to the published version of the manuscript.

Funding: All authors are members of the Healthy Food Retail Working Group leadership team, jointly supported by Healthy Eating Research (HER), a national program of the Robert Wood Johnson Foundation, and the Nutrition and Obesity Policy Research and Evaluation Network (NOPREN). NOPREN is supported by Cooperative Agreement No. 5U48DP00498-05 from the Centers for Disease Control and Prevention (CDC), Prevention Research Centers (PRCs) Program. All authors receive a stipend from HER for their leadership role with the working group. Support for MRW's effort was also provided by the National Heart, Lung, and Blood Institute (NHLBI), grant number K99HL144824 (Principal Investigator: MRW). Publication fees were supported by Healthy Eating Research, a national program of the Robert Wood Johnson Foundation. The findings in this study are solely the responsibility of the authors and do not necessarily represent the official views of CDC, HER, or NOPREN.

Acknowledgments: We would like to thank Alyssa Moran for reviewing this paper and providing feedback.

Conflicts of Interest: The authors declare no conflict of interest.

References

1. Popkin, B.M.; Siega-Riz, A.M.; Haines, P.S. A comparison of dietary trends among racial and socioeconomic groups in the United States. *N. Engl. J. Med.* **1996**, *335*, 716–720. [CrossRef] [PubMed]
2. Walker, R.E.; Keane, C.R.; Burke, J.G. Disparities and access to healthy food in the United States: A review of food deserts literature. *Health Place* **2010**, *16*, 876–884. [CrossRef] [PubMed]
3. Council for Agricultural Science and Technology. *Economic Impacts of COVID-19 on Food and Agricultural Markets*; Council for Agricultural Science and Technology: Ames, IA, USA, 2020.
4. Naja, F.; Hamadeh, R. Nutrition amid the COVID-19 pandemic: A multi-level framework for action. *Eur. J. Clin. Nutr.* **2020**, 1–5. [CrossRef]
5. Knoll, C. Panicked Shoppers Empty Shelves as Coronavirus Anxiety Rises. *The New York Times*, 2020.
6. McCarthy, K. Nearly 16,000 restaurants have closed permanently due to the pandemic, Yelp data shows. *ABC News*, 24 July 2020. Available online: https://abcnews.go.com/Business/16000-restaurants-closed-permanently-due-pandemic-yelp-data/story?id=71943970 (accessed on 22 July 2020).
7. Redman, R. Online grocery sales to grow 40% in 2020. *Supermarket News*, 11 May 2020. Available online: https://www.supermarketnews.com/online-retail/online-grocery-sales-grow-40-2020 (accessed on 22 July 2020).
8. Beshudi, A.; McCrimmon, R. Food goes to waste amid coronavirus crisis. *POLITICO*, 5 April 2020. Available online: https://www.politico.com/news/2020/04/05/food-waste-coronavirus-pandemic-164557 (accessed on 22 July 2020).
9. CDC. Meat and Poultry Processing Workers and Employers. Available online: http://www.cdc.gov/coronavirus/2019-ncov/community/organizations/meat-poultry-processing-workers-employers.html (accessed on 30 July 2020).
10. Lussenhop, J. Coronavirus at Smithfield pork plant: The untold story behind America's biggest outbreak. *BBC News*, 17 April 2020. Available online: https://www.bbc.com/news/world-us-canada-52311877 (accessed on 22 July 2020).
11. Parks, C.A.; Nugent, N.B.; Fleischhacker, S.E.; Yaroch, A.L. Food System Workers are the Unexpected but Under Protected COVID Heroes. *J. Nutr.* **2020**, *150*, 2006–2008. [CrossRef] [PubMed]
12. Soucheray, S. *US Food Processing Plants Become COVID-19 Hot Spots*; Center for Infectious Disease Research and Policy: Minneapolis, MN, USA, 2020.
13. Dunn, C.G.; Kenney, E.; Fleischhacker, S.E.; Bleich, S.N. Feeding Low-Income Children during the Covid-19 Pandemic. *N. Engl. J. Med.* **2020**, *382*, e40. [CrossRef] [PubMed]

14. Belanger, M.J.; Hill, M.A.; Angelidi, A.M.; Dalamaga, M.; Sowers, J.R.; Mantzoros, C.S. Covid-19 and Disparities in Nutrition and Obesity. *N. Engl. J. Med.* **2020**, *383*, e69. [CrossRef] [PubMed]
15. Eisenhauer, E. In poor health: Supermarket redlining and urban nutrition. *GeoJournal* **2001**, *53*, 125–133. [CrossRef]
16. Gould, E.; Wilson, V. *Black Workers Face Two of the Most Lethal Preexisting Conditions for Coronavirus—Racism and Economic Inequality*; Economic Policy Institute: Washington, DC, USA, 2020.
17. Coleman-Jensen, A.; Alisha, M.; Rabbitt, C.; Singh, A. *Household Food Security in the United States in 2018*; U.S. Department of Agriculture, Economic Research Service: Washington, DC, USA, 2019.
18. Schanzenbach, D.; Pitts, A. *How Much Has Food Insecurity Risen? Evidence from the Census Household Pulse Survey*; Northwestern University Institute for Policy Research Rapid Research Report: Evanston, IL, USA, 2020.
19. Bleich, S.; Fleischhacker, S.; Laska, M. Protecting hungry children during the fight for racial justice. *The Hill*, 2 June 2020. Available online: https://thehill.com/opinion/civil-rights/500656-protecting-hungry-children-during-the-fight-for-racial-justice (accessed on 22 July 2020).
20. Bauer, L. The COVID-19 Crisis Has Already Left Too Many Children Hungry in America. *The Hamilton Project*, 6 May 2020. Available online: https://www.brookings.edu/blog/up-front/2020/05/06/the-covid-19-crisis-has-already-left-too-many-children-hungry-in-america/ (accessed on 22 July 2020).
21. Bauer, L. About 14 million children in the US are not getting enough to eat. *Brookings*, 9 July 2020. Available online: https://www.brookings.edu/blog/up-front/2020/07/09/about-14-million-children-in-the-us-are-not-getting-enough-to-eat/ (accessed on 22 July 2020).
22. Harvard Law School. Promoting Food Donation during COVID-19. Available online: https://www.chlpi.org/food-law-and-policy/covid-19-response/promoting-food-donation-during-covid-19/ (accessed on 22 July 2020).
23. USDA. USDA Farmers to Families Food Box. Available online: https://www.ams.usda.gov/selling-food-to-usda/farmers-to-families-food-box (accessed on 22 July 2020).
24. University of Illinois. *Keeping Nourished When Not Feeling Well*; Illinois Extension: Urbana, IL, USA, 2020.
25. COVID-19: Resources for Your Families Health. Available online: http://ccesuffolk.org/community-nutrition-health/covid-19-resources-for-your-families-health (accessed on 5 October 2020).
26. University of Illinois. *How Safe Is My Food in a COVID-19 World?* Illinois Extension: Urbana, IL, USA, 2020.
27. USDA FNS. SNAP—Denial of Certain Requests to Adjust SNAP Regulations. Available online: https://www.fns.usda.gov/snap/covid-19/denial-certain-state-requests (accessed on 5 October 2020).
28. USDA FNS. Supplemental Nutrition Assistance Program Education (SNAP-Ed). Available online: https://www.fns.usda.gov/snap/SNAP-Ed (accessed on 5 October 2020).
29. Aussenberg, R.A.; Billings, K.C. *USDA Domestic Food Assistance Programs' Response to COVID-19: P.L. 116-127, P.L. 116-136, and Related Efforts*; Congressional Research Service: Washington, DC, USA, 2020; p. 4.
30. USDA. SNAP Online Purchasing to Cover 90% of Households. Available online: https://www.usda.gov/media/press-releases/2020/05/20/snap-online-purchasing-cover-90-households (accessed on 22 July 2020).
31. USDA. FNS FNS Launches the Online Purchasing Pilot. Available online: https://www.fns.usda.gov/snap/online-purchasing-pilot (accessed on 28 August 2020).
32. Bleich, S.; Dunn, C.; Fleischhacker, S. *The Impact of Increasing SNAP Benefits on Stabilizing the Economy, Reducing Poverty and Food Insecurity Amid COVID-19 Pandemic*; Healthy Eating Research: Minneapolis, MN, USA, 2020.
33. Chester, J.; Kopp, K.; Montgomery, K.C. *Does Buying Groceries Online Put SNAP Participants At Risk?* Center for Digital Democracy: Washington, DC, USA, 2020.
34. Jilcott Pitts, S.B.; Ng, S.W.; Blitstein, J.L.; Gustafson, A.; Niculescu, M. Online grocery shopping: Promise and pitfalls for healthier food and beverage purchases. *Public Health Nutr.* **2018**, *21*, 3360–3376. [CrossRef] [PubMed]
35. Malkan, S. Junk Food Makers Target Blacks, Latinos and Communities of Color, Increasing Risks From COVID. *U.S. Right to Know*, 2020.
36. Families First Coronavirus Response Act; H.R. 6201 116th Congress; Became Law 116-12 March 18, 2020. Available online: https://www.congress.gov/bill/116th-congress/house-bill/6201/text (accessed on 30 July 2020).

37. Gustafson, D.; Miller, J.; Gutknecht, K.; Phelps, B.; Chilcoat, J.; Gilland, J.; Duncan, A.; Seitel, T.; Ewing, T.; Rogness, M.; et al. *WIC/EWIC Pickup and Delivery Requirements*; National WIC Association: Washington, DC, USA, 2020; p. 8.
38. USDA. WIC—Electronic Benefits Transfer (EBT) Guidance and Resources. Available online: https://www.fns.usda.gov/wic/wic-electronic-benefits-transfer-ebt-guidance (accessed on 22 July 2020).
39. Dunn, C.; Kennedy, E.; Bleich, S.; Fleischhacker, S. *Strengthening WIC's Impact during and after the COVID-19 Pandemic*; Healthy Eating Research: Durham, NC, USA, 2020.
40. Harvard Law School. *COVID-19 Food-Related Policy Tracking*; Center for Health Law and Policy Innovation: Cambridge, MA, USA, 2020.
41. Healthy Food Policy Project Local Government Policies to Support Food Access During the COVID-19 Pandemic—An Index. Available online: https://healthyfoodpolicyproject.org/resources/index-of-local-government-policies-for-to-support-food-access-during-the-covid-19-pandemic (accessed on 22 July 2020).
42. McLoughlin, G.; Fleischhacker, S.; Hecht, A.; McGuirt, J.; Read, M.; Vega, C.; Colón-Ramos, U.; Dunn, C. Feeding students during COVID-19 related school closures: A nationwide assessment of initial responses. *J. Nutr. Educ. Behav.* Forthcoming.
43. Kinsey, E.; Hecht, A.; Dunn, C.; Levi, R.; Read, M.; Smith, C.; Niesen, P.; Seligman, H.; Hager, E. School Closures During COVID-19: Opportunities for Innovation in Meal Service. *Am. J. Public Health* **2020**, e1–e9. [CrossRef] [PubMed]
44. USDA. ERS Eating-Out Expenditures in March 2020 Were 28 Percent Below March 2019 Expenditures. Available online: http://www.ers.usda.gov/data-products/chart-gallery/gallery/chart-detail/?chartId=98556 (accessed on 22 July 2020).
45. Salaky, K. Grocery Stores Are Changing Their Hours and Policies Amid the Coronavirus Outbreak. Available online: https://www.delish.com/food-news/a31677621/grocery-stores-open-coronavirus/ (accessed on 22 July 2020).
46. Sainato, M. Retail workers at Amazon and Whole Foods coordinate sick-out to protest Covid-19 conditions. *The Guardian*, 2020.
47. IFIC. *2020 Food and Health Survey*; International Food Information Council: Washington, DC, USA, 2020.
48. Juntti, M. How COVID-19 has changed online grocery shopping for good. *New Hope Network*, 2020.
49. Thakker, K. Older millennials embrace traditional grocers, online shopping. *Grocery Dive*, 2020.
50. Whaley, J.; Hur, S.; Kim, Y.-K. Grocery Shopping Channels: Segmentation by Gender and Age Group. *J. Bus. Theory Pract.* **2019**, *7*, 124. [CrossRef]
51. Ryan, T. Will Boomers and Gen X keep shopping online post-pandemic? *RetailWire*, 2020.
52. Douglas, L. Most SNAP Recipients Can't Buy Groceries Online. Now, Some States Push for Change. Available online: https://thefern.org/ag_insider/most-snap-recipients-cant-buy-groceries-online-now-some-states-push-for-change/ (accessed on 28 August 2020).
53. Here's Who's Shopping Online for Groceries. *Marketing Charts*, 18 August 2017. Available online: https://www.marketingcharts.com/industries/cpg-and-fmcg-79612 (accessed on 22 July 2020).
54. Conduent Government Payment Solutions|EBT, WIC, EPC, & ECC. Available online: https://www.conduent.com/solution/public-sector-solutions/social-services/ (accessed on 30 July 2020).
55. Sweeney, E. How To Support Restaurants Without Putting Food Delivery Workers At Risk. Available online: https://www.huffpost.com/entry/support-restaurants-without-risking-food-delivery-workers_l_5e7a2e27c5b6f5b7c54bbda4 (accessed on 30 July 2020).
56. Haynes-Maslow, L. *Guidance for SNAP Authorized Retailers in North Carolina*; North Carolina State University: Raleigh, NC, USA, 2020.
57. Veggie Van Mobile Market COVID-19 Resources for Mobile Markets. Available online: https://www.myveggievan.org/covid-19.html (accessed on 30 July 2020).
58. Schmidt, C.; Goetz, S.; Rocker, S.; Tian, Z. Google Searches Reveal Changing Consumer Food Sourcing in the COVID-19 Pandemic. *J. Agric. Food Syst. Community Dev.* **2020**, *9*, 9–16. [CrossRef]
59. Bleich, S.N.; Fleischhacker, S. Hunger or Deportation: Implications of the Trump Administration's Proposed Public Charge Rule. *J. Nutr. Educ. Behav.* **2019**, *51*, 505–509. [CrossRef] [PubMed]
60. Tiku, N. Desperate workers rush to delivery app jobs to find low pay and punishing rules. *Washington Post*, 2020.

61. Lempert, P. We Say Supermarket Workers Are Essential Workers, But Oxfam Asks If They Are Being Treated That Way? *Forbes*, 24 June 2020.
62. From Pandemic to Protests: How Food Businesses Are Responding Bon Appétit. Available online: https://www.bonappetit.com/story/food-businesses-covid-19 (accessed on 24 July 2020).
63. Feldman, B. Farmers Markets Across Nation Face Potential Economic Crisis from COVID-19. Available online: https://farmersmarketcoalition.org/farmers-markets-across-the-nation-face-a-precarious-economic-situation-due-to-covid-19/ (accessed on 5 October 2020).
64. Galindo, E. How Carnicerias, Liquor Stores, Tienditas and Latino Supermarkets Are Feeding Their Neighborhoods. Available online: https://laist.com/2020/03/26/carnicerias_liquor_stores_tienditas_latino_supermarkets_feeding_la_neighborhoods.php (accessed on 22 July 2020).
65. Vaziri, A. Bay Area Corner Stores Become a Lifeline during the Coronavirus Crisis. Available online: https://www.sfchronicle.com/bayarea/article/Bay-Area-corner-stores-become-a-lifeline-during-15156886.php (accessed on 22 July 2020).
66. Wu, L. Grocery Stores and the Effect of the COVID-19 Pandemic. Available online: https://www.forbes.com/sites/lesliewu/2020/05/31/grocery-stores-and-the-effect-of-the-covid-19-pandemic/ (accessed on 22 July 2020).
67. Belarmino, E.H.; Bertmann, F.; Wentworth, T.; Biehl, E.; Neff, R.; Niles, M.T. Early COVID-19 Impacts on Food Retail and Restaurants: Consumer Perspectives from Vermont. (2020). College of Agriculture and Life Sciences Faculty Publications. 24. Available online: https://scholarworks.uvm.edu/calsfac/24 (accessed on 22 July 2020).
68. Grocery, Retail Workers Protest Pandemic Working Conditions. *NBC Boston*, 1 May 2020. Available online: https://www.nbcboston.com/news/coronavirus/grocery-retail-workers-protest-pandemic-working-conditions/2116892/ (accessed on 22 July 2020).
69. USDA. *Another Look at Availability and Prices of Food Amid the COVID-19 Pandemic*; U.S. Department of Agriculture: Washington, DC, USA, 2020.
70. Niles, M.T.; Bertmann, F.; Morgan, E.H.; Wentworth, T.; Biehl, E.; Neff, R. Food Access and Security During Coronavirus: A Vermont Study (2020). College of Agriculture and Life Sciences Faculty Publications. 21. Available online: https://scholarworks.uvm.edu/calsfac/21 (accessed on 22 July 2020).
71. Bureau of Labor Statistics. *Consumer Price Index—June 2020*; U.S. Department of Labor: Washington, DC, USA, 2020; p. 38.
72. Villarreal, D. Grocery stores are avoiding sales and discounts during coronavirus pandemic. *Newsweek*, 2020.
73. Lalou, C. Kraft Heinz and Kellogg temporarily halt some child-focused ads during pandemic. *Nutrition Insight*, 2020.
74. TED: The Economics Daily Consumer Prices for Food at Home Increased 4.8 Percent for Year Ended May 2020: U.S. Bureau of Labor Statistics. Available online: https://www.bls.gov/opub/ted/2020/consumer-prices-for-food-at-home-increased-4-point-8-percent-for-year-ended-may-2020.htm (accessed on 2 October 2020).
75. Hiller, S. Local food movement gains momentum under COVID-19. *High Country News*, 28 May 2020. Available online: https://www.hcn.org/articles/covid19-local-food-movement-gains-momentum-under-covid-19 (accessed on 22 July 2020).
76. Oaklander, M. Our Diets Are Changing Because of the Coronavirus Pandemic. Is It for the Better? *Time*, 2020.
77. Niles, M.T.; Bertmann, F.; Morgan, E.H.; Wentworth, T.; Biehl, E.; Neff, R. The Impact of Coronavirus on Vermonters Experiencing Food Insecurity. (2020). College of Agriculture and Life Sciences Faculty Publications. 19. Available online: https://scholarworks.uvm.edu/calsfac/19 (accessed on 22 July 2020).
78. Fleischhacker, S.E.; Evenson, K.R.; Rodriguez, D.A.; Ammerman, A.S. A systematic review of fast food access studies. *Obes. Rev.* **2011**, *12*, e460–e471. [CrossRef] [PubMed]
79. Aman, F.; Masood, S. How Nutrition can help to fight against COVID-19 Pandemic. *Pak. J. Med. Sci.* **2020**, *36*, S121–S123. [CrossRef] [PubMed]
80. Richardson, S.; Hirsch, J.S.; Narasimhan, M.; Crawford, J.M.; McGinn, T.; Davidson, K.W.; Barnaby, D.P.; Becker, L.B.; Chelico, J.D.; Cohen, S.L.; et al. Presenting Characteristics, Comorbidities, and Outcomes Among 5700 Patients Hospitalized With COVID-19 in the New York City Area. *JAMA* **2020**, *323*, 2052–2059. [CrossRef] [PubMed]
81. Redman, R. Weekly grocery shopping down 20% since COVID-19 outbreak. *Supermarket News*, 2020.

82. Fleischhacker, S.; Moran, A.; Bleich, S.N. Legislative and Executive Branch Developments Affecting the United States Department of Agriculture Supplemental Nutrition Assistance Program. *J. Food Law Policy* **2019**, *15*, 119.
83. Brinkley, C. The Small World of the Alternative Food Network. *Sustainability* **2018**, *10*, 2921. [CrossRef]
84. Lucker, J.; O'Dwyer, J.; Renner, R. The Scale Paradox: Analytics disrupts the size factor. *Deloitte Insights*, March 2013.
85. Maudrie, T.; Colón-Ramos, U.; Harper, K.; Jock, B.; Gittelsohn, J. A systematic review of the use of Indigenous food sovereignty principles for intervention and future directions. *Curr. Dev. Nutr.* Under review.

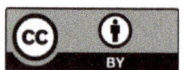 © 2020 by the authors. Licensee MDPI, Basel, Switzerland. This article is an open access article distributed under the terms and conditions of the Creative Commons Attribution (CC BY) license (http://creativecommons.org/licenses/by/4.0/).

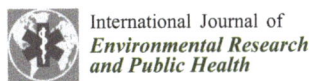

Review

Understanding the Intersection of Race/Ethnicity, Socioeconomic Status, and Geographic Location: A Scoping Review of U.S. Consumer Food Purchasing

Chelsea R. Singleton [1,*], Megan Winkler [2], Bailey Houghtaling [3], Oluwafikayo S. Adeyemi [1], Alexandra M. Roehll [1], JJ Pionke [4] and Elizabeth Anderson Steeves [5]

[1] Department of Kinesiology and Community Health, University of Illinois at Urbana-Champaign, Champaign, IL 61820, USA; oadey2@illinois.edu (O.S.A.); aroehll2@illinois.edu (A.M.R.)
[2] Division of Epidemiology and Community Health, School of Public Health, University of Minnesota, Minneapolis, MN 55455, USA; mwinkler@umn.edu
[3] School of Nutrition and Food Sciences, Louisiana State University (LSU) & LSU Agricultural Center, Baton Rouge, LA 70803, USA; bhoughtaling@agcenter.lsu.edu
[4] University Library, University of Illinois at Urbana-Champaign, Champaign, IL 61820, USA; pionke@illinois.edu
[5] Department of Nutrition, University of Tennessee, Knoxville, TN 37996, USA; eander24@utk.edu
* Correspondence: csingle1@illinois.edu; Tel.: +1-217-300-8139

Received: 1 September 2020; Accepted: 19 October 2020; Published: 21 October 2020

Abstract: Disparities in diet quality persist in the U.S. Examining consumer food purchasing can provide unique insight into the nutritional inequities documented by race/ethnicity, socioeconomic status (SES), and geographic location (i.e., urban vs. rural). There remains limited understanding of how these three factors intersect to influence consumer food purchasing. This study aimed to summarize peer-reviewed scientific studies that provided an intersectional perspective on U.S. consumer food purchasing. Thirty-four studies were examined that presented objectively measured data on purchasing outcomes of interest (e.g., fruits, vegetables, salty snacks, sugar-sweetened beverages, Healthy Eating Index, etc.). All studies were of acceptable or high quality. Only six studies (17.6%) assessed consumer food purchases at the intersection of race/ethnicity, SES, or geographic location. Other studies evaluated racial/ethnic or SES differences in food purchasing or described the food and/or beverage purchases of a targeted population (example: low-income non-Hispanic Black households). No study assessed geographic differences in food or beverage purchases or examined purchases at the intersection of all three factors. Overall, this scoping review highlights the scarcity of literature on the role of intersectionality in consumer food and beverage purchasing and provides recommendations for future studies to grow this important area of research.

Keywords: intersectionality; food purchasing; diet quality; race; ethnicity; socioeconomic status; urban; rural

1. Introduction

Most Americans' diets fall short of national dietary guidelines [1]. Nearly 75% of Americans consume too few fruits and vegetables, and more than 60% consume excess added sugar, saturated fat, and sodium [2]. Furthermore, most Americans' overall diet quality is rated moderate to poor [2]. Food purchasing is a critical behavior in shaping the overall nutritional quality of consumed diets [3,4]. Purchases made in full-service (e.g., supercenters, grocery stores, etc.) and limited-service (e.g., corner stores, gas stations, dollar stores, pharmacies, etc.) stores comprise upwards of 63% of an individual's total daily energy intake [5]; the remaining 37% is acquired from venues such as full-service and fast food restaurants. Additionally, more than 60% of the sugar-sweetened beverages (SSB) and discretionary foods consumed by U.S. adults come from retail food outlets [6].

Food retailer availability, adverse dietary behaviors, and the related health consequences are not distributed equally across the U.S. population [7–10]. Significant inequities in diet and health status have been, and continue to be, documented by race/ethnicity, socioeconomic status (SES), and geographic location (i.e., urban vs. suburban vs. rural) in the U.S. [8–10]. However, health disparities are often researched and described by experts in a way that can discount the complex identities of many marginalized individuals [11–13]. Intersectionality is a theoretical framework used to describe how multiple social categories measured at the individual level (e.g., race, ethnicity, SES) reflect interlocking systems of privilege and oppression at the societal level [11]. As these realities are experienced jointly, it is important to examine how these factors work together to influence health behaviors such as dietary intake and food purchasing.

Prior reviews of food and beverage purchasing have primarily focused on evaluating interventions aimed at improving purchasing behaviors [14–19], and recently, the use of commercial food purchasing datasets to discover specific purchasing trends [3]. Studies often present information on food and beverage purchasing behaviors at the individual or household-level by racial/ethnic group or SES [3,5]. However, there continues to be a limited synthesized understanding of how the intersectional nature of these factors influences trends in consumer food purchases. Filling this gap in knowledge can inform research and practice approaches to improve food purchasing environments and behaviors among populations with a long-standing history of oppression and marginalization.

Therefore, the primary aim of this scoping review was to identify and summarize scientific studies providing an intersectional perspective on U.S. consumer food purchasing. Specifically, we were interested in assessing food and/or beverage purchasing at the intersection of race/ethnicity, SES, and geographic location as these three factors are often considered in studies of nutritional inequities across populations [8–10]. Additional aims of this review included (1) summarize key findings from studies that assessed consumer food purchasing solely by race/ethnicity, SES, or geographic location and (2) identify areas for future research that will expand the field's understanding of how the intersection of these three factors influences food and beverage purchasing. Thus, findings from this review may significantly contribute to the work of public health researchers, policy makers, and individuals in the private sector seeking to gain a better understanding of food retail, purchasing, and marketing in the U.S. and develop solutions to address nutritional inequities.

2. Materials and Methods

2.1. Search Strategy and Inclusion Criteria

In December 2019, a systematic search of the literature was conducted to identify peer-reviewed papers on U.S. consumer food and beverage purchasing. A librarian (J. P.) searched the following six databases, selected based on lead sources for peer-reviewed literature among several disciplines including public health, medicine, psychology, sociology, and economics: PubMed, Scopus, PsycINFO, CINAHL, ScoINDEX, and Business Source Ultimate. The search strategy developed by the librarian based on preliminary testing in PubMed (See Supplementary Material Part I) was translated across all remaining databases for optimum article retrieval. All citations returned by the search were extracted and imported into an open-source citation management software.

The following inclusion criteria were used: (1) published in a peer-reviewed journal, (2) published in 2000 or later (up until December 2019), (3) available in English, (4) based in the U.S., (5) employed an observational study design (e.g., cross-sectional, longitudinal, etc.), (6) analyzed objectively measured food and/or beverage purchasing data collected at any level (i.e., individual, household, or store) from full-service or limited-service stores, and (7) presented findings on purchasing by race/ethnicity, SES, geographic location, or any combination of these three factors. Studies that examined purchasing intersections (i.e., explored interaction terms or reported stratified regression models) for two or more factors were labeled "intersectional". Studies that presented purchasing findings for a specific intersectional population (example: low-income non-Hispanic Black households living in an urban setting) were also included. These studies were labeled as "targeted". Since this review aimed to summarize observational data on consumer food purchasing, interventions, natural experiments, and policy evaluation studies were excluded. Furthermore, studies that solely analyzed self-reported food and/or beverage data were also excluded. A wide range of objectively measured purchasing data were considered including store-generated sales data, annotated receipt data, and customer intercept data. Given the large variability in food and beverage purchasing outcomes assessed by selected studies, the types of outcomes considered by the current study were narrowed to a specific list of categories (see *Data Extraction*).

2.2. Study Selection

A flow chart describing the study selection process is presented in (Figure 1). The search returned 1256 citations: PubMed (n = 430), Scopus (n = 354), PsycINFO (n = 140), CINAHL (n = 181), ScoINDEX (n = 28 results), and Business Source Ultimate (n = 123).

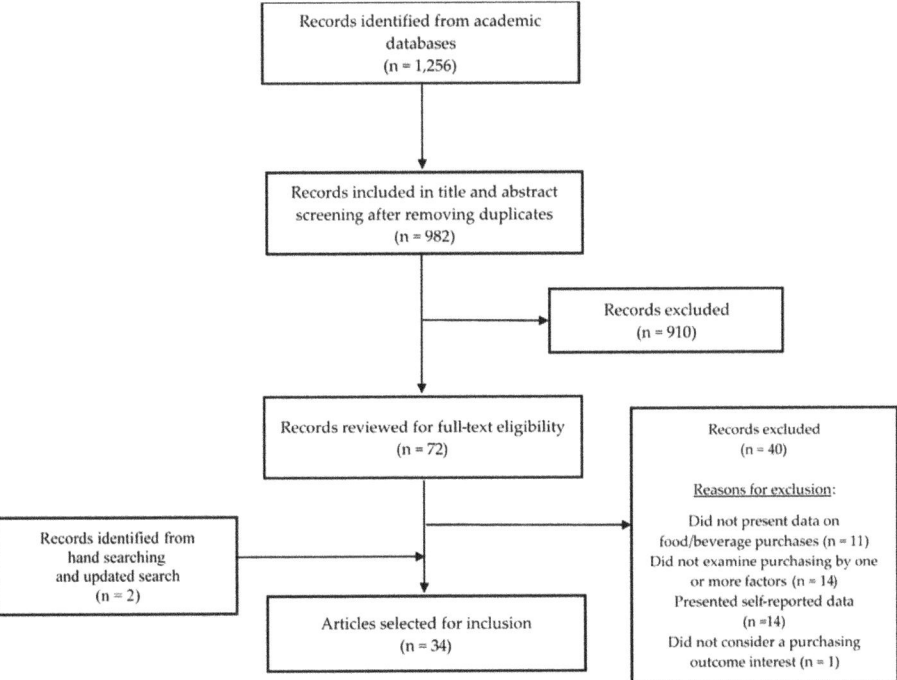

Figure 1. Flow chart for scoping review.

After removing duplicate citations, three reviewers (O. S. A., A. M. R., and C. R. S.) reviewed titles and abstracts among 982 unique studies. Titles and abstracts indicated that 910 studies did not meet inclusion criteria. The complete text was retrieved for citations appearing to meet inclusion criteria or were unclear (n = 72). Two independent reviewers (O. S. A. and A. M. R.) performed the full text review, and a third reviewer (C. R. S.) made the final decision on inclusion for any disagreements. Excluded studies were ineligible because they (1) did not present findings on food and/beverage purchases (n = 11), (2) used self-reported purchasing measures (n = 14), (3) did not present findings by one or more of the three factors of interest (n = 14), or (4) did not present findings on a purchasing outcome of interest (n = 1). Hand searching, specifically forward and backwards reference searching of intersectional papers, was performed to find intersectional studies not captured by the search strategy resulting in the identification of one additional paper. The search was repeated in September 2020 to identify additional intersectional papers published since December 2019. Again, one paper was identified bringing the final number of studies included in this scoping review to 34.

2.3. Data Extraction

All authors extracted data from an assigned subset of included studies using a standardized data extraction tool developed by research team members (C. R. S., M. W., B. H., and E. A. S.). Specifically, data on authors, study design, study population, sample size, and detailed information on measurement methods used to capture consumer food and/or beverage purchasing as well as variable definitions for race, ethnicity, SES, and geographic location were extracted. An additional team member performed a quality assessment for each source (see *Methodological Quality Assessment*).

Given the enormous diversity in customer purchasing outcomes examined across the included studies, team members (C. R. S., M. W., B. H., or E. A. S.) extracted food-at-home customer purchasing results for a pre-specified list of product and nutrition outcomes. These particular outcomes were selected because they are often the subject of U.S.-based policy and public health interventions [3,7]: (1) fruits, (2) vegetables, (3) whole grains, (4) salty snacks, (5) desserts, sweet snacks, and candy, (6) sugar-sweetened beverages (SSBs), including regular soda, juice drinks (<100% juice), sports drinks, and energy drinks, (7) non-sugar-sweetened beverages (non-SSBs), including water, diet/zero calorie soda, 100% juice, diet/zero calorie sports drinks, and diet/zero calorie energy drinks, (8) healthy eating index (HEI), (9) total energy (i.e., kilocalories/kcals), (10) specific nutrients, including sugar; saturated fat; and sodium. We extracted results on these outcomes in any form (e.g., weekly expenditures, proportion of weekly purchases, kilocalories/person/day purchased for household, etc.) and prioritized inferential results, although descriptive results were extracted if it was the only data available. Lastly, we extracted results for any study that examined intersections or presented inferential results by race/ethnicity, SES, or geographic location. A narrative format was used to describe review results and identify similarities/differences in population purchasing trends based on intersectionality.

2.4. Methodological Quality Assessment

Risk of bias was assessed using the National Heart, Lung, and Blood Institute's (NHLBI) Quality Assessment Tool for Observational Cohort and Cross-sectional Studies [20]. The tool allowed reviewers to evaluate internal validity across 14 criteria, four of which were deemed not applicable to the studies of consumer food purchasing included in this review (items 6, 7, 10, and 12). One reviewer (O.S.A. or A. M. R.) conducted this assessment, with a second reviewer (C. R. S.) reviewing for agreement. Reviewers recorded yes, no, or cannot determine for each item regarding a study's original aim/purpose and results. Thus, quality scores represent overall quality of study designs and not necessarily the quality of purchasing results extracted. "Yes" responses were tallied and the highest score a study could receive was a 10. Although the tool was not intended for use as a scoring scheme, we identified scores between 1–4 as low, 5–7 as acceptable, and 8–10 as high quality to assist our results interpretation.

3. Results

Thirty-four studies were included in this scoping review [21–54]. Information on customer purchasing assessment methodologies used across studies is shown in (Table 1). Most studies examined both food and beverage purchasing (n = 29; 85.3%) and collected data at the household level (n = 24, 70.6%). While several studies assessed purchases from all types of stores (n = 24, 70.6%), seven (21.2%) and three (9.1%) studies focused solely on purchasing at limited-service and full-service stores, respectively. A variety of data sources were used across studies with most using Nielsen Consumer Panel data (n = 11, 33.3%) or the USDA's Food Acquisition and Purchasing Survey (FoodAPS) dataset

(n = 5, 20.8%). Several data collection methods were used to study purchasing including customer intercepts, receipt collection, and Universal Product Code (UPC) scanning.

Descriptive characteristics of studies are provided in (Table 2). All studies were considered acceptable or high quality according to our interpretation of papers using the NHLBI Quality Assessment Tool for Observational Cohort and Cross-sectional Studies. The majority examined purchasing using a nationally representative sample of U.S. households (n = 18, 52.9%). All other studies assessed purchasing locally in a specific city or regionally in the Midwest or Northwest.

Key findings are described below by intersectional attributes. Studies that presented intersectional results on consumer food and beverage purchases are described first, followed by those that studied a single attribute (i.e., examined purchasing by race/ethnicity, SES, or geographic location alone). Finally, descriptive results from studies with targeted populations are provided.

3.1. Intersectional Results

Key findings from studies that assessed consumer food and/or beverage purchases at the intersection of race/ethnicity, SES, or geographic location are in (Table 3). Details on how each study measured each purchasing outcome of interest are also provided in (Table 3). Only six studies (17.6%) examined any intersection between our three factors of interest [29,34,35,45,47,54]. All six studies examined intersections between race/ethnicity and SES by using interaction terms or stratified regression models. We focused on results with significant interaction terms or with different associative patterns in the stratified models (e.g., association between race/ethnicity and purchasing was significant in opposite directions across SES groups or the association was statistically significant for one SES group and non-significant for the other).

Three studies examined fruit and vegetable purchasing and only one identified different associations between race/ethnicity and purchasing across SES [29,34,45]. Using specific market basket items and stratifying by SES, Palmer et al. (2019) reported more purchasers than non-purchasers of canned/bottled peaches and potatoes among White higher income households (>200% FPL), whereas no significant difference in proportion of purchasers to non-purchasers was observed among White low-income households [45]. In addition, there were significantly fewer purchasers than non-purchasers of potatoes among Black higher income households, which was not observed among Black low-income households [45]. No studies examined whole grain purchasing. Three studies examined salty snacks and desserts, sweet snacks, and candy purchasing [29,34,35], with only one identifying different associations between race/ethnicity and purchasing across stratified SES models [35]. Among households not participating in the Supplemental Nutrition Assistance Program (SNAP), Grummon and Taillie (2018) identified non-Hispanic Black households (henceforth NHB) purchased less salty snacks, desserts, and sweet snacks compared to non-Hispanic White households (henceforth NHW) [35]. In addition, Hispanic households purchased less candy, desserts, and sweet snacks compared to NHW households. These race/ethnicity differences were not observed among SNAP-participating households. Three studies examined SSBs and non-SSBs, but none found significant differences across intersections [29,34,35].

Table 1. Summary of Customer Purchasing Data Assessment Methodologies of Included Studies (n = 34).

Items Assessed	Purchasing Level	Retail Stores	Data Type	Data Source	Data Collection Method [a]
Beverages only (2) Foods only (3) Foods and Beverages (29)	Individual (8) Household (24) Store (2)	Full-service only (3) Limited-service only (7) All Stores (24)	Primary data collection (14) Secondary data analysis (19) Primary and secondary data (1)	Nielsen Consumer Panel (11) USDA FoodAPS (5) The STORE Study (3) The SHOPPER Study (3) National Food Stamp Program Survey (1) IRI Consumer Network Panel (1) Consumer Expenditure Survey (1) Other (9)	Retailer-scanner data (3) Customer store intercepts (7) Customers scanned UPCs (11) Customer receipt collection (5) Multiple methods/Other (8)

Note. USDA, United States Department of Agriculture; FoodAPS, Food Acquisition and Purchasing Survey; STORE, the Staple Food Ordinance Evaluation; SHOPPER, the Study of Household Purchasing Patterns, Eating, and Recreation; UPC, Universal Product Code. [a] Primary method used to collect information on purchases. Studies using multiple methods (e.g., receipt collection and barcode scanning) were categorized as multiple methods and one study used detailed diaries, which was categorized as other.

Table 2. Descriptive Characteristics of Included Studies (n = 34).

Author, Year	Study Purpose	Study Year(s) [a]	Study Location	Sample Size	Intersectional Attribute(s)	Sample Demographics [b]	Stores Assessed	QA [c]
Andreyeva, 2012	Describe supermarket beverage purchases of WIC and SNAP households.	2011	New England	39,172 Households	Targeted: Low-Income	100% WIC Participation, 54% SNAP Participation	Full-Service	6
Appelhans, 2017	Determine if household food purchases predict diet quality and nutrient density.	2014–2016	Chicago, IL	196 Households	Targeted: Urban	Mean age: 44; 83% female; 31% (NHW), 44% (NHB), 11% (Hisp), 13% (NHO); 38% (PIR: 0–1.99), 29% (2–3.99), 16% (4–5.99), 18% (≥ 6)	All Stores	9
Borradaile, 2009	Describe after-school corner stores purchases of low-income children.	2008	Philadelphia, PA	833 Shoppers	Targeted: Low-Income + Urban	Grade range: 4–6 grade; 54% (NHW), 11.6% (NHB), 22.9% (Hisp), 10.8% (NHA); 82.1% of students at participating schools eligible for free/reduced lunch.	Limited-Service	5

Table 2. Cont.

Author, Year	Study Purpose	Study Year(s) [a]	Study Location	Sample Size	Intersectional Attribute(s)	Sample Demographics [b]	Stores Assessed	QA [c]
Caspi, 2017 [1]	Examine differences in food and beverage purchases by type of limited-service store.	2014	Minneapolis, MN	661 Shoppers	Targeted: Urban	47% (NHW), 34% (NHB), 3% (Hisp), 3% (NHA), 3% (NHO); 38% ≤ high school diploma	Limited-Service	7
Caspi, 2017 [2]	Determine if food and beverage purchases at limited-service stores with health-promoting features are healthier.	2014	Minneapolis, MN	594 Shoppers	Targeted: Urban	Mean age: 40; 58% male; 48% (NHW), 36% (NHB), 3% (Hisp), 3% (NHA), 3% (NHO); 36% ≤ high school diploma	Limited-Service	9
Chrisinger, 2018 [1]	Compare high-calories and low-calorie food purchases of Black women by store type.	2012	Philadelphia, PA	35 Shoppers	Targeted: Black + Urban [d]	Mean age: 39; 100% female; 100% Black Identifying; 37% Annual Income ≤ FPL	All Stores	8
Chrisinger, 2018 [2]	Assess the healthfulness of household food purchases by SNAP and WIC participation status.	2012–2013	National	4962 Households	RE, SES	17.2% (30–39 years), 18.5% (40–49), 20.2% (50–59), 29.9% (60+); 64% female; 70% (NHW), 10.2% (NHB), 13.7% (Hisp), 6% (NHO); 13.1% (SNAP participant), 19.3% (SNAP-Eligible Non-Participant), 67.6% (Ineligible Non-Participant)	Full-Service	8
Crane, 2019	Identify gender differences in the nutrient quality of food purchases.	2014–2016	Midwest	202 Households	Targeted: Urban	29.9% (NHW), 45.6% (NHB), 5.9% (Hisp), 18.6% (NHO); 40.6% receive government food assistance benefits	All Stores	8

Table 2. Cont.

Author, Year	Study Purpose	Study Year(s) [a]	Study Location	Sample Size	Intersectional Attribute(s)	Sample Demographics [b]	Stores Assessed	QA [c]
Cullen, 2007	Characterize food purchases of households by educational level and ethnicity.	2004	Houston, TX	167 Households	RE x SES	45.8% (<40 years); 74.8% (female); 11.2% (NHW), 41.1% (NHB), 39.3% (Hisp), 2.8% (NHO); 46.7% (≤ High School Graduate), 28% (Some College), 14% (College Graduate), 6.5% (Advanced Degree)	All Stores	8
Ford, 2014	Examine trends in purchases of consumer packaged goods among households with children age 2–5 years old.	2000–2011	National	14,110 Households	RE, SES	68.3% (NHW), 10.3% (NHB), 16.8% (Hisp), 4.8% (NHO); 17.3% (<131% FPL), 14% (131–185% FPL), 68.3% (> 185% FPL)	All Stores	7
Frankle, 2017	Describe differences in the purchasing of SNAP-eligible foods by SNAP participation status.	2012–2014	New York, New England	188 Stores	SES	NR	Full-Service	7
French, 2019	Assess differences in the nutritional quality of foods and beverages purchased by household income level.	2014–2016	Chicago, IL	202 Households	SES	15.3% (18–24 years), 47.5% (30–49), 36.6% (50+); 83% (female); 29.7% (NHW), 43.1% (NHB), 24.7% (Hisp); 24.3% (PIR: 0–1.3), 38.6% (PIR: 1.4–3.4), 37.1 (3.5+)	All Stores	7

Table 2. Cont.

Author, Year	Study Purpose	Study Year(s) [a]	Study Location	Sample Size	Intersectional Attribute(s)	Sample Demographics [b]	Stores Assessed	QA [c]
Gorski Finding, 2018	Determine if neighborhood retail food access is associated with overweight/obesity in children.	2012–2013	National	3748 Children	SES	SNAP Participants: 32% (NHW), 31.6% (H), 29.7% (NHB), 6.7% (O); SNAP-Eligible Non-Participants: 33.5% (NHW), 41.2% (Hisp), 19.6% (NHB), 5.7% (NHO); Ineligible Non-Participants: 65.0% (NHW), 16.9% (Hisp), 9.8% (NHB), 8.3% (NHO)	All Stores	8
Grummon, 2017	Examine the nutritional profile of household food and beverage purchases by SNAP participation status.	2012–2013	National	70,477 Households	RE x SES [e]	SNAP Participants: Mean age: 55.5, 77% (NHW), 14% (NHB), 5% (Hisp), 4% (NHO); Income-Eligible Non-Participants: Mean age: 59.1, 82% (NHW), 8% (NHB), 4% (Hisp), 6% (NHO); Higher Income Non-Participants: Mean age: 59.3, 83% (NHW), 8% (NHW), 4% (Hisp), 5% (NHO).	All Stores	8
Grummon, 2018	Describe differences in the unhealthy food and beverage purchases by race/ethnicity and SNAP participation status.	2010–2014	National	30,403 Households	RE x SES	Mean age: 59.2; 87% (NHW), 8% (NHB), 5% (Hisp); 17.5% SNAP Participations; 16% (SNAP among NHW), 27% (SNAP among NHB), 21% (SNAP among Hisp)	All Stores	7

Table 2. *Cont.*

Author, Year	Study Purpose	Study Year(s) [a]	Study Location	Sample Size	Intersectional Attribute(s)	Sample Demographics [b]	Stores Assessed	QA [c]
Gustafson, 2017	Determine how neighborhood food store availability influences food stores choice and food store purchases.	2012–2013	National	2962 Households	SES	53% (SNAP Participants); 47% (SNAP-Eligible Non-Participants)	All Stores	6
Jones, 2003	Assess differences in food shopping behaviors and consumption patterns between grocery store customers in low-income and high-income areas.	2001	Columbus, OH	6 Stores	SES	Low-Income Areas: 76.2% (NHW), 21.7% (NHB), 2.0% (NHO); High-Income Areas: 93.6% (NHW), 3.5% (NHB), 3.0% (NHO)	Full-Service	6
Kiszko, 2015	Describe the food and beverage purchases of bodega shoppers in low-income communities.	2012	New York City	779 Shoppers	Targeted: Low-Income + Urban	Mean age: 39.1; 51.5% female; 57.0% (Hisp), 34.9% (NHB), 8.1% (NHO); 53% of shoppers had an annual income ≤ USD 25,000	Limited-Service	5
Lenk, 2018	Assess associations between customer characteristics, shopping patterns, and the healthfulness of purchases in limited-service stores.	2014	Minneapolis, MN	661 Shoppers	Targeted: Urban	47% (NHW), 36% (NHB), 17% (NHO); 38% ≤ high school, 37% (some college), 26% (≥college degree)	Limited-Service	6
Lent, 2014	Describe corner store purchases by age group in a low-income urban neighborhood.	2011	Philadelphia, PA	9283 Shoppers	Targeted: Low-Income + Urban	75.5% adults, 15.5% adolescents, 9.9% children; 41.4% female.	Limited-Service	6

Table 2. Cont.

Author, Year	Study Purpose	Study Year(s) [a]	Study Location	Sample Size	Intersectional Attribute(s)	Sample Demographics [b]	Stores Assessed	QA [c]
Lin, 2014	Examine the roles of food prices and supermarket accessibility in determining food purchases of low-income households.	1996–1997	National	882 Households	Targeted: Low-Income	100% SNAP Households	All Stores	8
Ng, 2016	Evaluate racial/ethnic and income trends in calories purchased in households with children.	2000–2013	National	64,709 Households	RE, SES	NR	All Stores	7
Ng, 2017	Estimate trends in added sugars in beverage purchases among US households by race/ethnicity and socioeconomic status.	2007–2012	National	110,539 Households	RE, SES	NR	All Stores	8
O'Malley, 2013	Determine the feasibility of increasing fruit and vegetable offerings in corner stores.	NR	New Orleans, LA	60 Shoppers	Targeted: Low-Income	48.3% female; 88.3% (AA); 63.3% Annual Income < USD 25,000	Limited-Service	6
Palmer, 2019	Explore food store selection and food purchases in the Northeast using 3 different data sources.	2012–2014	Northeast	IRI CNP: 12,770 Households CES: 3428 Households	SES	IRI Consumer Network Panel (CNP) data: 19.4% (low income), 80.6% (non-low income); Consumer Expenditure Survey (CES) data: 10% of households on SNAP	All Stores	7
Paulin, 2001	Compare food expenditure patterns of Hispanics to Non-Hispanics.	1995–1996	National	13,367 Households	RE	9.2% Hispanic Households, 90.8% Non-Hispanic Households	All Stores	8

Table 2. Cont.

Author, Year	Study Purpose	Study Year(s) [a]	Study Location	Sample Size	Intersectional Attribute(s)	Sample Demographics [b]	Stores Assessed	QA [c]
Poti, 2016	Examine associations between race/ethnicity, ready-to-eat, highly-processed food and beverage purchasing.	2000–2012	National	157,142 Households	RE × SES	81.3% (NHW), 9.3% (NHB), 7.1% (Hisp)	All Stores	7
Stern, 2016	Determine if food store selection is associated with the nutrient profile of package food purchases across racial/ethnic groups	2007–2012	National	356,611 Households	RE	81.8% (NHW), 8.7% (NHB, 5.1% (Hisp), 4.2% (NHO); 19.0% (≤185% FPL), 43.0% (185–400% FPL), 38% (≥400% FPL)	All Stores	7
Taillie, 2016	Assess the relationship between food retail chain type and the healthfulness of food purchases.	2000–2013	National	164,315 Households	RE, SES	81% (NHW), 9% (NHB), 5% (Hisp), 4% (NHO); 10% of households ≤ 130% FPL	All Stores	7
Taillie, 2017 [1]	Describe the prevalence of price promotions among food and beverage purchases of households with children.	2008–2012	National	90,046,893 Purchases	RE, SES	NR	All Stores	6
Taillie, 2017 [2]	Examine trends in the proportion of packaged food and beverage purchases with a low-nutrient or no-nutrient claim.	2008–2012	National	80,038,247 Purchases	RE, SES	NR	All Stores	7

Table 2. Cont.

Author, Year	Study Purpose	Study Year(s) [a]	Study Location	Sample Size	Intersectional Attribute(s)	Sample Demographics [b]	Stores Assessed	QA [c]
Taillie, 2018	Compare the nutritional profile of food and beverages of SNAP participants to non-participants.	2010–2014	National	76,458 Households	SES	SNAP Participants: Mean age: 54.5, 76.5% (NHW), 13.8% (NHB), 5.7% (Hisp), 4.0% (NHO); Income-Eligible Non-Participants: Mean age: 58.4, 82.0% (NHW), 8.3% (NHB), 4.5% (Hisp), 5.3% (NHO); Higher-Income Non-Participants: Mean age: 58.5, 82.9% (NHW), 7.9% (NHB), 4.4% (Hisp), 4.7% (NHO)	All Stores	7
Vadiveloo, 2019	Describe geographic differences in the diet quality of household food purchases.	2012–2013	National	3961 Households	RE	Mean age: 50.6; 70.2% female; 70.3% (NHW), 9.9% (NHB), 13.0% (Hisp), 6.8% (NHO); 16.9% (FPL <130%), 41.1% (130–349%), 42.0% (≥350%); 34.6% rural households	All Stores	7

Table 2. Cont.

Author, Year	Study Purpose	Study Year(s) [a]	Study Location	Sample Size	Intersectional Attribute(s)	Sample Demographics [b]	Stores Assessed	QA [c]
Vadiveloo, 2020	Evaluate racial/ethnic, socioeconomic, and weight-based differences in the diet quality of household food purchases.	2012–2013	National	3961 Households	RE × SES	Mean age: 50.6; 70.2% female; 70.3% (NHW), 9.9% (NHB), 13.0% (Hisp), 6.8% (NHO); 16.9% (FPL<130%), 41.1% (130–349%), 42.0% (≥350%); 57.8% high degree/some college; 12.7% SNAP participation; 34.6% rural households	All Stores	8

Note: AA, African American; FPL, Federal poverty limit; Hisp, Hispanic; NHA, non-Hispanic Asian; NHB, non-Hispanic Black; NHW, non-Hispanic White; NR, None Reported; NHO, non-Hispanic Other (according to the authors' definition); PIR, Poverty-to-Income ratio; QA, Quality Assessment; RE, Racial/ethnic differences; SES, Socioeconomic differences; SNAP, Supplemental Nutrition Assistance Program; WIC, Special Supplemental Nutrition Program for Women, Infants, and Children. [a] Study year (s) reflect the year the data was collected. If data collection dates were not provided, the date the statistical analysis was performed was recorded. [b] Demographic information on race/ethnicity, socioeconomic status, and urban/rural status are provided in the table. If socioeconomic information was not available, descriptive statistics for education level or employment status were recorded (if provided by authors). [c] The National Heart, Lung, and Blood Institute's (NHLBI) quality assessment tool for observational cohort and cross-sectional studies was used for quality assessment: https://www.nhlbi.nih.gov/health-topics/study-quality-assessment-tools. [d] This targeted study also assessed SES differences. [e] "X" indicates that intersectional information is provided on the two factors listed.

Table 3. Key Findings from Intersectional Studies ($n = 6$).

Authors (Year)	Intersection Groups	Purchasing Outcomes Examined									Key Findings ‡
		F&V	WG	SS	Dess.	SSB	Bev	HEI	Kcals	Nutri.	Other	
Cullen (2007)	Race × SES	X		X	X	X	X					Interactions between ethnicity of participant (Hisp versus non-Hispanic [NHW and NHB combined]) and SES (highest education of household: high school graduate or less versus some college or more) were explored. No significant interactions were identified for purchasing (percent of total grocery dollar spent on category) of fruit, vegetables, salty snacks, cakes/pies/desserts, candy, carbonated and sweetened drinks, 100% fruit juice, and water.

Table 3. *Cont.*

Authors (Year)	Intersection Groups	Purchasing Outcomes Examined									Key Findings ‡
		F&V	WG	SS	Dess.	SSB	Bev	HEI	Kcals	Nutri.	Other	
Grummon (2017)	Race × SES	X		X	X	X	X		X	X		Interactions between race/ethnicity of the head of household (NHW, Hisp, NHB, NHO) and SES (SNAP participant, income-eligible nonparticipant, higher income nonparticipant) were explored. After adjusting for multiple comparisons, no significant interactions were identified for purchasing (kcal/capita/day) of fruit, vegetables, salty snacks, desserts and sweet snacks, candy and gum, SSBs, 100% juice, total energy, sugar, saturated fat, and sodium.
Grummon (2018)	Race × SES			X	X	X			X	X		Differences by race/ethnicity (NHW, NHB, Hisp) tested in models stratified by SES (SNAP participant v. non-participant with household income <250% FPL). Significant race/ethnicity differences varied across SES: Among non-participants and comparing to NHW (ref), NHB had significantly less purchasing (kcals/capita/day) of desserts and sweet snacks and salty snacks and Hisp had less purchasing of desserts and sweet snacks and candy but more purchasing of sodium (mg/capita/day); no significant differences by race/ethnicity occurred for these outcomes among SNAP participants. Among SNAP participants and comparing to NHW, NHB had more purchasing of overall kcals and Hisp less purchasing of sugar (g/capita/day); no significant differences by race/ethnicity occurred for these outcomes among non-participants. Remaining outcomes (SSBs and saturated fat) either did not have significant differences across race/ethnicity or significant differences by race/ethnicity were in the same direction across SES groups.

Table 3. *Cont.*

Authors (Year)	Intersection Groups	Purchasing Outcomes Examined										Key Findings ‡
		F&V	WG	SS	Dess.	SSB	Bev	HEI	Kcals	Nutri.	Other	
Palmer (2019)	Race × SES	X										Proportion of purchasers compared to non-purchasers for specific market basket items examined across SES (household income <200% FPL [low] v. > 200% FPL [high]) and race (White, Black) and ethnicity (Hispanic) groups. Among White high income, there were significantly more purchasers than non-purchasers of canned/bottled peaches and potatoes; no significant differences identified among White low income. Among Black high income, there were significantly fewer purchasers than non-purchasers for potatoes; no significant difference identified among Black low income. Remaining outcomes (frozen broccoli) and groups (e.g., Hisp of low or high income) either did not have significant differences or were in the same direction across SES groups.
Poti (2016)	Race × SES										X	Interactions between race/ethnicity (NHW, Hisp, NHB) and SES (household income: <USD 25,000 [low], USD 25,000–USD 49,999, USD 50,000–USD 74,999 and > USD 75,000 [high]) were tested for other outcomes: Proportion of purchases (% of kcals) by 4 categories of degree of processing (minimally-, basic-, moderately- and highly-processed [HPI]) and 3 categories of ready-to-eat (requires cooking, ready-to-heat, ready-to-eat [RTE]). Small, though significant, differences identified for basic-processed and requires cooking. Basic-processed *food-only purchases*: NHB and Hisp had greater purchasing than NHW at low-income; at high income, differences narrowed and purchasing was more similar across groups. Requires-cooking *food-only purchases*: NHB and Hisp greater purchasing than NHW at low-income; at high income, differences narrowed and purchasing was similar across groups. No other significant interactions reported.

Table 3. *Cont.*

Authors (Year)	Intersection Groups	Purchasing Outcomes Examined									Key Findings ‡
		F&V	WG	SS	Dess.	SSB	Bev	HEI	Kcals	Nutri.	Other	
Vadiveloo (2020)	Race × SES							X				Interactions between race/ethnicity of primary respondent (NHW, NHB, Hisp, NHO) and family SES (<130% of FPL, 130–349% ≥350%) were explored. No significant interaction was identified for the overall quality of food-at-home purchases as measured by HEI-2015 total score.

Note: SES, socioeconomic status; NHW, non-Hispanic White; NHB, non-Hispanic Black; Hisp, Hispanic; NHO, non-Hispanic Other following author definition; SNAP, Supplemental Nutrition Assistance Program; FPL, Federal poverty limit; F&V, fruits and/or vegetables; WG, whole grains; SS, Salty Snacks; Dess., desserts, sweet snacks and candy; SSB, sugar-sweetened beverages; Bev, non-sweetened beverages; HEI, healthy eating index; Kcals, kilocalories; Nutri., sugar, saturated fat, and/or sodium; Other, other purchasing outcomes of interest; ref, reference group in modeling; HP, highly-processed; RTE, ready-to-eat; g, grams; mg, milligrams. ‡ Findings present results from adjusted models unless otherwise noted. Significant results follow the authors' definition (e.g., some use Bonferroni correction). Underline-bold highlights purchasing outcomes of interest in this review. *Underline-italics* indicates when results for kilocalories/energy density, sugar, saturated fat, sodium, or other category was examined among food purchases and beverage purchases separately.

One study examined the quality of household food purchases using HEI [54]. However, Vadiveloo et al. (2020) reported no significant interactions between race/ethnicity and family income. Two studies examined overall kilocalories purchased [34,35], with one identifying relevant results [35]. Among SNAP households, Grummon and Taillie (2018) identified that NHB purchased significantly more kilocalories compared to NHW, which was not observed among non-SNAP households. Two studies examined sugar, saturated fat, and sodium, and Grummon and Taillie (2018) reported significant intersectional results for sodium and sugar [34,35]. Hispanics had significantly greater purchasing of sodium compared to NHW among non-SNAP households, which was not observed in SNAP households. In addition, among SNAP households, Hispanics had significantly less purchasing of sugar than NHW, though this was not observed in non-SNAP households.

Poti et al. (2016) was the only study that examined purchasing outcomes that were not part of our primary outcomes of interest across intersectional attributes [47]. They explored whether household income moderated the association between race/ethnicity and purchasing products with different degrees of processing (e.g., highly processed, minimally processed) and ready-to-eat (e.g., requires cooking, ready-to-heat). Significant interactions between race/ethnicity and SES were identified for basic-processed and requires cooking food purchases. Greater purchasing of both outcomes was observed among NHB and Hispanics compared to NHW among low-income households.

3.2. Single Attribute Results

3.2.1. Race/Ethnicity

Fifteen studies (44.1%) examined purchasing outcomes across racial and/or ethnic groups [27,29,30,39,42,43,45–51,53,54]. All studies examined purchasing among NHW, 14 examined purchasing among NHB, 14 studied purchasing among Hispanic, nine examined purchasing among non-Hispanic Other (or a different author definition that collapsed multiple racial/ethnic groups), and three investigated purchasing among Asian (using the author definition). Key findings from studies that presented racial/ethnic differences in consumer food and/or beverage purchases are described in detail in Supplementary Material Part II (Table S1).

3.2.2. Socioeconomic Status

We identified 19 (55.9%) studies that examined purchasing outcomes across SES categories [26,27,29–34,36,37,39,42,43,45,49–52,54]. Ten studies evaluated SES by looking across household income levels, while seven studies used federal food assistance program participation status (i.e., SNAP status), four studies used education level, one study used employment status, and one study classified food retail stores based on income of the surrounding neighborhoods. In three studies, SES was examined in more than one way (e.g., both income and education levels were assessed). Supplementary Material Part II (Table S2) present key findings from the studies that evaluated SES differences in consumer food and/or beverage purchases.

3.2.3. Geographic Location

We did not identify any studies that examined differences in customer food and/or purchasing by geographic setting (i.e., urban vs. suburban vs. rural).

3.3. Targeted Population Results

3.3.1. Intersectional Targeted Populations

Eleven studies (33.3%) were labeled targeted [21–26,28,38,40,41,44]. Five examined consumer food purchases among an intersectional targeted population [23,26,38,40,44]. These populations were low-income individuals or households living in an urban city [23,38,40,44] and NHBs living in an urban city [26]. All studies with a low-income urban population focused solely on limited-service store purchasing. Three studies assessed fruit and vegetable purchasing while none examined whole grain purchasing [26,40,44]. Overall, fruit and vegetable purchasing was moderate to low. Chrisinger et al. (2018) reported that 14% of total food expenditures among a small sample of NHB women were spent on fruits and vegetables [26]. Lent et al. (2014) and O'Malley et al. (2013) found that fruits and vegetables comprised 2.3% and 5% of purchases from limited-service store shoppers in low-income urban communities, respectively [40,44]. All five studies examined purchasing of salty snacks, desserts, sweet snacks, and/or candy. While Chrisinger et al. (2018) reported that these items represented only 11% of food expenditures among NHB women, the other four articles found that these items represented a large percentage of customer purchases in limited-service stores (>20%). All five studies assessed SSB purchasing; only three assessed non-sweetened beverage purchasing [23,40,44]. SSB were the items most often purchased across all studies. No study examined the quality of purchases using HEI. Only Borradaile et al. (2009) and Lent et al. (2014) examined kilocalories, saturated fat, sugar, and sodium content of purchases [40,44]. Both studies reported high volumes of each nutrient among customer purchases from limited-service stores. Key findings from studies that assessed consumer food and/or beverage purchases with a targeted population are reported in (Table S3) of Supplementary Material Part III.

3.3.2. Single Factor Targeted Populations

The remaining six targeted studies reported purchasing for a single factor targeted population [21,22,24,25,28,41] including low-income individuals or households [21,41] and individuals or households residing in an urban city [22,24,25,28]. Low-income targeted populations focused on participants of federal food assistance programs such as SNAP and the Special Supplemental Nutrition Program for Women, Infants, and Children (WIC). Key findings from studies that focused on single factor targeted populations are also presented in Supplementary Material Part III (Table S3).

4. Discussion and Future Directions

We aimed to summarize peer-reviewed scientific studies that assessed U.S. food and/or beverage purchasing at the intersection of race/ethnicity, SES, and geographic location, and recommend future approaches to expand this area of research. Food purchasing behaviors have been reviewed previously [4,14–19], although this scoping review is the first to (1) synthesize findings on food and beverage purchases by race/ethnicity, SES, and geographic location and (2) examine the intersectional nature of these factors. Our main finding is a limited number of studies published since 2000 provide an intersectional perspective on food and/or beverage purchasing across our three factors of interest, which have been consistently linked with diet and health inequities [29,34,35,45,47,54]. Thus, the vast majority of studies evaluated purchasing by a single attribute or within a specific targeted population. Below, we describe the implications of our review findings by attribute and provide future recommendations for studies seeking to contribute to this literature. A comprehensive list of future directions is provided in (Table 4).

Table 4. Recommendations for Future Directions in Assessing U.S. Consumer Food and Beverage Purchasing.

Intersectional Attribute:	Future Directions:
General	• Compare food and beverage purchasing patterns among full-service and limited-service stores across racial/ethnic groups, SES, and urban/rural status. Specificity regarding purchasing decisions by store type within these broad categories is recommended to inform tailored public health interventions.
Two or More Factors: Race/Ethnicity, SES, and Geographic Location	• Prioritize examining U.S. consumer food and/or beverage purchases at the intersection of two or more factors (i.e., race/ethnicity, SES, and geographic location). • Determine how urban/rural status moderates racial/ethnic and SES differences in food and beverage purchasing.

Table 4. *Cont.*

Intersectional Attribute:	Future Directions:
Race/Ethnicity	• Prioritize evaluating consumer food and/or beverage purchases across a greater diversity of racial/ethnic groups: NHB, Hispanic, Asian, Native American, Pacific Islander, etc. • Examine heterogeneity of purchasing within racial and ethnic groups (example: Hispanic subcultures). • Move beyond assessing "race" as a risk factor and determine how systemic and structural racism influences food and beverage purchasing.
SES	• Consider SES differences in purchasing for food and beverage groups/items that are understudied (i.e., whole grains, non-sweetened beverages) • Assess the relationship between purchasing and community-level factors such as economic deprivation, gentrification displacement, crime, and blight.
Geographic Location Urban vs. Rural	• Examine U.S. consumer food and/or beverage purchases by geographic location at the national, regional, and local levels. • Evaluate urban vs. suburban vs. rural purchasing patterns by store type: full-service vs. limited service. • Prioritize perspectives from minority populations in rural areas regarding influences on food and beverage purchasing.
Targeted Populations	• Study consumer food and/or beverage purchasing among single factor targeted populations that represent populations beyond low-income and/or urban. • Assess consumer food and/or beverage purchasing among intersectional targeted populations that represent 2+ attributes (example: low-income Hispanic families living in a rural area).

Note. SES, Socioeconomic Status; NHW, non-Hispanic White; NHB, non-Hispanic Black.

4.1. Understanding the Intersection of Race/Ethnicity, SES, and Geographic Location

As mentioned, several studies have reported health and nutritional inequities by race/ethnicity, SES, and urban vs. rural status [8–10]. Assessing the intersectional nature of these factors may provide researchers new insight into food and beverage purchasing patterns to inform the design of policy, systems, and environmental change interventions that advance health equity [11–13]. Only six studies (17.6%) in this review examined the intersection of two attributes with all assessing race/ethnicity by SES differences [29,34,35,45,47,54]. Given the small number of studies and the inconsistency in food and beverage purchasing outcomes considered, specific patterns in purchasing could not be identified. Thus, we still have limited understanding of how measures reflecting SES moderate racial/ethnic differences in food purchasing. Future studies should examine U.S. consumer food and/or beverage purchases at the intersection of more than two factors. Since none of the intersectional studies considered geographic location, future studies should determine how urban vs. suburban vs. rural status moderates racial/ethnic and SES differences in purchasing. Moreover, since most studies included in this review (n = 18, 52.9%) examined purchasing using data collected from a nationally-representative sample of U.S. households, future studies could focus on providing an intersectional perspective on food and beverage purchasing at the local and regional levels, especially in the South and West regions of the country.

4.2. Race/Ethnicity

Several reviewed studies (n = 15, 44.1%) presented purchasing findings by race/ethnicity [27,29,30,39,42,43,46–51,53,54]. Despite the large number of studies conducted to date, inconsistencies exist. Across studies, we identified more consistent patterns between NHW and Hispanics regarding purchasing, with Hispanics exhibiting healthier purchasing patterns relative to NHW. For example, we found that most studies examining differences between NHW and Hispanics reported greater fruit and/or vegetable purchasing and less salty snack, dessert, and candy purchasing. Fewer consistencies were noted between NHB and NHW although several studies reported greater SSB and sugar purchasing among NHB compared to NHW. These findings align with the dietary consumption literature, which continues to highlight significant racial/ethnic differences in intake among adults and children [8,10,54–56]. Additional studies are needed to establish consistent patterns in food and beverage purchasing by racial/ethnic group. Future studies should evaluate consumer food and/or beverage purchases across a greater variety of racial/ethnic groups (i.e., non-Hispanic Asian, Native American, Pacific Islander, etc.). Given the heterogeneous composition of all races and ethnicities, future studies could conduct robust assessments of purchasing within groups, which will permit the study of characteristics such as acculturation and nativity—two factors that are often considered in studies of diet quality [55,56]. In recent years, public health research has placed greater emphasis on socio-political factors that create racial/ethnic inequities in health such as structural and systemic racism [57]. Future studies should consider how these important social factors impact food and beverage purchasing.

4.3. Socioeconomic Status

Most studies included in this review (n = 19, 55.9%) examined SES differences in consumer food and/or beverage purchases [26,27,29–34,36,37,39,42,43,45,49–52,54]. These findings underscore that identifying purchasing patterns by SES continues to be a major priority in the field; included studies generally showed a lower likelihood of fruit, vegetable, and whole grain purchases and a higher likelihood for discretionary product purchases (i.e., salty snacks, sweets, and SSB) among consumers with lower incomes compared to higher incomes [58]. Low-income consumers have been described as more likely to be targeted by marketing for food items high in kilocalories, saturated fat, added sugars, and sodium in retail food outlets [59–61], and the results of this review and reviews of diet quality differences by SES align with such observations given the poor quality of food and beverage purchases observed [62]. Furthermore, qualitative evidence has found that low-income consumers are more likely than consumers with higher incomes to purchase less costly, energy-dense and nutrient-poor products amid household financial constraints [63]. Approaches are needed to assess SES differences in purchasing using intersectional theory as a guiding framework to discern opportunities for tailored policy, systems, and environmental change interventions to improve the dietary quality of populations who experience diet-related health disparities [11]. Moreover, given the increase in studies that have evaluated the public health implications of community-level factors such as economic deprivation, blight, and gentrification displacement, future studies should also consider these factors in the context of consumer food and/or beverage purchasing [64,65].

4.4. Geographic Location

No studies included in this review examined geographic differences (i.e., urban vs. suburban vs. rural) regarding consumer food and/or beverage purchasing. This is particularly concerning because rural populations experience a higher burden of major diet-related diseases than urban populations (e.g., heart disease, cancer, stroke), which represent the leading causes of death in the U.S. [66]. The idea that more food environment research specific to rural people and places is needed is not new [67,68]. Rural residents have been shown to have few opportunities for choosing food and beverage options aligned with dietary guidelines in general when compared to residents of more urban areas [69,70]. It is unknown how food environment disparities influence differences in purchasing and dietary patterns between urban, suburban, rural populations, and how multiple socio-demographic factors such as race/ethnicity and SES to influence food purchasing disparities. This requires much more focus moving forward, in order to mitigate prominent health disparities in the U.S.

4.5. Targeted Populations

We included studies that targeted a specific population in order to provide greater context to findings from studies that evaluated consumer food and/or beverage purchases by race/ethnicity, SES, or geographic location [21–26,28,38,40,41,44]. While several studies were labeled targeted (n = 11, 33.3%), the variety of target populations considered was limited to primarily low-income individuals and households residing in an urban setting. No targeted study described purchasing in a rural population or specific racial/ethnic group that is often understudied in this area of research:

non-Hispanic Asian, Native American, etc. Thus, studies are needed to address this gap and contribute more knowledge on the food and beverage purchases of intersectional target populations that represent two or more attributes (example: low-income Hispanic families living in a rural setting).

4.6. Limitations

Several limitations should be considered alongside review results. First, like most reviews, there were limitations in the research strategy. While a trained research librarian (J.P.) guided the literature search process, we limited our search to six databases with a set combination of key words. There is the possibility that relevant studies available in other databases were not included in this review. The large variety of purchasing measures presented by included studies made it not feasible to extract all of the purchasing data. Data from included studies were extracted based upon pre-selected purchasing outcomes of interest such as food groups (fruits, vegetable, whole grains, etc.) and nutritional characteristics (HEI, kcals, etc.). Thus, some purchasing outcomes (e.g., meat, dairy products, etc.) were not examined because they fell outside the scope of our data extraction protocol. An "Other" category was included to allow for the extraction of specific results of interest (example: nutrient claims) that did not align with the pre-specified categories.

Interventions and natural experiments that aimed to modify food and/or beverage purchasing were excluded from the review. It is possible that baseline findings from these studies documented food and beverage purchasing by one or more of our factors of interest. Because this scoping review solely focused on U.S. consumer food and beverage purchasing, findings may not be generalizable to other countries. The methodological assessment tool was not designed to assess the quality of nutrition studies or studies of consumer food purchasing. As previously mentioned, quality scores reported in (Table 2) solely reflect study design and not the quality of the purchasing data presented in the paper. Finally, during the data extraction phase, statistical significance was relied on heavily to identify which results to include in this review. While this made data extraction practical for the research team, this method limits the ability to account for the magnitude of differences in the various analyses. Detailed descriptions of key findings from included studies presented in this paper and the supplemental tables allow the reader to explore consumer purchasing outcomes in more detail.

5. Conclusions

This scoping review found that few studies to date have examined consumer food and beverage purchasing in the U.S. at the intersection of race/ethnicity, SES, and geographic location, despite the large number of studies that assessed purchasing by one of these factors alone. To expand this area of research, future studies should use intersectional theory to guide efforts to evaluate consumer food and/or beverage purchasing in the U.S. at the intersection of race/ethnicity, SES, and geographic location rather than continuing to examine factors individually. Furthermore, future studies should select data collection and assessment methodologies that allow for the gathering of rich data on the relationship between intersectional identity and food purchasing [13]. For example, consumer purchasing intercepts coupled with qualitative interviews that elicit rich descriptions of factors influencing dietary purchasing decisions may be a useful approach to increase our knowledge base on the socio-political and cultural factors that create persistent inequities in food purchasing behavior, dietary intake, and health.

Supplementary Materials: The following are available online at http://www.mdpi.com/1660-4601/17/20/7677/s1, Supplementary Material Part I: Search Terms, Supplementary Material Part II: L Single Attribute Results, Table S1: Key Findings from Studies Examining Racial/Ethnic Differences, Table S2: Key Findings from Studies Examining Socioeconomic Differences, Supplementary Material Part III: Targeted Results, Table S3: Key Findings from Targeted Studies.

Author Contributions: C.R.S., E.A.S., M.W., and B.H. conceptualized the project and designed the data collection tools. J.J.P. developed the search strategy and performed the search. O.S.A. and A.M.R. performed the abstract and full text review. All authors extracted the data and synthesized the results. All authors participated in the writing of the manuscript and approved the final version for submission. All authors have read and agreed to the published version of the manuscript.

Funding: This research was funded by Healthy Eating Research, a national program of the Robert Wood Johnson Foundation. Support for MRW's effort was provided by the National Heart, Lung, and Blood Institute, grant number K99HL144824. BH's effort was supported by the USDA National Institute of Food and Agriculture, Hatch project 1024670. Funders had no role in review design, results, or conclusions. All authors have read and agreed to the published version of the manuscript.

Acknowledgments: The authors would like to acknowledge the guest editors (Alyssa Moran and Cristina Roberto), Mary Story, Kirsten Arm, and Megan Lott at Healthy Eating Research for their guidance and assistance.

Conflicts of Interest: The authors declare no conflict of interest.

References

1. Wilson, M.M.; Reedy, J.; Krebs-Smith, S.M. American Diet Quality: Where It Is, Where It Is Heading, and What It Could Be. *J. Acad. Nutr. Diet.* **2016**, *116*, 302–310. [CrossRef] [PubMed]
2. 2015–2020 Dietary Guidelines: Chapter 2–Current Eating Patterns in the United States. Available online: https://health.gov/our-work/food-nutrition/2015-2020-dietary-guidelines/guidelines/chapter-2/current-eating-patterns-in-the-united-states/ (accessed on 30 June 2020).
3. Volpe, R.; Okrent, A. Assessing the Healthfulness of Consumers' Grocery Purchases. U.S. Department of Agriculture, Economic Research Service 2012, EIB-102. Available online: https://ageconsearch.umn.edu/record/262129/ (accessed on 13 March 2020).
4. Bandy, L.; Adhikari, V.; Jebb, S.; Rayner, M. The use of commercial food purchase data for public health nutrition research: A systematic review. *PLoS ONE* **2019**, *14*, e0210192. [CrossRef] [PubMed]
5. Drewnowski, A.; Rehm, C.D. Energy Intakes of US Children and Adults by Food Purchase Location and by Specific Food Source. *Nutr. J.* **2013**, *12*, 59. [CrossRef] [PubMed]
6. An, R.; Maurer, G. Consumption of Sugar-Sweetened Beverages and Discretionary Foods among US Adults by Purchase Location. *Eur. J. Clin. Nutr.* **2016**, *70*, 1396–1400. [CrossRef] [PubMed]
7. Walker, R.; Keane, C.R.; Burke, J.G. Disparities and access to healthy food in the United States: A review of food deserts literature. *Health Place* **2010**, *16*, 876–884. [CrossRef]
8. Zhang, F.F.; Lui, J.; Rehm, C.D.; Wilde, P.; Mande, J.R.; Mozaffarian, D. Trends and Disparities in Diet Quality Among US Adults by Supplemental Nutrition Assistance Program Participation Status. *JAMA Netw. Open* **2018**, *1*, e180237. [CrossRef]
9. Lui, J.H.; Jones, S.J.; Sun, H.; Probst, J.C.; Merchant, A.T.; Cavicchia, P. Diet, physical activity, and sedentary behaviors as risk factors for childhood obesity: An urban and rural comparison. *Child. Obes.* **2012**, *8*, 440–448.
10. Hiza, H.A.B.; Casavale, K.O.; Guenther, P.M.; Davis, C.A. Diet Quality of Americans Differs by Age, Sex, Race/Ethnicity, Income, and Education Level. *J. Acad. Nutr. Diet.* **2013**, *113*, 297–306. [CrossRef]
11. Bowleg, L. The Problem with the Phrase Women and Minorities: Intersectionality—An Important Theoretical Framework for Public Health. *Am. J. Public Health* **2012**, *102*, 1267–1273. [CrossRef]
12. Bauer, G.R. Incorporating Intersectionality Theory into Population Health Research Methodology: Challenges and the Potential to Advance Health Equity. *Soc. Sci. Med.* **2014**, *110*, 10–17. [CrossRef]
13. Abrams, J.A.; Tabaac, A.; Jung, S.; Else-Quest, N.M. Considerations for employing intersectionality in qualitative health research. *Soc. Sci. Med.* **2020**, *258*, 113138. [CrossRef] [PubMed]
14. Hartmann-Boyce, J.; Bianchi, F.; Piernas, C.; Payne Riches, S.; Frie, K.; Nourse, R.; Jebb, S.A. Grocery store interventions to change food purchasing behaviors: A systematic review of randomized controlled trials. *Am. J. Clin. Nutr.* **2018**, *107*, 1004–1016. [CrossRef] [PubMed]
15. Gittelsohn, J.; Trude AC, B.; Kim, H. Pricing Strategies to Encourage Availability, Purchase, and Consumption of Healthy Foods and Beverages: A Systematic Review. *Prev. Chronic Dis.* **2017**, *14*, E107. [CrossRef] [PubMed]
16. Liberato, S.C.; Bailie, R.; Brimblecombe, J. Nutrition interventions at point-of-sale to encourage healthier food purchasing: A systematic review. *BMC Public Health* **2014**, *14*, 919. [CrossRef]
17. Epstein, L.H.; Jankowiak, N.; Nederkoorn, C.; Raynor, H.A.; French, S.A.; Finkelstein, E. Experimental research on the relation between food price changes and food-purchasing patterns: A targeted review. *Am. J. Clin. Nutr.* **2012**, *95*, 789–809. [CrossRef]
18. An, R. Effectiveness of subsidies in promoting healthy food purchases and consumption: A review of field experiments. *Public Health Nutr.* **2013**, *16*, 1215–1228. [CrossRef]

19. Abeykoon, A.H.; Engler-Stringer, R.; Muhajarine, N. Health-related outcomes of new grocery store interventions: A systematic review. *Public Health Nutr.* **2017**, *20*, 2236–2248. [CrossRef]
20. National Heart Lung and Blood Institute (NHBLI). Study Quality Assessment Tools. Available online: https://www.nhlbi.nih.gov/health-topics/study-quality-assessment-tools (accessed on 20 February 2020).
21. Andreyeva, T.; Luedicke, J.; Henderson, K.E.; Tripp, A.S. Grocery Store Beverage Choices by Participants in Federal Food Assistance and Nutrition Programs. *Am. J. Prev. Med.* **2012**, *43*, 411–418. [CrossRef]
22. Appelhans, B.; French, S.A.; Tangney, C.C.; Powell, L.M.; Wang, Y. To what extent do food purchases reflect shoppers' diet quality and nutrient intake? *Int. J. Behav. Nutr. Phys. Act.* **2017**, *14*, 46. [CrossRef]
23. Borradaile, K.E.; Sherman, S.; Vander Veur, S.S.; McCoy, T.; Sandoval, B.; Nachmani, J.; Karpyn, A.; Foster, G.D. Snacking in Children: The Role of Urban Corner Stores. *Pediatrics* **2009**, *124*, 1293–1298. [CrossRef]
24. Caspi, C.; Lenk, K.; Pelletier, J.E.; Barnes, T.L.; Harnack, L.; Erickson, D.J.; Laska, M.N. Food and beverage purchases in corner stores, gas-marts, pharmacies and dollar stores. *Public Health Nutr.* **2017**, *20*, 2587–2597. [CrossRef]
25. Caspi, C.; Lenk, K.; Pelletier, J.E.; Barnes, T.L.; Harnack, L.; Erickson, D.J.; Laska, M.N. Association between store food environment and customer purchases in small grocery stores, gas-marts, pharmacies and dollar stores. *Int. J. Behav. Nutr. Phys. Act.* **2017**, *14*, 76. [CrossRef] [PubMed]
26. Chrisinger, B.W.; Isselman DiSantis, K.; Hillier, A.E.; Kumanyika, S.K. Family food purchases of high- and low-calorie foods in full-service supermarkets and other food retailers by Black women in an urban US setting. *Prev. Med. Rep.* **2018**, *10*, 136–143. [CrossRef]
27. Chrisinger, B.W.; Kallan, M.J.; Whiteman, E.S.; Hillier, A.E. Where do U.S. households purchase healthy foods? An analysis of food-at-home purchases across different types of retailers in a nationally representative dataset. *Prev. Med.* **2018**, *112*, 15–22. [CrossRef]
28. Crane, M.M.; Tangney, C.C.; French, S.A.; Wang, Y.; Appelhans, B. Gender Comparison of the Diet Quality and Sources of Food Purchases made by Urban Primary Household Food Purchasers. *J. Nutr. Educ. Behav.* **2019**, *51*, 199–204. [CrossRef]
29. Cullen, K.; Baranowski, T.; Watson, K.; Nicklas, T.; Fisher, J.; O'Donnell, S.; Baranowski, J.; Islam, N.; Missaghian, M. Food Category Purchases Vary by Households Education and Race/Ethnicity: Results from Grocery Receipts. *J. Am. Diet. Assoc.* **2007**, *107*, 1747–1752. [CrossRef]
30. Ford, C.N.; Ng, S.W.; Popkin, B.M. Are food and beverage purchases in households with preschoolers changing? A longitudinal analysis from 2000–2011. *Am. J. Prev. Med.* **2014**, *47*, 275–282. [CrossRef] [PubMed]
31. Franckle, R.L.; Moran, A.; Hou, T.; Blue, D.; Greene, B.A.; Thorndike, A.; Polacsek, M.; Rimm, E.B. Transactions at a Northeastern Supermarket Chain: Differences by Supplemental Nutrition Assistance Program Use. *Am. J. Prev. Med.* **2017**, *53*, e131–e138. [CrossRef]
32. French, S.A.; Tangney, C.C.; Crane, M.M.; Wang, Y.; Appelhans, B. Nutrition quality of 1food purchases varies by household income: The SHoPPER study. *BMC Public Health* **2019**, *19*, 231. [CrossRef] [PubMed]
33. Gorski Findling, M.T.; Wolfson, J.A.; Rimm, E.B.; Bleich, S.N. Differences in the Neighborhood Retail Food Environment and Obesity Among US Children and Adolescents by SNAP Participation. *Obesity* **2018**, *26*, 1063–1071. [CrossRef]
34. Grummon, A.H.; Taillie, L.S. Nutritional Profile of Supplemental Nutrition Assistance Program Household Food and Beverage Purchases. *Am. J. Clin. Nutr.* **2017**, *105*, 1433–1442. [CrossRef] [PubMed]
35. Grummon, A.H.; Taillie, L.S. Supplemental Nutrition Assistance Program participation and racial/ethnic disparities in food and beverage purchases: SNAP and Racial/Ethnic Disparities. *Public Health Nutr.* **2018**, *21*, 3377–3385. [CrossRef] [PubMed]
36. Gustafson, A. Shopping pattern and food purchase differences among Supplemental Nutrition Assistance Program (SNAP) households and Non-supplemental Nutrition Assistance Program households in the United States. *Prev. Med. Rep.* **2017**, *7*, 152–157. [CrossRef] [PubMed]
37. Jones, E.; Akbay, C.; Roe, B.; Chern, W.S. Analyses of Consumers' Dietary Behavior: An Application of the AIDS Model to Supermarket Scanner Data. *Agribusiness* **2003**, *19*, 203–221. [CrossRef]
38. Kisko, K.; Cantor, J.; Abrams, C.; Ruddock, C.; Moltzen, K.; Devia, C.; McFarline, B.; Singh, H.; Elbel, B. Corner store purchases in a low-income urban community in NYC. *J. Community Health* **2015**, *40*, 1084–1090. [CrossRef]

39. Lenk, K.M.; Caspi, C.E.; Harnack, L.; Laska, M.N. Customer characteristics and shopping patterns associated with healthy and unhealthy purchases at small and non-traditional food stores. *J. Community Health* **2018**, *43*, 70–78. [CrossRef]
40. Lent, M.R.; Vander Veur, S.; Mallya, G.; McCoy, T.A.; Sanders, T.A.; Colby, L.; Rauchut Tewksbury, C.; Lawman, H.G.; Sandoval, B.; Sherman, S.; et al. Corner store purchases made by adults, adolescents and children: items, nutritional characteristics and amount spent. *Public Health Nutr.* **2014**, *18*, 1706–1712. [CrossRef]
41. Lin, B.; Ver Ploeg, M.; Kasteridis, P.; Yen, S.T. The roles of food prices and food access in determining food purchases of low-income households. *J. Policy Modeling* **2014**, *36*, 938–952. [CrossRef]
42. Ng, S.W.; Poti, J.M.; Popkin, B.M. Trends in racial/ethnic and income disparities in foods and beverages consumed and purchased from stores among US households with children, 2000–2013. *Am. J. Clin. Nutr.* **2016**, *104*, 750–759. [CrossRef]
43. Ng, S.W.; Ostrowski, J.D.; Li, K. Trends in added sugars from packaged beverages available and purchased by US households, 2007–2012. *Am. J. Clin. Nutr.* **2017**, *106*, 179–188. [CrossRef]
44. O'Malley, K.; Gustat, J.; Rice, J.; Johnson, C.C. Feasibility of Increasing Access to Healthy Foods in Neighborhood Corner Stores. *J. Community Health* **2013**, *38*, 741–749. [CrossRef] [PubMed]
45. Palmer, A.; Bonanno, A.; Clancy, K.; Cho, C.; Cleary, R.; Lee, R. Enhancing understanding of food purchasing patterns in the Northeast US using multiple datasets. *Renew. Agric. Food Syst.* **2019**, 1–15. [CrossRef]
46. Paulin, G.D. Variation in Food Purchases: A Study of Inter-Ethnic and Intra-Ethnic Group Patterns Involving the Hispanic Community. *Fam. Consum. Sci. Res. J.* **2001**, *29*, 336–381. [CrossRef]
47. Poti, J.M.; Mendez, M.A.; Ng, S.W.; Popkin, B.M. Highly Processed and Ready-to-Eat Packaged Food and Beverage Purchases Differ by Race/Ethnicity among US Households. *J. Nutr.* **2016**, *146*, 1722–1730. [CrossRef] [PubMed]
48. Stern, D.; Poti, J.M.; Ng, S.W.; Robinson, W.R.; Gordon-Larsen, P.; Popkin, B. Where people shop is not associated with the nutrient quality of packaged foods for any racial-ethnic group in the United States. *Am. J. Clin. Nutr.* **2016**, *103*, 1125–1134. [CrossRef]
49. Taillie, L.S.; Ng, S.W.; Popkin, B.M. Walmart and Other Food Retail Chains Trends and Disparities in the Nutritional Profile of Packaged Food Purchases. *Am. J. Prev. Med.* **2016**, *50*, 171–179. [CrossRef]
50. Taillie, L.S.; Ng, S.W.; Xue, Y.; Busey, E.; Harding, M. No Fat, No Sugar, No Salt... No Problem? Prevalence of "Low-Content" Nutrient Claims and Their Associations with the Nutritional Profile of Food and Beverage Purchases in the United States. *J. Acad. Nutr. Diet.* **2017**, *117*, 1366–1374. [CrossRef]
51. Taillie, L.S.; Ng, S.W.; Xue, Y.; Harding, M. Deal or no deal? The prevalence and nutritional quality of price promotions among U.S. food and beverage purchases. *Appetite* **2017**, *117*, 365–372. [CrossRef]
52. Taillie, L.S.; Grummon, A.H.; Miles, D.R. Nutritional Profile of Purchases by Store Type: Disparities by Income and Food Program Participation. *Am. J. Prev. Med.* **2018**, *55*, 167–177. [CrossRef]
53. Vadiveloo, M.; Perraud, E.; Parker, H.W.; Parekh, N. Geographic Differences in the Dietary Quality of Food Purchases among Participants in the Nationally Representative Food Acquisition and Purchase Survey (FoodAPS). *Nutrients* **2019**, *11*, 1233. [CrossRef]
54. Vadiveloo, M.; Parker, H.W.; Juul, F.; Parekh, N. Sociodemographic Differences in the Dietary Quality of Food-at-Home Acquisitions and Purchases among Participants in the U.S. Nationally Representative Food Acquisition and Purchase Survey (FoodAPS). *Nutrients* **2020**, *12*, 2354. [CrossRef] [PubMed]
55. Bleich, S.N.; Vercammen, K.A.; Wyatt Koma, J.; Li, Z. Trends in Beverage Consumption among Children and Adults, 2003–2014. *Obesity* **2018**, *26*, 432–441. [CrossRef] [PubMed]
56. Di Noia, J.; Monica, D.; Cullen, K.W.; Pérez-Escamilla, R.; Gray, H.L.; Sikorskii, A. Differences in Fruit and Vegetable Intake by Race/Ethnicity and by Hispanic Origin and Nativity Among Women in the Special Supplemental Nutrition Program for Women, Infants, and Children, 2015. *Prev. Chronic Dis.* **2016**, *13*, E115. [CrossRef]
57. Bailey, Z.D.; Krieger, N.; Agenor, M.; Graves, J.; Linos, N.; Bassett, M.T. Structural racism and health inequities in the USA: Evidence and interventions. *Lancet* **2017**, *389*, 8–14. [CrossRef]
58. Thompson, C.; Cummins, S.; Brown, T.; Kyle, R. Understanding Interactions with the Food Environment: An Exploration of Supermarket Food Shopping Routines in Deprived Neighbourhoods. *Health Place* **2013**, *19*, 116–123. [CrossRef] [PubMed]

59. Cohen, D.A. Obesity and the Built Environment: Changes in Environmental Cues Cause Energy Imbalances. *Int. J. Obes.* **2008**, *32*, S137–S142. [CrossRef]
60. Cohen, D.A.; Babey, S.H. Contextual Influences on Eating Behaviours: Heuristic Processing and Dietary Choices. *Obes. Rev.* **2012**, *13*, 766–779. [CrossRef]
61. Cohen, D.A.; Collins, R.; Hunter, G.; Ghosh-Dastidar, B.; Dubowitz, T. Store Impulse Marketing Strategies and Body Mass Index. *Am. J. Public Health* **2015**, *105*, 1446–1452. [CrossRef]
62. Andreyeva, T.; Tripp, A.S.; Schwartz, M.B. Dietary Quality of Americans by Supplemental Nutrition Assistance Program Participation Status: A Systematic Review. *Am. J. Prev. Med.* **2015**, *49*, 594–604. [CrossRef]
63. Fielding-Singh, P. A Taste of Inequality: Food's Symbolic Value across the Socioeconomic Spectrum. *Sociol. Sci.* **2017**, *4*, 424–448. [CrossRef]
64. Gibbons, J.; Barton, M.S. The Association of Minority Self-Rated Health with Black Versus White Gentrification. *J. Urban Health* **2016**, *93*, 909–922. [CrossRef] [PubMed]
65. Woolf, S.H.; Braveman, P. Where Health Disparities Begin: The Role of Social And Economic Determinants—And Why Current Policies May Make Matters Worse. *Health Aff.* **2011**, *30*, 1852–1859. [CrossRef] [PubMed]
66. Garcia, M.C.; Faul, M.; Massetti, G.; Thomas, C.C.; Hong, Y.; Bauer, U.E.; Iademarco, M.F. Reducing Potentially Excess Deaths From the Five Leading Causes of Death in the Rural United States. *MMWR Surveill. Summ.* **2017**, *66*, 1–7. [CrossRef] [PubMed]
67. Pinard, C.A.; Byker Shanks, C.; Harden, S.M.; Yaroch, A.L. An integrative literature review of small food store research across urban and rural communities in the U.S. *Prev. Med. Rep.* **2016**, *3*, 324–332. [CrossRef]
68. Houghtaling, B.; Serrano, E.L.; Kraak, V.I.; Harden, S.M.; Davis, G.C. A Systematic Review of Factors That Influence Food Store Owner and Manager Decision Making and Ability or Willingness to Use Choice Architecture and Marketing Mix Strategies to Encourage Healthy Consumer Purchases in the United States, 2005–2017. *Int. J. Behav. Nutr. Phys. Act.* **2019**, *16*, 5. [CrossRef]
69. Shikany, J.; Carson, T.L.; Hardy, C.M.; Li, Y.; Sterling, S.; Hardy, S.; Walker, C.M.; Baskin, M.L. Assessment of the nutrition environment in rural counties in the Deep South. *J. Nutr. Sci.* **2018**, *7*, e27. [CrossRef]
70. Byker Shanks, C.; Ahmed, S.; Smith, T.; Houghtaling, B.; Jenkins, M.; Margetts, M.; Schultz, D.; Stephens, L. Availability, Price, and Quality of Fruits and Vegetables in 12 Rural Montana Counties, 2014. *Prev. Chronic Dis.* **2015**, *12*, 150158. [CrossRef]

Publisher's Note: MDPI stays neutral with regard to jurisdictional claims in published maps and institutional affiliations.

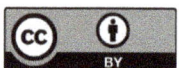

© 2020 by the authors. Licensee MDPI, Basel, Switzerland. This article is an open access article distributed under the terms and conditions of the Creative Commons Attribution (CC BY) license (http://creativecommons.org/licenses/by/4.0/).

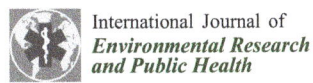 International Journal of
Environmental Research and Public Health

Review

Improving Consumption and Purchases of Healthier Foods in Retail Environments: A Systematic Review

Allison Karpyn [1],*, Kathleen McCallops [1], Henry Wolgast [1] and Karen Glanz [2]

1. Center for Research in Education and Social Policy, University of Delaware, Pearson Hall, 125 Academy Street, Newark, DE 19716, USA; kamcca@udel.edu (K.M.); hnrywlg@udel.edu (H.W.)
2. Perelman School of Medicine and School of Nursing, University of Pennsylvania, Philadelphia, 3400 Civic Center Blvd, PA 19104, USA; kglanz@pennmedicine.upenn.edu
* Correspondence: karpyn@udel.edu; Tel.: +1-302-831-6428

Received: 21 August 2020; Accepted: 10 October 2020; Published: 16 October 2020

Abstract: This review examines current research on manipulations of U.S. food retail environments to promote healthier food purchasing and consumption. Studies reviewed use marketing strategies defined as the 4Ps (product, price, placement, promotion) to examine results based on single- and multi-component interventions by study design, outcome, and which of the "Ps" was targeted. Nine electronic databases were searched for publications from 2010 to 2019, followed by forward and backward searches. Studies were included if the intervention was initiated by a researcher or retailer, conducted in-store, and manipulated the retail environment. Of the unique 596 studies initially identified, 64 studies met inclusion criteria. Findings show that 56 studies had at least one positive effect related to healthier food consumption or purchasing. Thirty studies used single-component interventions, while 34 were multi-component. Promotion was the most commonly utilized marketing strategy, while manipulating promotion, placement, and product was the most common for multi-component interventions. Only 14 of the 64 studies were experimental and included objective outcome data. Future research should emphasize rigorous designs and objective outcomes. Research is also needed to understand individual and additive effects of multi-component interventions on sales outcomes, substitution effects of healthy food purchases, and sustainability of impacts.

Keywords: food access; nutrition; healthier food; dietary behaviors; review; retail food environment; dietary intake

---

1. Introduction

The promotion of healthy purchasing in shopping environments is a focal point of public health and research efforts aimed at reducing obesity and improving health outcomes. In the U.S., 71.2% percent of adults and 41.0% of children ages 2–19 have overweight or obesity, a condition that increases risk for cardiovascular disease, cancer, and diabetes [1,2]. Recent examination of American diets found most Americans eat more total calories, saturated fat, salt, and added sugar than they need, and do not consume enough fruits and vegetables, and whole grain products [3]. The majority of food purchasing occurs in supermarkets, which are uniquely positioned between the consumer and food purchasing decisions [4]. In addition to providing access to food, the in-store food retail environment is recognized for its influential role in dietary outcomes [5]. In-store, food retail interventions influencing the food purchasing decisions of consumers have grown in popularity over the past 10 years. This shift is in part due to the popularity of behavioral economics as a foundation by which customers may be "nudged", though indirect suggestions, toward healthier products [6,7]. Most commonly, research on in-store approaches is characterized by the 4Ps of marketing (product, price, promotion, and place) and approaches targeting consumer purchasing habits toward "better-for-you" products [8,9]. Such products are often lower-calorie, lower-sugar, lower-salt, or include more whole grains. Better-for-you products have been promoted in food retail settings to reach those at highest risk for diet-related disease [10].

Despite growing research, increasing recognition of the importance of marketing in the food retail environment and the popularizing practice of multi-component interventions, which manipulate more than one of the four Ps [11], there remain many unanswered questions about best practices for implementing effective in-store interventions. Food marketing and consumer behavior research is cross-disciplinary by nature, with outcomes published in outlets unique to industry, business, agriculture as well as public health, creating an aggregation challenge for practitioners.

This review seeks to update and build on prior reviews which terminate with studies published on or around 2010 [9,12,13] by analyzing U.S.-specific interventions occurring within the past 10 years with the goal of examining the extent to which contemporary manipulations of U.S. food retail environments (i.e., grocery and supermarket) specifically intended to promote healthier food purchasing and consumption are effective. Findings were synthesized and organized based on whether the intervention was a single-component intervention, which manipulates one of the four Ps, or a multi-component intervention, which manipulates more than one of the four Ps, and further broken down into the 4Ps of marketing and study design: Experimental, quasi-experimental, pre-experimental, and time series. An emphasis is placed on the marketing techniques utilized in study interventions in order to determine which strategies have been found to be most and least effective using different research designs and outcome measures.

2. Materials and Methods

This review used the Preferred Reporting Items for Systematic Reviews and Meta-analyses (PRISMA) guidelines [14].

2.1. Search Strategy

The authors used several methods to ensure a thorough and comprehensive review of the literature on in-store marketing interventions for healthy food promotion. First, a list of inclusion criteria was created to identify papers to be included in the review sample. Second, a list of key terms was created to search for studies. Third, appropriate databases were identified for the search based on the database topics. Finally, the database search was conducted to identify inclusion articles, and forward and backward searches were conducted for each inclusion article. Below are the processes used to identify studies for this review.

2.2. Inclusion Criteria

The studies included are original empirical research published between 2010 and 2019, in English, and from the United States. Studies were researcher- or retailor-initiated, conducted inside the retail environment, and manipulated the retail environment. Evaluations could be quantitative or mixed methods and all interventions had to include at least one of the following outcomes: (1) Purchasing-related (i.e., objective store sales data, objective food purchasing data, customer receipts, and survey self-reported purchases or expenditures, store sales, or intent to purchase), and/or (2) consumption-related (i.e., food frequency questionnaire (FFQ), 24-h dietary recall, food diary, Veggie Meter^{TM} or other biometrics, or other survey self-reported diet/consumption or intent to eat).

2.3. Exclusion Criteria

Interventions were excluded if they were implemented by an entity other than a researcher or retailer (e.g., price intervention at the wholesale level or front-of-pack labels initiated by a food company), if they did not occur inside the retail environment (e.g., restaurants, schools, mobile food trucks, online, and laboratory), or if they did not manipulate the retail environment (e.g., grocery store tours).

2.4. Search Terms and Databases

Nine databases (i.e., Academic OneFile, Business Source Premier, CAB Abstracts, Communication and Mass Media Complete, Family and Society Studies Worldwide, PsycINFO, PubMed, Sociological Abstracts, and Web of Science) from a variety of sectors (i.e., agriculture, business, communication, health, and psychology) were searched. Key terms were constructed based on three concepts: (1) Healthier food, (2) study design, and (3) setting. A variety of search terms were used to ensure articles would be included with nuanced differences in terms (e.g., healthy food vs. better-for-you) across sectors. The following key terms were used in all databases:

Healthier food	"health* food*" OR "healthy eating" OR "fruit*" OR "vegetable*" OR "low* fat" OR "low* sodium" OR "low* sugar" OR "low-fat" OR "low-sodium" OR "low-sugar" OR "better for you" OR "nutritio*"
Study design	"intervention" OR "pilot" OR "experiment*"
Setting	"supermarket*" OR "grocery store*" OR "corner store*" OR "bodega*" OR "retail environment"

2.5. Procedure of Article Search

RefWorks database was used to organize all articles. The searches were conducted by two authors and yielded 1231 studies (see Figure 1). After excluding 635 duplicate articles, two authors reviewed each full-text article to determine eligibility and excluded 548 studies. This review yielded 42 articles that met all inclusion criteria. Then, citation and bibliography searches were conducted with all 42 articles identifying an additional 22 articles for a final total of 64 articles (see Table 1).

After removing duplicates, two reviewers independently screened the title, abstract, and full text of the remaining 596 articles. Reviewers discussed any differences and consulted a third reviewer, when necessary, and a consensus was reached. One reviewer conducted forward and backward searches of the included articles. Titles and then full texts were reviewed to assess eligibility. Articles were abstracted and coded independently with two coders; discrepancies were discussed until a consensus was reached. Article abstractions included participants, study design, intervention description, 4 Ps, intervention setting, duration of intervention, data collection methods, outcome variables, and key findings. Our research reviewed studies and categorized them according to the 4 Ps: Product, price, promotion, and/or placement. Examples of interventions that were classified as product included determining how many and how much variety of a product to stock. Interventions that examined price included strategies such as price reductions and coupons. Furthermore, examples of interventions classified as promotion included shelf labels, recipe cards, and taste tests, and examples of placement strategies included altering the in-store location of products, such as moving to an endcap or to eye level. Our review included an examination for biases, with a focus on research design (eliminating confounders) and measures (i.e., self-report vs. objective data). Bias was assessed using the principles laid out in the Cochrane risk of bias tool [15].

Table 1. Study design characteristics for inclusion articles.

Factor		n	%
Intervention Setting (n = 64) [1]			
	Supermarket	28	43.8%
	Corner Store (including tiendas, bodegas, and small food stores)	20	31.3%
	Grocery Store (including small markets, country stores, and local independent owned stores)	17	26.6%
	Convenience Store	6	9.4%
	Supercenter	2	3.1%
	Trading Post	2	3.1%
	Other (including large food retail stores and local food co-ops)	8	12.5%
Research Design (n = 65) [2]			
	Experiment	23	35.4%
	Quasi-experiment	18	27.7%
	Pre-experiment	22	33.8%
	Time Series	2	3.1%
Outcome Measures (n = 64) [3]			
Purchasing-Related Measures			
	Objective Store Sales Data	29	45.3%
	Objective Food Purchasing Data	6	9.4%
	Customer Receipts	5	7.8%
	Self-Report Purchases or Expenditures	25	39.1%
	Self-Report Store Sales	2	3.1%
	Self-Report Intent to Purchase	8	12.5%
Consumption-Related Measures			
	FFQ	2	3.1%
	24-h Dietary Recall	3	4.7%
	Veggie Meter™ or other biometrics	1	1.6%
	Self-Report Intent to Eat	1	1.6%
	Other Self-Report Diet/Consumption Survey	12	18.8%
	Food Diary	0	–
Duration of intervention (n = 64)			
	1 min to 24 h	4	6.2%
	>24 h to 1 week	2	3.1%
	>1 week to 1 month	6	9.4%
	>1 month to 3 months	12	18.8%
	>4 months to 6 months	15	23.4%
	>6 months to 1 years	9	14.1%
	>1 year	15	23.4%
	Not reported	1	1.6%
Duration of follow-up (n = 66) [4]			
	No follow-up (i.e., collected data while intervention was being implemented)	24	36.4%
	Immediately following the intervention	15	22.7%
	Not reported	4	6.1%
	≤1 week	1	1.5%
	>1 week to 1 month	6	9.1%
	>1 month to 3 months	3	4.5%
	>3 months to 1 year	10	15.2%
	>1 year	3	4.5%

Table 1. Cont.

Factor		n	%
Participant sample size at follow-up (n = 64)			
	Not reported or indeterminate	17	26.6%
	≤100	10	15.6%
	101–500	23	35.9%
	501–1000	8	12.5%
	>1000	6	9.4%
Store sample size at follow-up (n = 64)			
	Not reported, not applicable, or indeterminate	21	32.8%
	≤2	13	20.3%
	3–10	19	29.7%
	11–20	4	6.3%
	>20	7	10.9%
Participant response rate at follow-up (n = 64)			
	Not reported, not applicable, or indeterminate	41	64.1%
	<50%	3	4.7%
	50% to 75%	12	18.8%
	76% to 90%	4	6.2%
	>90%	4	6.2%

[1] Percentages do not add up to 100 because multiple intervention settings were used in some studies; [2] One intervention had two study designs; [3] Percentages do not add up to 100 because multiple outcomes were used in some studies; [4] Two interventions have different follow-up periods for difference stores.

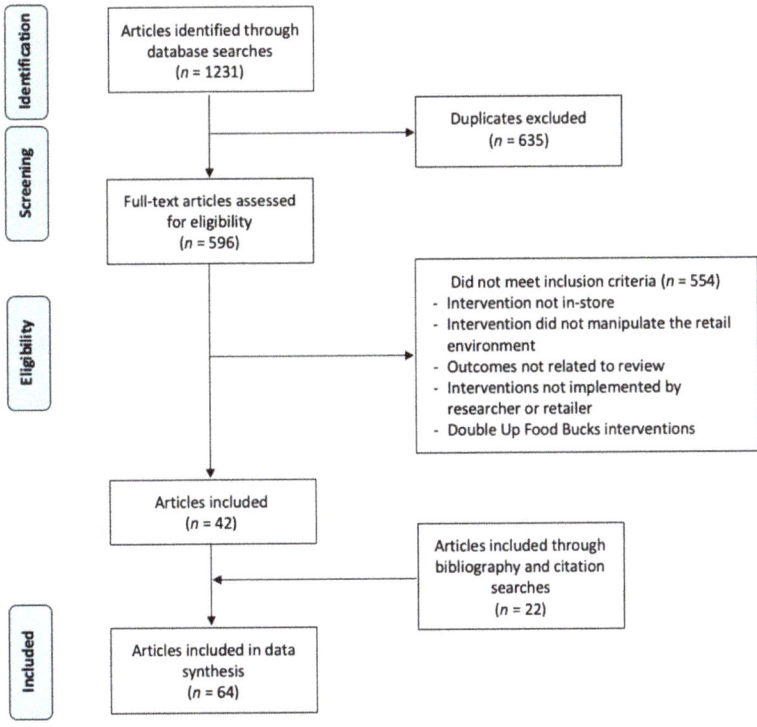

Figure 1. Article inclusion flow chart.

3. Results

3.1. Features of Included Articles

The primary intervention sites varied in terms of store size and included supermarkets (43.8%), corner stores (31.3%), grocery stores (26.6%), and/or convenience stores (9.4%) (see Table 1). Experimental designs accounted for about one-third (35.4%) of available studies, while the remaining were pre-experimental (33.8%), quasi-experimental (27.7%), or time series (3.1%). The most frequently used objective outcome data were store sales data (46.9%), while self-reported purchasing or expenditures was the most frequently used self-report measure (40.6%). Intervention length varied from 22 min to 3.5 years. Most studies (89%) incorporated promotion as a key component of the intervention, although efforts to address product (34%) and placement (31%) were also prominent. Relatively few interventions focused on price (16%). A total of 56 of 64 studies (87.5%) had at least one positive effect. When considering only objective measures of sales and more rigorous methods of determining dietary intake (i.e., 24 h recalls or biometric data), 100% (14 out of 14) had at least one positive effect.

3.2. Single- and Multi-Component Interventions

Thirty interventions were classified as single-component interventions because they only manipulated one of the four Ps, while 34 interventions were classified as multi-component. Over the past 10 years, the number of single- and multi-component interventions have both slightly increased (see Figure 2).

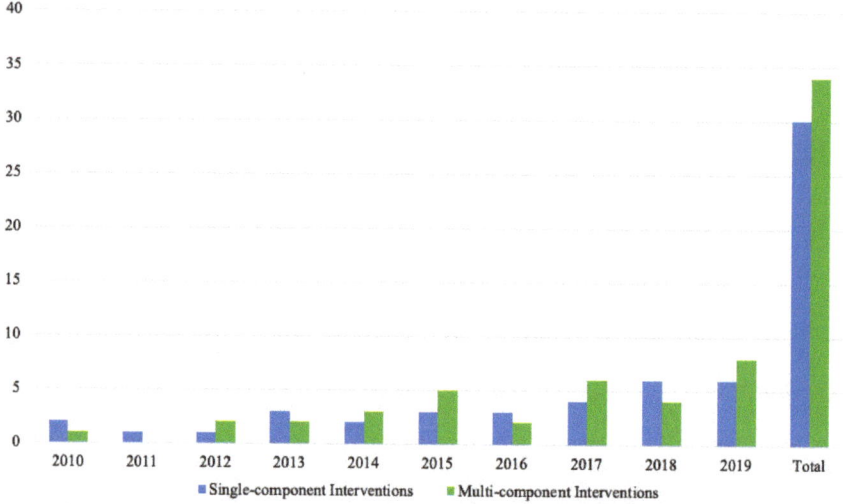

Figure 2. Number of single- and multi-component interventions by year.

3.3. Single-Component Interventions

Among the 30 single-component interventions, 27 had at least one positive effect on improving consumption and purchasing of healthier foods. Promotion was the most commonly utilized marketing P and was the focus of 23 studies. Overall, 1 study had mixed effects (positive + negative) [16], 5 had mixed effects (positive + null) [17–21], 8 had mixed effects (positive + null + negative) [22–29], 1 had negative effects [30], 2 had null effects [31,32], and 13 had positive effects [33–45], (see Table 2).

Table 2. Summary of included single-component interventions: Design, focus, and effects.

References	Study Design	Price	Prod	Prom	Place	Other	Intervention Name & Length	Outcome Measures	Food Categories	Effect
Milliron et al., A point-of-purchase intervention featuring in-person supermarket education affects healthful food purchases. (2012) [17].	EXP			P			*EatSmart* program, 4 months	Customer receipts [+] Objective food purchasing data (digital photographs) [+, null]	Fruits and vegetables (fresh)	Mixed~~
Geliebter et al., Supermarket discounts of low-energy density foods: Effects on purchasing, food intake, and body weight. (2013) [33].	EXP	P					Supermarket discounts intervention, 8 weeks	Objective store sales data [+] 24-h dietary recall [+]	Fruits and vegetables	Positive
Kiesel & Villas-Boas, Can information costs affect consumer choice? nutritional labels in a supermarket experiment. (2013) [22].	EXP			P			Nutritional labelling intervention, 4 weeks	Objective store sales data [+, −, null]	Salty snacks (popcorn)	Mixed~~~
Tal & Wansink, An apple a day brings more apples your way: Healthy samples prime healthier choices. (2015) [34].	EXP			P			Healthy and indulgent food samples, Not reported	Objective food purchasing data (bag checks) [+]	Fruits and vegetables	Positive
Bernales-Korins et al., Psychosocial influences on fruit and vegetable intake following a NYC supermarket discount. (2017) [18].	EXP	P					Supermarket discount intervention, 8 weeks	Objective store sales data [+, null] 24-h dietary recall [+, null]	Fruits and vegetables	Mixed~~
Liu et al., The Sales Impact of Featuring Healthy Foods, Indulgent Foods, or Both: Findings from a Large-Scale Retail Field Study. (2018) [23].	EXP				P		Endcap food displays, 2 months	Objective store sales data [+, −, null]	Nuts Protein (protein bars) Salty snacks (granola bars) Sweets (candy and cookies)	Mixed~~~
Palacios et al., Effectiveness of the Nutritional App "MyNutriCart" on Food Choices Related to Purchase and Dietary Behavior: A Pilot Randomized Controlled Trial. (2018) [24].	EXP			P			"MyNutricart" smartphone application, 8 weeks	Customer receipts [+] FFQ [+, null] 24-h dietary recall [+, −]	Beverages (100% juice) Dairy Fruits and vegetables Grains Legumes Proteins (meats) Salty Snacks Sweets	Mixed~~~

125

Table 2. Cont.

References	Study Design	Price	Prod	Prom	Place	Other	Intervention Name & Length	Outcome Measures	Food Categories	Effect
Biswas et al., Sounds like a healthy retail atmospheric strategy: effects of ambient music and background noise on food sales. (2019) [16].	EXP					P	Retail atmosphere intervention, 2 weekdays	Objective store sales data [+, −]	Dairy (yogurt and eggs) Fruits and vegetables Grains (bread) Protein (ham and pork) Salty snacks (chips) Soup Sweets (candy, cakes, and cookies)	Mixed^
Biswas & Szocs, The smell of healthy choices: Cross-modal sensory compensation effects of ambient scent on food purchases. (2019) [35].	EXP					P	Ambient scent 1 h	Customer receipts [+]	Dairy (milk) Fruits and vegetables (including fried potatoes) Grains (crackers) Protein (chicken) Salty snacks (chips) Sweets (Rice Krispy treats and fruit cobbler)	Positive
Berning et al., Do positive nutrition shelf labels affect consumer behavior? findings from a field experiment with scanner data. (2011) [30].	QE			P			Positive nutrition shelf labels, 4 weeks	Objective store sales data [−]	Salty snack (popcorn)	Negative
Rahkovsky et al., Effects of the Guiding Stars Program on purchases of ready-to-eat cereals with different nutritional attributes. (2013) [36].	QE			P			Guiding Stars, 20 months	Objective store sales data [+]	Grains (cereal)	Positive
Nikolova & Inman, Healthy choice: The effect of simplified point-of-sale nutritional information on consumer food choice behavior. (2015) [37].	QE			P			NuVal Nutritional Scoring System, 6 months	Objective store sales data [+]	Dairy (yogurt and ice cream) Frozen meals (pizza) Salty snacks (granola bars) Sauces and dressing Soup	Positive
Schultz & Litchfield, Evaluation of traditional and technology-based grocery store nutrition education. (2016) [38].	QE			P			Aisle demonstrations and technology-based education treatments, 4 months	Other self-report diet/consumption survey [+]	Fruits and vegetables Grains (whole grains) Protein (lean meats and seafood)	Positive

Table 2. Cont.

References	Study Design	Price	Prod	Prom	Place	Other	Intervention Name & Length	Outcome Measures	Food Categories	Effect
Finnell et al., 1% low-fat milk has perks!: An evaluation of a social marketing intervention. (2016) [25].	QE			P			1% Low-Fat Milk Has Perks!, 12 weeks	Objective store sales data [+, −, null]	Dairy (milk)	Mixed~~~
Zhen & Zheng, The impact of NuVal shelf nutrition labels on food purchase. (2017) [39].	QE			P			NuVal Nutritional Scoring System, 4 months	Objective store sales data [+]	Dairy [yogurt]	Positive
Bachman & Arigo, Reported influences on restaurant-type food selection decision making in a grocery store chain. (2018) [26].	QE			P			Calorie labelling intervention, 1 month	Self-report purchases [+, −, null]	Deli and bakery prepared foods	Mixed~~~
Jilcott Pitts et al., One-year follow-up examination of the impact of the North Carolina Healthy Food Small Retailer Program on healthy food availability, purchases, and consumption. (2018) [31].	QE			P			North Carolina Healthy Food Small Retailer Program, 6 months	Objective food purchasing data (bag checks) [null] Veggie Meter™ [null] Other self-report diet/consumption survey [null]	Beverages (SSBs) Fruits and vegetables (fresh, canned, and frozen)	Null
Jetter & Cassady, Increasing fresh fruit and vegetable availability in a low-income neighborhood convenience store: A pilot study. (2010) [40].	PE		P				Produce availability intervention, 7 months	Objective store sales data [+]	Fruits and vegetables (fresh)	Positive
Sutherland et al., Guiding Stars: The effect of a nutrition navigation program on consumer purchases at the supermarket. (2010) [41].	PE			P			Guiding Stars, 2 years	Objective store sales data [+]	Grains (cereal)	Positive
Bangia & Palmer-Keenan, Grocery store podcast about omega-3 fatty acids influences shopping behaviors: A pilot study. (2014) [42].	PE			P			Podcast, 5 min	Self-report purchases [+] Self-report intent to purchase [+]	Protein (N-3-rich foods)	Positive
Cawley et al., The impact of a supermarket nutrition rating system on purchases of nutritious and less nutritious foods. (2015) [19].	PE			P			Guiding Stars, 15 months	Objective store sales data [+, null]	All food categories	Mixed~~~

Table 2. Cont.

References	Study Design	Price	Prod	Prom	Place	Other	Intervention Name & Length	Outcome Measures	Food Categories	Effect
Weiss et al., Consumer taste tests and milk preference in low-income, urban supermarkets. (2015) [43].	PE			P			Healthy Retail Solutions milk taste testing intervention, 2 min >>note same study as Foster et al., 2014	Self-report intent to purchase [+]	Dairy (milk)	Positive
Bangia et al., A point-of-purchase intervention using grocery store tour podcasts about omega-3s increases long-term purchases of omega-3-rich food items. (2017) [20].	PE			P			Podcast, 22 min	Objective store sales data [+] Self-report intent to purchase [null]	Protein (N-3-rich foods)	Mixed~
Lopez et al., Development and evaluation of a nutritional smartphone application for making smart and healthy choices in grocery shopping. (2017) [44].	PE			P			Smartphone nutrition application, 8 weeks	Self-report purchases [+]	Fruits and vegetables	Positive
Gustafson & Zeballos, The effect of ingredient-specific calorie information on calories ordered. (2018) [27].	PE			P			Ingredient specific calorie labeling, 8 months	Customer receipts [+, −, null]	Dairy (cheese) Grains (bread) Protein (deli meats) Vegetables	Mixed~~~
Finkelstein et al., Identifying the effect of shelf nutrition labels on consumer purchases: results of a natural experiment and consumer survey. (2018) [21].	PE			P			NuVal Nutritional Scoring System, 138 weeks	Objective store sales data [+, null]	Dairy (miscellaneous dairy, milk, and yogurt)	Mixed~
Gustafson et al., Community-wide efforts to improve the consumer food environment and physical activity resources in rural Kentucky. (2019) [45].	PE			P			Plate it Up Kentucky Proud (PIUKP), 12 months	Other self-report diet/consumption survey [+]	Fruits and vegetables	Positive
Melo et al., Does point-of-sale nutrition information improve the nutritional quality of food choices? (2019) [28].	PE			P			NuVal Nutritional Scoring System, 14 months	Objective store sales data [+, −, null]	Dairy (yogurt) Frozen meals Grains (cereal)	Mixed~~~

Table 2. *Cont.*

References	Study Design	Price	Prod	Prom	Place	Other	Intervention Name & Length	Outcome Measures	Food Categories	Effect
Privitera et al., Impact of price elasticity on the healthfulness of food choices by gender. (2019) [29].	PE	P					Price elasticity conditions, 1 week	Self-report purchases [+, null] Self-report expenditures [+, −, null]	Fruits and vegetables	Mixed^^^^
Sutton et al., Healthy food marketing and purchases of fruits and vegetables in large grocery stores. (2019) [32].	PE			P			Nutrition Education and Obesity Prevention program, 5 months	Self-report purchases [null]	Fruits and vegetables	Null

EXP = experimental; QE = quasi-experiment; PE = pre-experiment; Mixed^ = positive + negative; Mixed^^ = positive + null; Mixed^^^^ = positive + null + negative; 'P' indicates that the intervention utilized this marketing approach.

3.3.1. Product

Of the 30 single-component interventions, only one intervention manipulated product [40]. The study utilized a pre-experimental design and found positive effects on produce sales after increasing stocking and availability of fresh produce [40].

3.3.2. Placement

One study implemented a placement-only intervention [23]. This experimental study had mixed effects (positive + null + negative). Positive effects were found such that featuring healthy products in aisle endcaps increased sales of these healthy products. However, when healthy products and indulgent products were featured together in aisle endcaps, sales of indulgent products increased while healthy products did not increase [23].

3.3.3. Price

Three studies implemented price-only interventions [18,29,33]. One study had mixed effects (positive + null + negative) [29], while another had mixed effects (positive + null) [18] and one study had only positive effects [33]. Both experimental studies provided a 50% discount for fruits and vegetables [18,33] and found that customers who received the discount purchased significantly more fruits and vegetables than customers who did not receive the discount [18,33]. However, one study also found no sustained effect on participants' spending on fruits and vegetables from baseline to follow-up period [18]. In addition, one study used a pre-experimental design [29].

3.3.4. Promotion

Twenty-three studies used a promotion strategy [17,19–22,24–28,30–32,34,36–39,41–45] as the sole intervention approach. Ten promotion interventions had positive effects [34,36–39,41–45], four reported mixed effects (positive + null) [17,19–21], six reported mixed effects (positive + null + negative) [22,24–28], two reported null effects [31,32], and one reported negative effects [30].

Four studies used experimental designs [17,18,22,34]. The interventions focused on nutrition shelf labeling [18], food samples [34], nutrition education [17], and a smartphone app [24]. One study found positive effects on fruit and vegetables purchases [34], while another study found mixed effects (positive + null) on food purchasing (e.g., positive effects on servings of fruit and no effect on servings of vegetables) [17]. Two studies found mixed effects (positive + null + negative) for the change in consumption and purchases of products authors classified as healthier (e.g., fruits, vegetables, and whole grains) as compared to products identified as less healthy (e.g., higher calorie products and sweets) [24] and for change in the sale of popcorn using different nutrition shelf labels [22]. One example of a study with largely positive results used a combination of shelf labels (e.g., "healthier option," "low sodium") in combination with education about the labels [17]. Positive effects were found such that customers purchased more servings of fruits and dark-green/bright-yellow vegetables. However, there were no significant differences between the groups on saturated fat, trans fat, and servings of vegetables [17].

Eight studies focused only on promotion, utilizing quasi-experimental designs [25,26,30,31,36–39]. Of these, four studies tested shelf labels [30,36,37,39], one examined the effectiveness of nutrition information labeling [26], one utilized a mass media campaign [25], one tested food demonstrations [38], and one examined the ability of increased stocking and promotions to sell healthy items [31]. Three found positive effects on purchases of healthier products [36,37,39] and one found positive effects regarding self-reported fruit and vegetable consumption [38]. One study had null effects on healthy food purchases and consumption, using both self-report measures and a skin carotenoid test [31]. Another study found negative effects on the demand for healthy popcorn [30]. Two studies found mixed effects (positive + null + negative) on sales of milk and the influence of caloric information on purchases [25,26].

Pre-experimental study designs reflected the majority of single-component intervention studies employing promotion [19–21,27,28,32,41–45]. Five implemented shelf labels [19,21,27,28,41], two used mass media social marketing campaigns [32,45], two implemented podcasts [20,42], one used taste tests [43], and one used a smartphone app [44].

3.3.5. Other

In addition to the 4Ps, two studies did not fit into the standard 4P framework and therefore were classified as "other" [16,35]. Both utilized experimental study designs. One examined the effects of ambient music [16] and the other study analyzed effects of ambient scents [35]. Findings showed mixed effects (positive + negative) as lower volume music increased healthier purchasing patterns and higher volume music increased unhealthier purchases [16]. Additionally, findings showed positive effects when using an in-store indulgent scent (i.e., chocolate chip cookies), which led to increased purchasing of healthier foods, and decreased purchasing of unhealthy foods [35].

3.4. Multi-Component Interventions

Out of the 34 multi-component interventions, 13 interventions included two Ps [46–58], 20 interventions included three Ps [59–78], and one intervention included all four Ps [79]. All of the multi-component interventions included promotion. Overall, 8 had positive effects [57,58,65,66,71,73,75,76], 2 studies had mixed effects (positive + negative) [68,78], 13 had mixed effects (positive + null) [46,47,49,51–53,56,59–62,64,72], 4 had mixed effects, (positive + null + negative) [50,55,63,77], and 7 had null effects [48,54,67,69,70,74,79] (see Table 3).

Table 3. Summary of included multi-component interventions: Design, focus, and effects.

References	Study Design	Price	Prod	Prom	Place	Other	Intervention Name & Length	Outcome Measures	Food Categories	Effect
Ayala et al., Efficacy of a store-based environmental change intervention compared with a delayed treatment control condition on store customers' intake of fruits and vegetables. (2013). [46]	EXP			P	P		Food marketing campaign 4 months	Other self-report diet/consumption survey [+, null]	Fruits and vegetables (fresh, canned, and frozen)	Mixed~~
Gittelsohn et al., A food store-based environmental intervention is associated with reduced BMI and improved psychosocial factors and food-related behaviors on the Navajo nation. (2013) [47].	EXP		P	P			Navajo Healthy Stores 14 months	Self-report intent to purchase [+, null] Self-report intent to eat [+, null] Self-report purchases [+, null]	41 healthy food items and 12 unhealthy food items: Beverages (soda) Grains (whole-wheat bread)	Mixed~~
Foster et al., Placement and promotion strategies to increase sales of healthier products in supermarkets in low-income, ethnically diverse neighborhoods: A randomized controlled trial. (2014) [59].	EXP		P	P	P		In-store marketing strategies intervention 6 months	Objective store sales data [+, null]	Beverages Dairy (milk) Frozen meals Grains (cereal)	Mixed~~
Lent et al., A randomized controlled study of a healthy corner store initiative on the purchases of urban, low-income youth. (2014) [48].	EXP		P	P			Snackin' Fresh Intervention 2 years	Self-report purchases [null]	Beverages Grains (bread) Protein (deli meat) Salty snacks (chips) Sweets (candy)	Null
Martinez-Donate et al., Evaluation of a pilot healthy eating intervention in restaurants and food stores of a rural community: A randomized community trial. (2015) [49].	EXP		P	P			Waupaca Eating Smart 10 months	Self-report purchases [+, null]	Fruits and vegetables	Mixed~~
Shin et al., Impact of Baltimore healthy eating zones: An environmental intervention to improve diet among African American youth. (2015) [50].	EXP		P	P			Baltimore Healthy Eating Zones 8 months	Self-report purchases [+, −, null] Self-report intent to purchase [+, −]	Fruits and vegetables Grains (whole wheat bread and cereal) Salty snacks (trail mix) Nuts and seeds	Mixed~~

Table 3. Cont.

References	Study Design	Price	Prod	Prom	Place	Other	Intervention Name & Length	Outcome Measures	Food Categories	Effect
Gittelsohn et al., The impact of a multi-level multi-component childhood obesity prevention intervention on healthy food availability, sales, and purchasing in a low-income urban area. (2017) [51].	EXP		P	P			B'more Healthy Communities for Kids (BHCK), 2 years	Objective store sales data [+, null] Self-report purchases [null]	Beverages (soda, energy drinks, water, 100% fruit juice, and unsweetened tea) Dairy (milk and yogurt) Fruits and vegetables (fresh and dried) Grains (cereals and bread) Nuts and seeds Protein (canned tuna and dried beans) Salty snacks (pretzels, and chips)	Mixed^
Thorndike et al., Choice architecture to promote fruit and vegetable purchases by families participating in the special supplemental program for women, infants, and children (WIC): Randomized corner store pilot study. (2017) [66].	EXP		P	P	P		Choice architecture intervention 5 months	Objective store sales data [+] Self-report purchases [+, null]	Fruits and vegetables	Mixed^
Banerjee & Nayak, Believe it or not: Health education works. (2018) [52].	EXP			P			Healthy food consumption education 2 weeks	Objective store sales data [+, null]	Fruits and vegetables (fresh) Grains (whole grain)	Mixed^
Trude et al., A multilevel, multicomponent childhood obesity prevention group-randomized controlled trial improves healthier food purchasing and reduces sweet-snack consumption among low-income African-American youth. (2018) [61].	EXP		P	P	P		BHCK 14 months	Self-report purchases [+, null]	Dairy (string cheese, yogurt, and ice cream) Fruits and vegetables (fresh and canned) Grains (cereals) Salty snacks (popcorn, chips, and pretzels) Sweets (candy, cookies, cakes, pies, and donuts)	Mixed^
Bird Jernigan et al., A Healthy Retail Intervention in Native American Convenience Stores: The THRIVE Community-Based Participatory Research Study. (2019) [79].	EXP	P	P	P	P		Tribal Health and Resilience in Vulnerable Environments study 9–12 months	Other self-report diet/consumption survey [null]	Fruits and vegetables (including fried potatoes) Protein (meat) Salty snacks (chips)	Null

133

Table 3. *Cont.*

References	Study Design	Price	Prod	Prom	Place	Other	Intervention Name & Length	Outcome Measures	Food Categories	Effect
Trude et al., The impact of a multilevel childhood obesity prevention intervention on healthful food acquisition, preparation, and fruit and vegetable consumption on African-American adult caregivers. (2019) [62].	EXP		P	P	P		BHCK 14 months	Other self-report diet/consumption survey [+, null] Self-report purchases [null]	Fruits and vegetables	Mixed~~
Wensel et al., B'more healthy corner stores for moms and kids: Identifying optimal behavioral economic strategies to increase WIC redemptions in small urban corner stores. (2019) [63].	EXP		P	P	P		B'more Healthy Corner Stores 4 Moms and Kids 1 year	Objective store sales data [+, −, null]	Beverages (juice) Dairy Fruits and vegetables (fresh) Grain (miscellaneous grains and cereal) Infant foods and formula Protein	Mixed~~~
Gittelsohn et al., An urban food store intervention positively affects food-related psychosocial variables and food behaviors. (2010) [64].	QE	P	P	P			Baltimore Healthy Stores 10 weeks	FFQ [+, null] Self-report intent to purchase [+]	26 healthy food items: Beverages Dairy (milk) Fruits and vegetables Grains (cereal and pretzels)	Mixed~~
Steeves et al., A rural small food store pilot intervention creates trends toward improved healthy food availability. (2015) [65].	QE		P	P	P		Maryland Healthy Stores 4 months	Self-report store sales data [+]	Dairy (milk and cheese) Fruits and vegetables Grains (whole wheat bread) Salty snacks (baked chips)	Positive
Surkan et al., Eat Right-Live Well! supermarket intervention impact on sales of healthy foods in a low-income neighborhood. (2016) [66].	QE	P	P	P			Eat Right-Live Well! (ERLW), 3 months	Objective store sales data [+]	Beverages (sugar-sweetened beverages [SSBs]) Dairy Fruits and vegetables Grains Salty snacks Sweets	Positive

Table 3. Cont.

References	Study Design	Price	Prod	Prom	Place	Other	Intervention Name & Length	Outcome Measures	Food Categories	Effect
Ortega et al., Substantial improvements not seen in health behaviors following corner store conversions in two Latino food swamps. (2016) [67].	QE		P	P	P		Proyecto Mercado FRESCO 2 years	Self-report expenditures [null] Other self-report diet/consumption survey [null]	Fruits and vegetables	Null
Adjoian et al., Healthy checkout lines: A study in urban supermarkets. (2017) [68].	QE			P	P		Healthy checkout lanes 2 weeks	Objective food purchasing data (checkout line observations) [+, −]	Beverages (water and seltzer) Fruits (fresh and dried) Nuts and seeds Salty snacks (granola bars, trail mix, and chips)	Mixed^
Albert et al., A corner store intervention to improve access to fruits and vegetables in two Latino communities. (2017) [69].	QE		P	P	P		Proyecto MercadoFRESCO 3.5 years	Self-report purchases [null] Other self-report diet/consumption survey [null] Self-report expenditure [null]	Fruits and vegetables (fresh, canned, and frozen)	Null
Payne & Niculescu, Can healthy checkout end-caps improve targeted fruit and vegetable purchases? evidence from grocery and SNAP participant purchases. (2018) [53].	QE			P	P		Healthy checkout aisle end-caps 1 month	Objective store sales data [+, null]	Fruits and vegetables	Mixed^^
Gustafson et al., The association between the "Plate it Up Kentucky" supermarket intervention and changes in grocery shopping practices among rural residents. (2019) [70].	QE	P		P	P		Plate it Up Kentucky 3 months	Customer receipts [null] Other self-report diet/consumption survey [null]	Beverages (SSBs) Fruits and vegetables	Null
Moran et al., Make It Fresh, for Less! A supermarket meal bundling and electronic reminder intervention to promote healthy purchases among families with children. (2019) [54].	Study 1: QEStudy 2:EXP			P	P		Study 1: Make it Fresh for Less! Study 2: Electronic reminders 16 weeks	Objective store sales data [null] Self-report purchases [null]	Various meal recipe ingredients with and without fruits and vegetables	Null

Table 3. Cont.

References	Study Design	Price	Prod	Prom	Place	Other	Intervention Name & Length	Outcome Measures	Food Categories	Effect
Holmes et al., Effect of a grocery store intervention on sales of nutritious foods to youth and their families. (2012) [55].	Time series			P	P		Healthy Kids Campaign, 12 weeks	Objective food purchasing data (cart checks) [+] Objective store sales data [+, −, null]	Dairy (milk and string cheese) Fruits and vegetables (fresh) Grains (whole wheat bagels) Nuts and seeds (sunflower seeds) Salty snacks (chips)	Mixed~~
Chapman et al., Evaluation of three behavioural economics 'nudges' on grocery and convenience store sales of promoted nutritious foods. (2019) [56].	Time series			P	P		Behavioral economic nudges 6 months	Objective store sales data [+, null] Self-report intent to purchase [+]	Fruits and vegetables (fresh) Salty snack (granola bars)	Mixed~~
Dannefer et al., Healthy bodegas: Increasing and promoting healthy foods at corner stores in New York City. (2012) [71].	PE		P	P	P		Healthy Bodegas Initiative 5 months	Self-report purchases [+] Self-report store sales data [+]	Dairy (milk) Fruits and vegetables (fresh and canned) Grain (whole-grain bread) Salty Snacks	Positive
Paek et al., Assessment of a healthy corner store program (FIT store) in low-income, urban, and ethnically diverse neighborhoods in Michigan. (2014) [72].	PE	P	P	P			Fit Store Program 6 months	Other self-report diet/consumption survey [+, null] Self-report purchases [+]	Beverages (100% fruit juice) Dairy (low-fat milk) Fruits and vegetables (fresh) Grains (whole grain bread and brown rice) Salty snacks Nuts and seeds Legumes	Mixed~~
Gudzune et al., Increasing access to fresh produce by pairing urban farms with corner stores: a case study in a low-income urban setting. (2015) [73].	PE		P	P	P		Farmers and corner store intervention, 9 weeks	Objective store sales data [+]	Fruits and vegetables (fresh)	Positive

Table 3. *Cont.*

References	Study Design	Price	Prod	Prom	Place	Other	Intervention Name & Length	Outcome Measures	Food Categories	Effect
Lawman et al., Changes in quantity, spending, and nutritional characteristics of adult, adolescent and child urban corner store purchases after an environmental intervention. (2015) [74].	PE		P	P	P		Healthy Corner Store Initiative, 12 months	Objective food purchasing data (bag checks) [null] Self-report expenditure [null]	Beverages Grains (bread) Protein (deli meat) Salty Snacks (chips) Sweets (candy)	Null
Davis et al., Employee and customer reactions to a healthy in-store marketing intervention in supermarkets. (2016) [57].	PE			P	P		Healthy in-store marketing intervention 6 months	Self-report purchases [+]	Dairy (milk) Frozen meals Grains	Positive
Liu et al., Marketing strategies to encourage rural residents of high-obesity counties to buy fruits and vegetables in grocery stores. (2017) [75].	PE	P		P	P		PIUKP 4 months	Other self-report diet/consumption survey [+]	Fruits and vegetables	Positive
Rushakoff et al., Evaluation of Healthy2Go: a country store transformation project to improve the food environment and consumer choices in Appalachian Kentucky. (2017) [76].	PE		P	P	P		Healthy2Go 18 months	Self-report purchases [+] Self-report intent to purchase [+] Other self-report diet/consumption survey [+]	Beverages (water, soda, and 100% juice) Dairy (milk) Fruits and vegetables (fresh, canned, and frozen) Grains Salty snacks (chips) Nuts and seeds	Positive
Woodward-Lopez et al., Changes in consumer purchases in stores participating in an obesity prevention initiative. (2018) [77].	PE		P	P	P		Kaiser Permanente Healthy Eating and Active Living, 1 year (Zones 1 and 3) and 3 years (Zone 2)	Objective store sales data [+, −, null] Self-report purchases [+]	Beverages (SSBs) Fruits and vegetables Salty snacks (chips) Sweets (candy)	Mixed^
MacKenzie et al., Healthy Stores Initiative Associated with Produce Purchasing on Navajo Nation. (2019) [58].	PE			P	P		Healthy Navajo Stores Initiative 1 year	Self-report purchases [+]	Fruits and vegetables (fresh and frozen)	Positive
Paluta et al., Evaluating the impact of a healthy corner store initiative on food access domains. (2019) [78].	PE		P	P	P		Fresh Foods Here 10 months	Objective store sales data [+]	Healthy items which were classified as low sodium, low fat, and low sugar	Mixed^

EXP = experimental; QE = quasi-experiment; PE = pre-experiment; Mixed^ = positive + negative; Mixed^^ = positive + null; Mixed^^^ = positive + null + negative; 'P' indicates that the intervention utilized this marketing approach.

3.4.1. Interventions Including 2 Ps

Promotion and Placement

Seven studies examined the impact of interventions that used both promotion and placement strategies [46,53–58]. Two studies found positive effects [57,58], one found null effects [54], one found mixed (positive + null + negative) [55], and three found mixed effects (positive + null) [46,53,56].

An experimental design was used in only one study [46]. The intervention included a food marketing campaign (inclusive of food demonstrations, recipe cards, and an audio novella) featuring fruit and vegetable characters in tiendas [46]. Positive effects were found on daily fruit and vegetable intake but not variety [46].

Three studies employed quasi-experimental designs [53,54,58]. One intervention manipulated the in-store location of produce (i.e., moving pre-packaged produce near checkout lines), added shelf labels, and distributed recipe cards [58]. Another intervention focused on the effects of promoting meal bundles through in-store displays [54], while another examined the effects of pre-packaged produce packs moved to aisle endcaps packages [53]. One study found that shoppers who were exposed to the intervention were more likely to purchase produce [58], and another found that moving the pre-packaged produce near checkout lines increased healthy purchasing [53]. However, displaying meal bundles was ineffective in increasing healthy item sales [54]. One study used a pre-experimental design [57].

Two studies with time series designs addressed the effects of using behavioral nudges [56] and implementing a healthy food kiosk coupled with food sampling [55]. Results showed positive effects for healthy food sales when multiple behavioral nudges were implemented simultaneously [56] and when food sampling was combined with featured food kiosks [55]. Null and negative effects were found for healthy item sales when intervention tactics were isolated as well as among certain foods [55,56].

Promotion and Product

Five studies examined the impact of promotion and product interventions [47–51]. Three studies had mixed effects (positive + null) [47,49,51], one study had mixed effects (positive + null + negative) [50], and one had null effects [48].

All five studies utilized an experimental design [51,59–62] and included components related to increased stock of healthier items. Promotional strategies varied: One incorporated food demonstrations [47], one used social marketing campaigns [48], and all five used point-of-purchase promotions (e.g., taste testing, shelf labels, educational displays, food samples, and signage) [47–51]. All studies found at least one null effect on healthy food consumption and purchasing [47–51]. However, positive effects were shown in four of five studies as participants' intent to purchase healthier foods increased with exposure to the interventions [47,49–51].

Promotion and Price

Only one study examined the effects of promotion and price and it used an experimental design [52]. The intervention examined the effects of healthy food consumption education and coupons with mixed effects (positive + null) on healthier purchases. Combining education and coupons was the most effective intervention group for increasing healthier purchases while null effects were largely observed for education and coupon only groups [52].

3.4.2. Interventions Including 3 Ps

Promotion, Product, and Placement

Fifteen studies implemented interventions with promotion, product, and placement strategies [59–63,65,67–69,71,73,74,76–78]. Out of the 15, 2 had mixed effects (positive + negative) [68,78], 4 had mixed effects (positive + null) [59–62], 2 had mixed effects (positive + negative + null) [63,77], 3 had null effects [67,69,74], and 4 had positive effects [65,71,73,76].

Five studies were experimental [59–63]. The interventions included adding point-of-purchase promotions, changing the store structure and environment (e.g., adding a buffet bar or refrigerator, grouping products in a display), and altering the in-store location of products (e.g., multiple facings, prime placement, secondary placement, checkout aisle end-caps), and increased stocking of healthier products [59–63]. All five studies found mixed effects for improving the purchasing and consumption of healthy food. For example, Foster and colleagues (2014) implemented an intervention to increase the purchases of specific healthier foods through shelf tagging promotions and by altering the shelf placement of products [59]. In intervention stores, sales of 2% milk, whole milk, two targeted cereals, and one of three promoted frozen meals remained the same, while sales of skim milk, 1%, and two out of three frozen meals increased [59].

Four studies utilized quasi-experimental designs [65,67–69]. Two studies added point-of-purchase promotions, changed store structure and environment, altered in-store location, and increased stock of fresh produce [67,69]. Another study introduced healthier products to checkout lanes and added point-of-purchase promotions [68], and another changed store structure, increased media coverage about healthier choices, and offered in-store education sessions. Two studies found null effects on consumption and purchasing of fruits and vegetables [67,69], one found mixed effects (positive + negative) on consumer purchasing of healthy foods in healthy vs. standard checkout lanes [68], and one found positive effects of store owners' perceptions of changes in sales of promoted healthy foods [65]. Of these four quasi-experimental studies, two interventions were Proyecto MercadoFRESCO [67,69]. Both studies found null effects, such that there were no significant differences in consumption of and dollars spent on fruit and vegetables [67,69].

Six studies in this category used a pre-experimental [71,73,74,76–78] design. Similar to previous studies, strategies added point-of-purchase promotions, changed store structure and environment, altered in-store location, and increased stock of fresh produce [71,74,76–78]; one study implemented these strategies and paired urban farms with corner stores such that corner stores sold products obtained from urban farms [73]. Three studies found positive effects on purchases, sales, consumption, and intent to purchase healthy food [71,73,76].

Promotion, Product, and Price

Three studies utilized promotion, product, and price marketing strategies [64,66,72]. One study found positive effects [66] and two found mixed effects (positive + null) [64,72].

Of the three studies, two studies used a quasi-experimental design [64,66]. Both were multifaceted interventions that included increased stocking of healthy foods, point-of-purchase promotions, and price reductions/incentive cards [64,66]. One of the studies found when shelf labels were consistently used (high fidelity), positive effects on sales of the promoted, healthy items were found [66]. The second quasi-experimental study found mixed effects (positive + null): shelf labels on healthy items led to participants purchasing more promoted foods but did not change consumption. However, the study authors did not observe changes in healthy food consumption. Finally, one study used a pre-experimental design [72], with mixed results.

Promotion, Placement, and Price

Two studies examined the effects of promotion, placement, and price strategies [70,75]. One study found null effects [70] and the other found positive effects [75]. Both studies used similar interventions, Plate It Up Kentucky Proud [75] and Plate It Up [70], which added point-of-purchase promotions, altered product placement, and offered coupons and discounts [70,75].

One study used a quasi-experimental design [70]. The results showed null effects on fruit and vegetable consumption. The study authors found no difference in the percent of food purchasing dollars spent on fruits and vegetables between control and intervention groups [70]. In addition, Liu and colleagues (2017) used a pre-experimental design [75] and found that recipe cards had a positive effect on customers' purchases of recipe ingredients and increased consumption of fruits and vegetables [75].

3.4.3. Intervention Including 4 Ps

Finally, only one study utilized all four Ps [79]. The study used an experimental, participatory design and found null effects for fruit and vegetable consumption. However, there was a significant decrease in the consumption of some unhealthy foods (e.g., chips) [79]. The intervention increased stocking of healthy foods, altered the in-store environment, added point-of-purchase promotions, and included discounts [79].

4. Discussion

This review, which examined the scope and impact of in-store marketing strategies related to healthy food sales, purchasing, and measures of diet, yields several important conclusions. One key finding of this recent review of literature is that both single- and multi-component interventions have become equally common focal points of research. Approaches provide evidence that increasing access to healthy food products in stores, particularly while utilizing promotion strategies, increases healthy food sales, purchasing, or improves dietary outcomes. While prior reviews found that positive outcomes were more common in studies utilizing multiple Ps [12,13], ours found more parity, even when considering the level of rigor applied to research designs and outcome measures. Overall, positive results were found in 27 of 30 single-component interventions as compared to 29 of 34 multi-component interventions, despite that multi-component interventions reported results related to a higher quantity of outcome measures.

Promotion efforts, including shelf labels, call out messages, and sampling products, continue to show promise as an important mechanism to improve purchasing. In-store promotion interventions are increasingly common, often with positive effects, either in combination with other approaches, or used alone. Previous reviews have found that older interventions, specifically those prior to 2008, were more likely to manipulate promotion, most often in single-component interventions [9,11]. In the more recent studies examined in this review, promotional interventions were frequently paired with placement and product strategies in multi-component interventions, for example including the coupling of a shelf labeling intervention with an end of aisle display, yielding positive effects.

Prior literature has identified multi-component interventions' added complexities in deciphering effects of its individual components [4,11]. There are two reasons for this complexity. One is the layered nature of multi-component interventions which by definition result in activities such as taste-testing, coupled with an end-cap placement and a shelf tagging, which make it difficult to decipher how components work together or separately to influence purchasing. It is possible for example that similar effects could be seen from just a single-component intervention, rather than multiple, though such impacts are difficult to decipher. Future multi-component interventions should consider alternative research designs where elements of the intervention are incorporated at different times and in different combinations, and then removed and then incorporated again in order to understand collective and individual effects, such a 2×2 factorial design or an ABA design [80].

Limitations and Future Directions

Of 64 studies reviewed, 24 in total (38%) were conducted without a control or comparison group. Only 14 of the 64 studies were experimental and included objective outcome measure data. The lack of a control group in more than one-third of studies displays the limitations of food environment research. Studies conducted with control groups, using store sales outcome data, and using rigorous dietary outcome measures are needed. Further research is also needed to better understand the individual and additive effects of multi-component interventions on outcomes like product sales.

The literature is limited in its ability to capture the extent to which increased healthy food sales results in overall less healthy food purchases. While several studies examine interventions in terms of specific product substitutions, for example by testing whether promoting a healthier item in a category results in changed sales in that product and a less healthy alternative (e.g., replacing higher fat popcorn with low-fat popcorn), few studies examine how targeted product sales relate to sales in other product categories (i.e., a spillover effect; e.g., increase in fruit sales associated with increase in low-fat dairy sales). Future research is needed to understand how increases in healthy food purchases do or do not serve to substitute for less healthy foods.

In addition to better understanding the marketing mechanisms that work best to shift purchasing, future research should examine the extent to which interventions yield sustained effects. Our review found that less than 20% of studies examined impacts beyond three months and only 4.5% considered impacts beyond one year.

It is unclear how the current COVID-19 context will continue to impact in-person food sales as compared to online sales and the extent to which product promotion and placement strategies can, or will, translate into online environments. Future work should seek to better understand how online food purchasing environments, including virtual supermarkets and real-world e-commerce platforms, can incorporate the four Ps to increase access to affordable foods.

5. Conclusions

Efforts to improve consumption and purchases of healthier foods in retail environments are diverse, even within the framework of the 4Ps. Considering these marketing strategies, this review found that promotion was the most commonly utilized strategy for single-component interventions, and manipulating promotion, placement, and product was the most common strategy used for multi-component intervention. In addition, interventions included in the review often employed pre-experimental or quasi-experimental research designs and relied more on self-report data rather than objective data. New research should implement interventions using rigorous designs and objective outcomes in order to advance the field. Further, given the large proportion of studies that implemented multi-component interventions, research is also needed to understand the individual and additive effects of approaches that use more than one of the 4Ps on objective sales outcomes, substitution effects of healthy food purchases, and the sustainability of impacts.

Author Contributions: A.K. contributed to the study concept and design. K.M. was responsible for screening. K.M. and H.W. extracted and coded the data, analyzed the data, and drafted the manuscript. A.K. critically reviewed all drafts. A.K. and K.G. approved the final version submitted for publication. All authors have read and agreed to the published version of the manuscript.

Funding: This research was funded by the National Institute of Health and Johns Hopkins Center for a Livable Future. Publication fees were supported by Healthy Eating Research, a national program of the Robert Wood Johnson Foundation.

Conflicts of Interest: The authors declare no conflict of interest.

References

1. Fryer, C.D.; Carroll, M.D.; Ogden, C.L. *Prevalence of Overweight, Obesity, and Severe Obesity among Children and Adolescents Aged 2–19 Years: United States, 1963–1965 through 2015–2016*; National Center for Health Statistics: Hyattsville, MD, USA, 2018.
2. Fryer, C.D.; Carroll, M.D.; Ogden, C.L. *Prevalence of Overweight, Obesity and Severe Obesity among Adults Aged 20 and over: United States, 1960–1962 through 2015–2016*; National Center for Health Statistics: Hyattsville, MD, USA, 2018.
3. Dietary Guidelines Advisory Committee. *Scientific Report of the 2020 Dietary Guidelines Advisory Committee: Advisory Report to the Secretary of Agriculture and the Secretary of Health and Human Services*; U.S. Department of Agriculture, Agricultural Research Service: Washington, DC, USA, 2020.
4. Cameron, A.J.; Charlton, E.; Ngan, W.W.; Sacks, G. A systematic review of the effectiveness of supermarket-based interventions involving product, promotion, or place on the healthiness of consumer purchases. *Curr. Nutr. Rep.* **2016**, *5*, 129–138. [CrossRef]
5. Caspi, C.E.; Sorensen, G.; Subramanian, S.V.; Kawachi, I. The local food environment and diet: A systematic review. *Health Place* **2012**, *18*, 1172–1187. [CrossRef] [PubMed]
6. Thaler, R.H.; Sunstein, C.R. *Nudge: Improving Decisions about Health, Wealth, and Happiness*, 6th ed.; Penguin Books: New York, NY, USA, 2009; pp. 115–179.
7. Wayman, E.; Madhvanath, S. Nudging Grocery Shoppers to Make Healthier Choices. In Proceedings of the 9th ACM Conference on Recommender Systems, Vienna, Austria, 16–20 September 2015; pp. 289–292. [CrossRef]
8. Kotler, P.; Armstrong, G. *Principles of Marketing*, 13th ed.; Prentice Hall Inc.: Upper Saddle River, NJ, USA, 2010.
9. Glanz, K.; Bader, M.D.; Iyer, S. Retail grocery store marketing strategies and obesity: An integrative review. *Am. J. Prev. Med.* **2012**, *42*, 503–512. [CrossRef] [PubMed]
10. Hudson Institute. *Better-For-You Foods: It's Just Good Business*; Hudson Institute's Obesity Solutions Initiative: Washington, DC, USA, 2011.
11. Mah, C.L.; Luongo, G.; Hasdell, R.; Taylor, N.G.; Lo, B.K. A systematic review of the effect of retail food environment interventions on diet and health with a focus on the enabling role of public policies. *Curr. Nutr. Rep.* **2019**, *8*, 411–428. [CrossRef] [PubMed]
12. Gittelsohn, J.N.; Rowan, M.; Gadhoke, P. Interventions in small food stores to change the food environment, improve diet, and reduce risk of chronic disease. *Prev. Chronic Dis.* **2012**, *9*, 1–15. [CrossRef]
13. Escaron, A.L.; Meinen, A.M.; Nitzke, S.A.; Martínez-Donate, A.P. Supermarket and grocery store–based interventions to promote healthful food choices and eating practices: A systematic review. *Prev. Chronic Dis.* **2013**, *10*, 1–20. [CrossRef] [PubMed]
14. Liberati, A.; Altman, D.G.; Tetzlaff, J.; Mulrow, C.; Gøtzsche, P.C.; Ioannidis, J.P.; Clarke, M.; Devereaux, P.J.; Kleijnen, J.; Moher, D. The PRISMA statement for reporting systematic reviews and meta-analyses of studies that evaluate health care interventions: Explanation and elaboration. *Ann. Intern. Med.* **2009**, *151*, 64–94. [CrossRef]
15. Higgins, J.P.; Altman, D.G.; Gøtzsche, P.C.; Jüni, P.; Moher, D.; Oxman, A.D.; Savović, J.; Schulz, K.F.; Weeks, L.; Sterne, J.A. The Cochrane Collaboration's tool for assessing risk of bias in randomised trials. *BMJ* **2011**, *343*, d5928. [CrossRef]
16. Biswas, D.; Lund, K.; Szocs, C. Sounds like a healthy retail atmospheric strategy: Effects of ambient music and background noise on food sales. *J. Acad. Mark.* **2019**, *47*, 37–55. [CrossRef]
17. Milliron, B.J.; Woolf, K.; Appelhans, B.M. A point-of-purchase intervention featuring in-person supermarket education affects healthful food purchases. *J. Nutr. Educ. Behav.* **2012**, *44*, 225–232. [CrossRef]
18. Bernales-Korins, M.; Ang, I.Y.H.; Khan, S.; Geliebter, A. Psychosocial influences on fruit and vegetable intake following a NYC supermarket discount. *Obes. Res.* **2017**, *25*, 1321–1328. [CrossRef]
19. Cawley, J.; Sweeney, M.J.; Sobal, J.; Just, D.R.; Kaiser, H.M.; Schulze, W.D.; Wansink, B. The impact of a supermarket nutrition rating system on purchases of nutritious and less nutritious foods. *Public Health Nutr.* **2015**, *18*, 8–14. [CrossRef] [PubMed]

20. Bangia, D.; Shaffner, D.W.; Palmer-Keenan, D. A point-of-purchase intervention using grocery store tour podcasts about omega-3s increases long-term purchases of omega-3-rich food items. *J. Nutr. Educ. Behav.* **2017**, *49*, 475–480. [CrossRef]
21. Finkelstein, E.A.; Li, W.; Melo, G.; Strombotne, K.; Zhen, C. Identifying the effect of shelf nutrition labels on consumer purchases: Results of a natural experiment and consumer survey. *Am. J. Clin. Nutr.* **2018**, *107*, 647–651. [CrossRef] [PubMed]
22. Kiesel, K.; Villas-Boas, S. Can information costs affect consumer choice? Nutritional labels in a supermarket experiment. *Int. J. Ind. Organ.* **2013**, *31*, 153–163. [CrossRef]
23. Liu, P.J.; Dallas, S.K.; Harding, M.; Fitzsimons, G.J. The Sales Impact of Featuring Healthy Foods, Indulgent Foods, or Both: Findings from a Large-Scale Retail Field Study. *J. Consum. Res.* **2018**, *3*, 346–363. [CrossRef]
24. Palacios, C.; Torres, M.; López, D.; Trak-Fellermeier, M.; Coccia, C.; Pérez, C. Effectiveness of the Nutritional App "MyNutriCart" on Food Choices Related to Purchase and Dietary Behavior: A Pilot Randomized Controlled Trial. *Nutrients* **2018**, *10*, 1967. [CrossRef]
25. Finnell, K.J.; John, R.; Thompson, D.M. 1% low-fat milk has perks! An evaluation of a social marketing intervention. *Prev. Med. Rep.* **2016**, *5*, 144–149. [CrossRef]
26. Bachman, J.L.; Arigo, D. Reported influences on restaurant-type food selection decision making in a grocery store chain. *J. Nutr. Educ. Behav.* **2018**, *50*, 555–563. [CrossRef]
27. Gustafson, C.R.; Zeballos, E. The effect of ingredient-specific calorie information on calories ordered. *Prev. Med. Rep.* **2018**, *12*, 186–190. [CrossRef]
28. Melo, G.; Zhen, C.; Colson, G. Does point-of-sale nutrition information improve the nutritional quality of food choices? *Econ. Hum. Biol.* **2019**, *35*, 133–143. [CrossRef]
29. Privitera, G.J.; Gillespie, J.J.; Zuraikat, F.M. Impact of price elasticity on the healthfulness of food choices by gender. *Health Educ. J.* **2019**, *78*, 428–440. [CrossRef]
30. Berning, J.P.; Chouinard, H.H.; McCluskey, J.J. Do positive nutrition shelf labels affect consumer behavior? Findings from a field experiment with scanner data. *Am. J. Agric. Econ.* **2011**, *93*, 364–369. [CrossRef]
31. Jilcott Pitts, S.; Wu, Q.; Truesdale, K.; Haynes-Maslow, L.; McGuirt, J.; Ammerman, A.; Laska, M. One-Year Follow-Up Examination of the Impact of the North Carolina Healthy Food Small Retailer Program on Healthy Food Availability, Purchases, and Consumption. *Int. J. Environ. Res. Public Health* **2018**, *15*, 2681. [CrossRef] [PubMed]
32. Sutton, K.; Caldwell, J.; Yoshida, S.; Thompson, J.; Kuo, T. Healthy food marketing and purchases of fruits and vegetables in large grocery stores. *Prev. Med. Rep.* **2019**, *14*, 100861. [CrossRef] [PubMed]
33. Geliebter, A.; Ang, I.Y.H.; Bernales-Korins, M.; Hernandez, D.; Ochner, C.N.; Ungredda, T.; Kolbe, L. Supermarket discounts of low-energy density foods: Effects on purchasing, food intake, and body weight. *Obes Res.* **2013**, *21*, E542–E548. [CrossRef] [PubMed]
34. Tal, A.; Wansink, B. An apple a day brings more apples your way: Healthy samples prime healthier choices. *Psychol. Mark.* **2015**, *32*, 575–584. [CrossRef]
35. Biswas, D.; Szocs, C. The smell of healthy choices: Cross-Modal sensory compensation effects of ambient scent on food purchases. *J. Mark. Res.* **2019**, *56*, 123–141. [CrossRef]
36. Rahkovsky, I.; Lin, B.H.; Lin, C.T.J.; Lee, J.Y. Effects of the Guiding Stars Program on purchases of ready-to-eat cereals with different nutritional attributes. *Food Policy* **2013**, *43*, 100–107. [CrossRef]
37. Nikolova, H.D.; Inman, J.J. Healthy choice: The effect of simplified point-of-sale nutritional information on consumer food choice behavior. *J. Mark. Res.* **2015**, *52*, 817–835. [CrossRef]
38. Schultz, J.; Litchfield, R. Evaluation of traditional and technology-based grocery store nutrition education. *Am. J. Health Educ.* **2016**, *47*, 355–364. [CrossRef]
39. Zhen, C.; Zheng, X. The impact of NuVal shelf nutrition labels on food purchase. *Appl. Econ. Perspect. Policy* **2017**, 1–15. [CrossRef]
40. Jetter, K.M.; Cassady, D.L. Increasing fresh fruit and vegetable availability in a low-income neighborhood convenience store: A pilot study. *Health Promot. Pract.* **2010**, *11*, 694–702. [CrossRef] [PubMed]
41. Sutherland, L.A.; Kaley, L.A.; Fischer, L. Guiding Stars: The effect of a nutrition navigation program on consumer purchases at the supermarket. *Am. J. Clin. Nutr.* **2010**, *91*, 1090S–1094S. [CrossRef]
42. Bangia, D.; Palmer-Keenan, D. Grocery store podcast about omega-3 fatty acids influences shopping behaviors: A pilot study. *J. Nutr. Educ. Behav.* **2014**, *46*, 616–620. [CrossRef]

43. Weiss, S.; Davis, E.; Wojtanowski, A.C.; Foster, G.D.; Glanz, K.; Karpyn, A. Consumer taste tests and milk preference in low-income, urban supermarkets. *Public Health Nutr.* **2015**, *18*, 1419–1422. [CrossRef]
44. Lopez, D.; Torres, M.; Velez, J.; Grullon, J.; Negron, E.; Perez, C.M.; Palacios, C. Development and evaluation of a nutritional smartphone application for making smart and healthy choices in grocery shopping. *Healthc. Inform. Res.* **2017**, *23*, 16–24. [CrossRef]
45. Gustafson, A.; McGladrey, M.; Stephenson, T.; Kurzynske, J.; Mullins, J.; Peritore, N.; Vail, A. Community-wide efforts to improve the consumer food environment and physical activity resources in rural Kentucky. *Prev. Chronic Dis.* **2019**, *16*. [CrossRef]
46. Ayala, G.X.; Baquero, B.; Laraia, B.A.; Ji, M.; Linnan, L. Efficacy of a store-based environmental change intervention compared with a delayed treatment control condition on store customers' intake of fruits and vegetables. *Public Health Nutr.* **2013**, *16*, 1953–1960. [CrossRef]
47. Gittelsohn, J.; Kim, E.M.; He, S.; Pardilla, M. A food store-based environmental intervention is associated with reduced BMI and improved psychosocial factors and food-related behaviors on the Navajo nation. *J. Nutr.* **2013**, *143*, 1494–1500. [CrossRef]
48. Lent, M.R.; Vander Veur, S.S.; McCoy, T.A.; Wojtanowski, A.C.; Sandoval, B.; Sherman, S.; Foster, G.D. A randomized controlled study of a healthy corner store initiative on the purchases of urban, low-income youth. *Obes. Res.* **2014**, *22*, 2494–2500. [CrossRef] [PubMed]
49. Martinez-Donate, A.P.; Riggall, A.J.; Meinen, A.M.; Malecki, K.; Escaron, A.L.; Hall, B.; Nitzke, S. Evaluation of a pilot healthy eating intervention in restaurants and food stores of a rural community: A randomized community trial. *BMC Public Health* **2015**, *15*, 136–147. [CrossRef]
50. Shin, A.Y.; Surkan, P.J.; Coutinho, A.J.; Suratkar, S.R.; Campbell, R.K.; Rowan, M.; Gittelsohn, J. Impact of Baltimore Healthy Eating Zones: An environmental intervention to improve diet among African American youth. *Health Educ. Behav.* **2015**, *42*, 97–105. [CrossRef] [PubMed]
51. Gittelsohn, J.; Trude, A.C.; Poirier, L.; Ross, A.; Ruggiero, C.; Schwendler, T.; Anderson Steeves, E. The impact of a multi-level multi-component childhood obesity prevention intervention on healthy food availability, sales, and purchasing in a low-income urban area. *Int. J. Environ. Res. Public Health* **2017**, *14*, 1371. [CrossRef]
52. Banerjee, T.; Nayak, A. Believe it or not: Health education works. *Obes. Res. Clin. Pract.* **2018**, *12*, 116–124. [CrossRef]
53. Payne, C.; Niculescu, M. Can healthy checkout end-caps improve targeted fruit and vegetable purchases? Evidence from grocery and SNAP participant purchases. *Food Policy* **2018**, *79*, 318–323. [CrossRef]
54. Moran, A.J.; Khandpur, N.; Polacsek, M.; Thorndike, A.N.; Franckle, R.L.; Boulos, R.; Rimm, E.B. Make it fresh, for less! A supermarket meal bundling and electronic reminder intervention to promote healthy purchases among families with children. *J. Nutr. Educ. Behav.* **2019**, *51*, 400–408. [CrossRef]
55. Holmes, A.S.; Estabrooks, P.A.; Davis, G.C.; Serrano, E.L. Effect of a grocery store intervention on sales of nutritious foods to youth and their families. *J. Acad. Nutr. Diet.* **2012**, *112*, 897–901. [CrossRef]
56. Chapman, L.E.; Sadeghzadeh, C.; Koutlas, M.; Zimmer, C.; De Marco, M. Evaluation of three behavioural economics 'nudges' on grocery and convenience store sales of promoted nutritious foods. *Public Health Nutr.* **2019**, *22*, 3250–3260. [CrossRef]
57. Davis, E.L.; Wojtanowski, A.C.; Weiss, S.; Foster, G.D.; Karpyn, A.; Glanz, K. Employee and customer reactions to a healthy in-store marketing intervention in supermarkets. *J. Food Res.* **2016**, *5*, 107–113. [CrossRef]
58. MacKenzie, O.W.; George, C.V.; Pérez-Escamilla, R.; Lasky-Fink, J.; Piltch, E.M.; Sandman, S.M.; Shin, S.S. Healthy Stores Initiative Associated with Produce Purchasing on Navajo Nation. *CDN* **2019**, *3*, nzz125. [CrossRef] [PubMed]
59. Foster, G.D.; Karpyn, A.; Wojtanowski, A.C.; Davis, E.; Weiss, S.; Brensinger, C.; Glanz, K. Placement and promotion strategies to increase sales of healthier products in supermarkets in low-income, ethnically diverse neighborhoods: A randomized controlled trial. *Am. J. Clin. Nutr.* **2014**, *99*, 1359–1368. [CrossRef] [PubMed]
60. Thorndike, A.N.; Bright, O.J.M.; Dimond, M.A.; Fishman, R.; Levy, D.E. Choice architecture to promote fruit and vegetable purchases by families participating in the special supplemental program for women, infants, and children (WIC): Randomized corner store pilot study. *Public Health Nutr.* **2017**, *20*, 1297–1305. [CrossRef] [PubMed]

61. Trude, A.C.; Surkan, P.J.; Cheskin, L.J.; Gittelsohn, J. A multilevel, multicomponent childhood obesity prevention group-randomized controlled trial improves healthier food purchasing and reduces sweet-snack consumption among low-income African-American youth. *Nutr. J.* **2018**, *17*, 96. [CrossRef]
62. Trude, A.C.; Surkan, P.J.; Steeves, E.A.; Porter, K.P.; Gittelsohn, J. The impact of a multilevel childhood obesity prevention intervention on healthful food acquisition, preparation, and fruit and vegetable consumption on African-American adult caregivers. *Public Health Nutr.* **2019**, *22*, 1300–1315. [CrossRef]
63. Wensel, C.R.; Trude, A.C.B.; Poirier, L.; Alghamdi, R.; Trujillo, A.; Steeves, E.A.; Gittelsohn, J. B'more healthy corner stores for moms and kids: Identifying optimal behavioral economic strategies to increase WIC redemptions in small urban corner stores. *Int. J. Env. Res. Public Health* **2019**, *16*, 64. [CrossRef]
64. Gittelsohn, J.; Song, H.J.; Suratkar, S.; Kumar, M.B.; Henry, E.G.; Sharma, S.; Anliker, J.A. An urban food store intervention positively affects food-related psychosocial variables and food behaviors. *Health Educ. Behav.* **2010**, *37*, 390–402. [CrossRef]
65. Steeves, E.A.; Penniston, E.; Rowan, M.; Steeves, J.; Gittelsohn, J. A rural small food store pilot intervention creates trends toward improved healthy food availability. *J. Hunger Environ. Nutr.* **2015**, *10*, 259–270. [CrossRef]
66. Surkan, P.J.; Tabrizi, M.J.; Lee, R.M.; Palmer, A.M.; Frick, K.D. Eat right-live well! Supermarket intervention impact on sales of healthy foods in a low-income neighborhood. *J. Nutr. Educ. Behav.* **2016**, *48*, 112–121. [CrossRef]
67. Ortega, A.N.; Albert, S.L.; Chan-Golston, A.M.; Langellier, B.A.; Glik, D.C.; Belin, T.R.; Prelip, M.L. Substantial improvements not seen in health behaviors following corner store conversions in two Latino food swamps. *BMC Public Health* **2016**, *16*, 389. [CrossRef]
68. Adjoian, T.; Dannefer, R.; Willingham, C.; Brathwaite, C.; Franklin, S. Healthy checkout lines: A study in urban supermarkets. *J. Nutr. Educ. Behav.* **2017**, *49*, 615–622. [CrossRef]
69. Albert, S.L.; Langellier, B.A.; Sharif, M.Z.; Chan-Golston, A.; Prelip, M.L.; Garcia, R.E.; Ortega, A.N. A corner store intervention to improve access to fruits and vegetables in two Latino communities. *Public Health Nutr.* **2017**, *20*, 2249–2259. [CrossRef]
70. Gustafson, A.; Ng, S.W.; Jilcott Pitts, S. The association between the "Plate it Up Kentucky" supermarket intervention and changes in grocery shopping practices among rural residents. *Transl. Behav. Med.* **2019**, *9*, 865–874. [CrossRef]
71. Dannefer, R.; Williams, D.A.; Baronberg, S.; Silver, L. Healthy bodegas: Increasing and promoting healthy foods at corner stores in New York City. *Am. J. Public Health* **2012**, *102*, 27–31. [CrossRef] [PubMed]
72. Paek, H.; Oh, H.J.; Jung, Y.; Thompson, T.; Alaimo, K.; Risley, J.; Mayfield, K. Assessment of a healthy corner store program (FIT store) in low-income, urban, and ethnically diverse neighborhoods in Michigan. *Fam. Community Health* **2014**, *37*, 86–99. [CrossRef] [PubMed]
73. Gudzune, K.A.; Welsh, C.; Lane, E.; Chissell, Z.; Steeves, E.A.; Gittelsohn, J. Increasing access to fresh produce by pairing urban farms with corner stores: A case study in a low-income urban setting. *Public Health Nutr.* **2015**, *18*, 2770–2774. [CrossRef]
74. Lawman, H.G.; Veur, S.V.; Mallya, G.; McCoy, T.A.; Wojtanowski, A.; Colby, L.; Foster, G.D. Changes in quantity, spending, and nutritional characteristics of adult, adolescent and child urban corner store purchases after an environmental intervention. *Prev. Med.* **2015**, *74*, 81–85. [CrossRef]
75. Liu, E.; Stephenson, T.; Houlihan, J.; Gustafson, A. Marketing strategies to encourage rural residents of high-obesity counties to buy fruits and vegetables in grocery stores. *Prev. Chronic Dis.* **2017**, *14*, 1–6. [CrossRef]
76. Rushakoff, J.A.; Zoughbie, D.E.; Bui, N.; DeVito, K.; Makarechi, L.; Kubo, H. Evaluation of Healthy2Go: A country store transformation project to improve the food environment and consumer choices in Appalachian Kentucky. *Prev. Med. Rep.* **2017**, *7*, 187–192. [CrossRef]
77. Woodward-Lopez, G.; Kao, J.; Kuo, E.S.; Rauzon, S.; Taylor, A.C.; Goette, C.; Williamson, D. Changes in consumer purchases in stores participating in an obesity prevention initiative. *Prev. Med.* **2018**, *54*, 160–169. [CrossRef]
78. Paluta, L.; Kaiser, M.L.; Huber-Krum, S.; Wheeler, J. Evaluating the impact of a healthy corner store initiative on food access domains. *Eval. Program. Plan.* **2019**, *73*, 24–32. [CrossRef]

79. Bird Jernigan, V.B.; Salvatore, A.L.; Williams, M.; Wetherill, M.; Taniguchi, T.; Jacob, T.; Tingle Owens, J.A. Healthy Retail Intervention in Native American Convenience Stores: The THRIVE Community-Based Participatory Research Study. *Am. J. Public Health* **2019**, *109*, 132–139. [CrossRef] [PubMed]
80. Karpyn, A.; Sawyer-Morris, G.; Grajeda, S.; Tilley, K.; Wolgast, H. Impact of Animal Characters at a Zoo Concession Stand on Healthy Food Sales. *J. Nutr. Educ. Behav.* **2019**, *52*, 80–86. [CrossRef] [PubMed]

Publisher's Note: MDPI stays neutral with regard to jurisdictional claims in published maps and institutional affiliations.

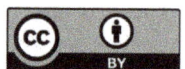

© 2020 by the authors. Licensee MDPI, Basel, Switzerland. This article is an open access article distributed under the terms and conditions of the Creative Commons Attribution (CC BY) license (http://creativecommons.org/licenses/by/4.0/).

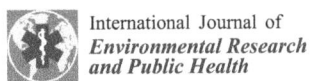

Review

Associations between Governmental Policies to Improve the Nutritional Quality of Supermarket Purchases and Individual, Retailer, and Community Health Outcomes: An Integrative Review

Alyssa J. Moran [1,*], Yuxuan Gu [2], Sasha Clynes [2], Attia Goheer [1], Christina A. Roberto [3] and Anne Palmer [4,5]

[1] Department of Health Policy and Management, Johns Hopkins Bloomberg School of Public Health, Baltimore, MD 21205, USA; agoheer1@jhu.edu
[2] Department of International Health, Johns Hopkins Bloomberg School of Public Health, Baltimore, MD 21205, USA; yuxuangreen@gmail.com (Y.G.); sclynes1@jhmi.edu (S.C.)
[3] Department of Medical Ethics and Health Policy, Perelman School of Medicine at the University of Pennsylvania, Philadelphia, PA 19104, USA; croberto@pennmedicine.upenn.edu
[4] Department of Health Behavior and Society, Johns Hopkins Bloomberg School of Public Health, Baltimore, MD 21205, USA; apalmer6@jhu.edu
[5] Center for a Livable Future, Johns Hopkins Bloomberg School of Public Health, Baltimore, MD 21202, USA
* Correspondence: amoran10@jhu.edu

Received: 7 September 2020; Accepted: 30 September 2020; Published: 15 October 2020

Abstract: Supermarkets are natural and important settings for implementing environmental interventions to improve healthy eating, and governmental policies could help improve the nutritional quality of purchases in this setting. This review aimed to: (1) identify governmental policies in the United States (U.S.), including regulatory and legislative actions of federal, tribal, state, and local governments, designed to promote healthy choices in supermarkets; and (2) synthesize evidence of these policies' effects on retailers, consumers, and community health. We searched five policy databases and developed a list of seven policy actions that meet our inclusion criteria: calorie labeling of prepared foods in supermarkets; increasing U.S. Department of Agriculture (USDA) Supplemental Nutrition Assistance Program (SNAP) benefits; financial incentives for the purchase of fruit and vegetables; sweetened beverage taxes; revisions to the USDA Special Supplemental Nutrition Program for Women, Infants, and Children (WIC) food package; financial assistance for supermarkets to open in underserved areas; and allowing online purchases with SNAP. We searched PubMed, Econlit, PsycINFO, Web of Science, and Business Source Ultimate to identify peer-reviewed, academic, English-language literature published at any time until January 2020; 147 studies were included in the review. Sweetened beverage taxes, revisions to the WIC food package, and financial incentives for fruits and vegetables were associated with improvements in dietary behaviors (food purchases and/or consumption). Providing financial incentives to supermarkets to open in underserved areas and increases in SNAP benefits were not associated with changes in food purchasing or diet quality but may improve food security. More research is needed to understand the effects of calorie labeling in supermarkets and online SNAP purchasing.

Keywords: food purchase; policy; retail food environment; food and beverage; grocery; federal nutrition assistance programs; beverage tax; menu labeling; financial incentives; health disparities

1. Introduction

Poor diet is widely considered a public health crisis, contributing to many of the leading causes of morbidity and mortality in the United States (U.S.) and globally [1,2]. There is growing recognition that dietary behaviors are shaped by the environments in which people live, learn, work, and play, and public health interventions increasingly target these settings [3]. Compared to nutrition interventions aimed at individuals or groups, upstream interventions designed to alter the environments in which people make food and beverage choices may be more effective for improving health, and are less costly to implement in the long-term [4,5]. For example, environmental interventions to treat obesity, such as sugary drink taxes and reductions in child-directed television advertising, are shown to be more cost-effective than commonly reimbursed clinical interventions, such as nutrition counseling or bariatric surgery [5].

In the U.S., supermarkets are natural and important settings for implementing environmental interventions to improve healthy eating. These stores, which generate more than $2 million annually in sales volume, are the primary retail store choice for the vast majority of U.S. households [6]. According to data from the U.S. Department of Agriculture (USDA) Food Acquisition and Purchase Survey, in 2012–2013, 89% of households did their primary shopping at supermarkets or other large grocers, with only 5% doing their primary shopping at other stores (e.g., convenience or dollar stores) [7]. During this time, supermarket purchases made up the majority of calories purchased by U.S. households (65%) and accounted for between 56% (households participating in the USDA Supplemental Nutrition Assistance Program [SNAP]) and 64% (higher income non-participating households) of household food expenditures [6]. Restaurant closures necessitated by the COVID-19 pandemic have likely increased reliance on supermarkets as a primary food source for many households.

The in-store environment is a well-recognized and powerful driver of dietary behaviors in supermarkets. Prior work has documented the important role of in-store food and beverage marketing, including availability, affordability, prominence, and promotion, in shaping consumer choices [8]. While these strategies hold promise for promoting healthy choices, they are often used to increase purchases of ultra-processed, nutritionally-poor products. A study of nearly 70 food retailers in three states found that sugary drinks were the most commonly promoted beverage, displayed in an average of 25 locations throughout the store [9]. National survey data show that the nutritional quality of purchases from supermarkets is generally poor, with diet quality scores (measured using the Healthy Eating Index 2010) closely mirroring those from national surveys of dietary intake [6,10].

Prior research has assessed the effectiveness of in-store promotions for healthy foods, finding that changes to product pricing, availability, packaging, display, signage, and labels are associated with consumer purchasing in the short-term [8]. Implementing these interventions long-term and scaling them across the nation's more than 30,000 supermarkets, however, has proven challenging [11]. Grocery stores operate at low margins and rely on trade fees and discounts from food and beverage companies for revenue [12]. These fees often favor the largest manufacturers and distributors, allowing them to control which products are stocked and how items are promoted in the store. It is estimated that supermarkets collect more than $50 billion a year in trade fees and discounts, with fees accounting for a large proportion of total grocery revenue relative to sales (although fees vary greatly by product, manufacturer, and store type) [11,12]. These exorbitant financial incentives make voluntary interventions to promote healthy purchases difficult to implement in supermarkets without food and beverage company buy-in.

In the absence of widespread and sustained voluntary action, governmental policies could help increase healthy purchases and decrease unhealthy purchases in the supermarket setting. To this end, several policies have been implemented across the U.S., and many studies have been conducted to evaluate their effects. This integrative review aims to synthesize the academic literature on this topic by: (1) identifying U.S. governmental policies, including regulatory and legislative actions of federal, tribal, state, and local governments, designed to promote healthy choices in supermarkets; and (2) summarizing the available evidence related to these policies' effects on retailers, consumers, and community health via changes to the supermarket environment. The objective of this review is to provide researchers and policymakers with information on existing policy options, their relative effectiveness in improving dietary behaviors, co-benefits or unintended consequences (e.g., impacts on retailer revenues or community economic development), and areas in need of further research. Although previous reviews have examined the effects of some of these policies, in isolation, on individual dietary or health outcomes, this will be the first, to our knowledge, to compare a wide range of outcomes across multiple policy approaches.

2. Methods

This review sought to answer two research questions: (1) which governmental policies in the U.S. aim to promote healthy choices in supermarkets; and (2) what is known about the effects of these policies on retailers, consumers, and communities? To answer these questions, we conducted searches of the peer-reviewed, academic, English-language literature published until January 2020. We searched PubMed, Econlit, PsycINFO, Web of Science, and Business Source Ultimate to identify papers spanning the economics, public health, marketing, consumer behavior, and business literature. Methods used to select and analyze results were consistent with the Preferred Reporting Items for Systematic Reviews and Meta-Analyses (PRISMA) guidelines (Figure 1) [13].

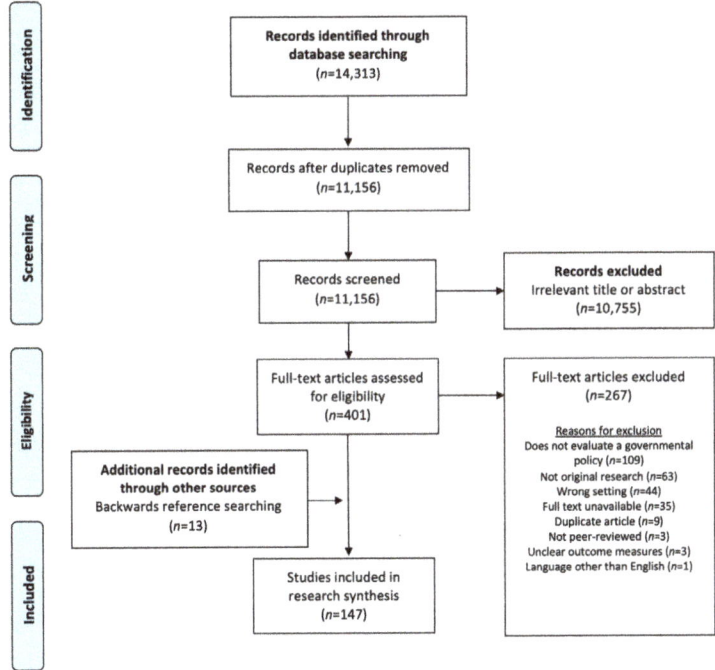

Figure 1. Preferred Reporting Items for Systematic Reviews and Meta-Analyses (PRISMA) Flow Diagram.

2.1. Policy Identification

To answer the first research question, we reviewed five nutrition policy databases: (1) World Cancer Research Fund International's NOURISHING Database [14]; (2) The World Health Organization Global Database on the Implementation of Nutrition Action [15]; (3) Healthy Food Access Portal [16]; (4) Growing Food Connections Local Government Policy Database [17]; and (5) Healthy Food Policy Project [18]. From each database, two authors (Y.G. and S.C.) recorded the name, brief summary, date of enactment, and locale of government regulatory or legislative actions, meeting the following inclusion criteria: (1) implemented in a supermarket setting; (2) enacted in the U.S. as of 26 September 2019; and (3) intended to promote healthy food purchases (with policy intent inferred by the authors based on subject matter expertise). Policies that had been proposed but not enacted; policies that may influence food or beverage choices without changes to retailer practices (e.g., food formulation or front-of-package labeling policies); policies affecting only small stores or other non-supermarket settings (e.g., a healthy staple food ordinance); or policies that may affect food and beverage purchases, but were not designed with such intent (e.g., small sales taxes on soda or federal mandates requiring states to issue Supplemental Nutrition Assistance Program [SNAP] benefits no more than once monthly) were not included.

2.2. Search Strategy and Inclusion Criteria

Policies identified in this initial search were used to define our search terms, which were developed in collaboration with an informationist with expertise in public health policy (Appendix A). Papers were included if they met all of the following criteria: (1) peer-reviewed, original research; (2) conducted in the U.S.; (3) written in English; (4) evaluated a governmental policy, as defined above; and (5) assessed outcomes related to retailers (e.g., supermarket or manufacturer sales, revenue, or employment), consumers (e.g., dietary intake, food purchases, food security, body mass index), or communities (e.g., healthcare costs). In addition to quantitative evaluations, implementation, mixed methods, and qualitative research were included. Studies were excluded if they: (1) only assessed outcomes in small stores or other non-supermarket settings (e.g., availability of healthful foods in convenience stores); (2) described policy development but did not evaluate policy effects; or (3) described public comments or public opinion prior to policy enactment. After each search, duplicates were removed and titles, abstracts, and full texts were independently screened for inclusion by two authors (Y.G. and S.C.) using Covidence, a software for evidence synthesis (Covidence, Melbourne, Australia). Backward reference searching of included articles and reviews was conducted to identify additional papers. A third author (A.J.M.) was available to resolve disagreements (Figure 1).

2.3. Evidence Synthesis

Research was catalogued in alignment with the NOURISHING framework, which classifies policies into specific actions (e.g., posting calories on menu boards) within ten broad approaches (e.g., nutrition labeling). Three authors (Y.G., S.C., and A.J.M.) read each article and abstracted data on study setting (U.S. census region and urbanicity); design (controlled experimental, controlled quasi-experimental, descriptive (quantitative, including uncontrolled interventions, microsimulations, and modeling studies); descriptive (qualitative), or mixed/multiple methods); and population (adults, children, households, or other (e.g., stores, prices, benefit redemptions)). For each study, one study design was selected, but multiple settings and populations could be selected. Given the large and varied amount of research reviewed, additional quantitative or meta-analysis was not possible. Instead, a summary of findings, including outcomes, approaches, and research gaps, was generated using thematic analysis and narrative synthesis. Results are presented by policy action and approach.

3. Results

We identified 147 peer-reviewed academic research studies for inclusion in this review. These studies evaluated seven policy actions within three policy approaches (Table 1). The majority of studies used a descriptive, quantitative (52%) or controlled, quasi-experimental design (37%); were conducted among adults (48%); and used national data (44%) or were set in the Northeast (30%) (Table 2). Few studies used experimental (7%), qualitative (4%), or mixed/multiple methods designs (3%); were conducted among children (24%); or were set in the south (6%), Midwest (7%), or rural areas (6%).

Table 1. Description of policy actions included in the review.

Policy Approach	Policy Action	Policy Description
Nutrition Label Standards and Regulations on The Use of Claims and Implied Claims on Food	Require Calorie Labeling of Prepared Food in Supermarkets (n = 3)	The 2010 Affordable Care Act mandated restaurants and similar food retail establishments with 20 or more locations nationwide disclose the number of calories in prepared foods on menus, menu boards, or in close proximity to food items ("calorie labeling") (P.L. 111-148, §4205) [19]. Food retailers are also required to display a statement about daily calorie intake ("2000 calories a day is used for general nutrition advice, but calorie needs vary") and must alert consumers that nutrition information for standard menu items is available upon request. The federal calorie labeling law differed from previously implemented state and local policies in that it expanded covered food retail establishments to include not only restaurants, but also supermarkets and other venues selling prepared foods. The Food and Drug Administration (FDA) published their final menu labeling rule in December 2014, issued draft industry guidance in 2017, and the law took effect on 7 May 2018. The following year, the FDA launched a consumer-facing nutrition education campaign to encourage the use of calorie information when eating out [20].
Use Economic Tools to Address Food Affordability and Purchase Incentives	Increase SNAP Benefits (n = 13)	SNAP provides monthly food benefits to approximately 36 million low-income Americans [21]. The majority (83%) of SNAP benefits are spent in supermarkets, totaling about $46 billion annually [21,22]. SNAP benefits are calculated on the assumption that households will spend 30% of their incomes on food, with SNAP bridging the gap between that contribution and the cost of the Thrifty Food Plan (a very low cost healthy diet, as determined by the USDA) [23]. Congressional action can increase the monthly SNAP benefit amount, and Congress has approved benefit increases in response to economic downturns. For example, in response to the great recession, the American Recovery and Reinvestment Act increased SNAP benefits by an average of 13.6% (about $80/month for a family of four) from April 2009 until November 2013 (P.L.111-5, §101). Benefit increases could also be provided by expanding Summer EBT for Children (Summer EBT), which provides benefits to families of students eligible for free or reduced-price lunch during the summer months, when school is not in session. Additionally, several policies may increase SNAP benefits indirectly, by reducing the number of meals provided to school-aged children by low-income households each week [24]. For example, policies that increase school participation in the Community Eligibility Provision, which allows schools or districts serving a certain percentage of eligible students to provide all students with free breakfast and lunch, may indirectly increase SNAP benefits among households with children by increasing student participation in school meal programs [25].
	Provide Financial Incentives for Fruits and Vegetables to Low-Income Households (n = 19)	The 2014 Farm Bill provided $100 million in mandatory funding for the Food Insecurity and Nutrition Incentive grant program to support programs that provide SNAP participants with financial incentives for the purchase of fruits and vegetables (P.L. 113-79, §4208) [26]. The 2018 Farm Bill expanded and permanently reauthorized this program, renamed the Gus Schumacher Nutrition Incentive Program (GusNIP), and increased funding to $250 million over five years (P.L. 115-334, §4205). Through GusNIP, the USDA also authorized the Produce Prescription Program, which provides funding to organizations to partner with healthcare providers to provide financial incentives for fresh fruits and vegetables to low-income people at risk of diet-related health conditions.

Table 1. Cont.

Policy Approach	Policy Action	Policy Description
Use Economic Tools to Address Food Affordability and Purchase Incentives	Tax Sweetened Beverages ($n = 48$)	In 2014, the city of Berkeley, California became the first U.S. city to pass a sweetened beverage excise tax of $0.01 per ounce [27]. Since then, a total of seven U.S. cities and the Navajo Nation have implemented similar taxes. All taxes except that of the Navajo Nation range from $0.01 to $0.02 per ounce. Sweetened beverage taxes typically apply to beverages with added sugar, but may also include drinks with low- or no-calorie sweeteners (e.g., the city of Philadelphia, Pennsylvania taxes both calorically and non-calorically sweetened beverages). Compared to a sales tax, which does not affect the posted retail price, excise taxes on beverage distributors can be passed on to consumers through retail price increases ("pass-through").
	Revise the WIC Food Package ($n = 44$)	In October 2009, as required under the Child Nutrition Act (P.L. 111-296, §17), the USDA reviewed and revised the WIC food package to better align with the 2005 Dietary Guidelines for Americans, American Academy of Pediatrics Infant Feeding Guidelines, and 2006 Institute of Medicine recommendations [28–30]. The revisions included cash-value vouchers for fruits and vegetables, expanded whole grain and low-fat dairy options, reductions in whole milk, juice, eggs, and cheese, and additional incentives for breastfeeding [31]. WIC-authorized stores were required to stock a minimum variety of fruits, vegetables, and whole grain products. States have flexibility to determine which specific foods are included in the food package (within federal guidelines) and may require stricter minimum stocking standards for authorized stores.
Set Incentives and Rules to Create a Healthy Retail and Food Service Environment	Provide Financial Assistance to Supermarkets to Locate in Underserved Areas ($n = 22$)	The Healthy Food Financing Initiative (HFFI) was launched in 2011 and formally established at the USDA as part of the 2014 Farm Bill (P.L. 113-79, §4206) [32]. The goal of the program was to improve access to healthy foods in low-income communities by building supermarkets or farmers' markets and improving the quality of foods offered in small stores through grants, loans, and tax incentives. Between 2011 and 2015, the HFFI awarded $195 million to community development organizations for nearly 1000 healthy food access projects in 35 states. Many municipalities operate similar programs at the state or local level [33].
	Allow Payment with SNAP for Online Grocery Purchases ($n = 4$)	The 2014 Farm Bill mandated the USDA Online Purchasing Pilot Program, which tests accepting SNAP/EBT for online grocery transactions (P.L. 113-79, §4011) [34]. In 2017, the USDA Food and Nutrition Service announced the selection of seven retailers in seven states to participate in the program, which was launched in Amazon, Shoprite, and Walmart in select zip codes in New York in April 2019. The program was meant to roll out among the remaining selected states and retailers over the next several years, but has rapidly expanded due to the COVID-19 pandemic. At the time of writing, forty states and five retailers were participating.

Note: The number of studies across all policy actions exceeds 147 because some studies addressed more than one policy action. Abbreviations: SNAP (Supplemental Nutrition Assistance Program); WIC (Supplemental Nutrition Program for Women, Infants, and Children); EBT (Electronic Benefits Transfer); HFFI (Healthy Food Financing Initiative); USDA (United States Department of Agriculture).

Table 2. Study design features of included articles, by policy action area.

Study Design Feature	Total (n = 147)	Calorie Labeling (n = 3)	SNAP Benefit Increase (n = 13)	Fruit and Vegetable Incentives (n = 19)	Sweetened Beverage Tax (n = 48)	WIC Food Package Revisions (n = 44)	Financial Assistance for Supermarkets (n = 22)	Online SNAP/EBT (n = 4)
Study Design								
Experimental	11 (7%)	0 (0%)	2 (15%)	9 (47%)	0 (0%)	0 (0%)	0 (0%)	0 (0%)
Quasi-experimental	55 (37%)	1 (33%)	8 (62%)	2 (11%)	17 (35%)	14 (32%)	13 (59%)	0 (0%)
Descriptive (Quantitative)	76 (52%)	2 (67%)	3 (23%)	7 (37%)	31 (65%)	25 (57%)	7 (32%)	1 (25%)
Descriptive (Qualitative)	6 (4%)	0 (0%)	0 (0%)	0 (0%)	0 (0%)	4 (9%)	1 (5%)	1 (25%)
Mixed or multiple methods	5 (3%)	0 (0%)	0 (0%)	1 (5%)	0 (0%)	1 (2%)	1 (5%)	2 (50%)
Population								
Adults	70 (48%)	2 (67%)	7 (54%)	13 (68%)	20 (42%)	12 (27%)	13 (59%)	3 (75%)
Children	35 (24%)	0 (0%)	3 (23%)	1 (5%)	10 (21%)	19 (43%)	2 (9%)	0 (0%)
Households	38 (26%)	0 (0%)	5 (38%)	9 (47%)	13 (27%)	8 (18%)	3 (14%)	0 (0%)
Other (e.g., stores)	33 (22%)	1 (33%)	1 (8%)	2 (11%)	13 (27%)	10 (23%)	5 (23%)	1 (25%)
U.S. Census Region								
National	64 (44%)	1 (33%)	11 (85%)	7 (37%)	26 (54%)	13 (30%)	5 (23%)	1 (25%)
Northeast	44 (30%)	1 (33%)	2 (15%)	8 (42%)	12 (25%)	9 (20%)	11 (50%)	1 (25%)
South	9 (6%)	0 (0%)	0 (0%)	0 (0%)	0 (0%)	5 (11%)	3 (14%)	1 (25%)
Midwest	10 (7%)	0 (0%)	1 (8%)	3 (16%)	2 (4%)	3 (7%)	1 (5%)	0 (0%)
West	30 (20%)	1 (33%)	1 (8%)	1 (5%)	10 (21%)	14 (32%)	2 (9%)	1 (25%)
Urban/Rural *								
Urban	54 (37%)	1 (33%)	1 (8%)	9 (47%)	18 (38%)	15 (34%)	11 (50%)	3 (75%)
Rural	9 (6%)	0 (0%)	0 (0%)	6 (32%)	0 (0%)	2 (5%)	1 (5%)	0 (0%)
Not specified or applicable	91 (62%)	2 (67%)	12 (92%)	8 (42%)	31 (65%)	27 (61%)	10 (45%)	1 (25%)

Note: The number of studies across all policy actions exceeds 147 because some studies addressed more than one policy action. Study design categories were mutually exclusive, but some studies addressed more than one geographic area and/or population. * As described in study ("cities" considered urban).

3.1. Nutrition Labeling

Require Calorie Labeling of Prepared Food in Supermarkets

Few ($n = 3$) studies examined outcomes related to calorie labeling of prepared foods in supermarkets [35–37] and only one estimated the effects of calorie labels on food choices in a real-world supermarket setting [35]. Bachman et al. studied 393 women before and after calorie labeling in nine locations of a regional supermarket using a quasi-experimental design. Only 16% of study participants exposed to calorie labeling reported noticing the labels, and calorie labels did not influence food choices, although the sample size was small. In two studies, people trying or wanting to lose weight were more likely to rate calorie labels as important than people who were satisfied with their current weight [35,37]. Both studies used self-reported measures of consumer perceptions to assess the impact of calorie labeling; no studies have measured outcomes using validated dietary assessment surveys or objective food purchase data.

3.2. Economic Tools to Address Food Affordability and Purchase Incentives

3.2.1. Increase Supplemental Nutrition Assistance Program (SNAP) Benefits

Thirteen studies assessed the effect of increased SNAP benefits (see Table 1 for description of policy) on household expenditures [38–41], food security [24,40,42,43], dietary behaviors [24,40,43–47], obesity [25], and healthcare utilization [48], with the majority using experimental ($n = 2$) or quasi-experimental ($n = 8$) designs. Studies indicate that increasing SNAP during the American Recovery and Reinvestment Act (ARRA) increased food-at-home expenditures but not food-away-from home expenditures [39,41,47], increased the share of benefits spent at superstores versus small stores [38], and increased spending on other necessary goods and services, including housing (mortgage, rent, utilities), transportation, and educational tuition [41]. Studies consistently demonstrated improvements in food security resulting from the ARRA benefit increase and Summer Electronic Benefits Transfer (EBT), as well as decreases in food security when the ARRA benefit increase ended [24,40,42,43]. Two studies found that benefit increases resulting from ARRA significantly reduced, but did not eliminate, declines in energy intake at the end of the benefit month [44,45], and one study found that ARRA was associated with a 65% reduction in outstanding medication needs due to cost among SNAP-eligible children [48].

The evidence for improving dietary behaviors and obesity is mixed. Most studies have found null or limited effects of a SNAP benefit increase on adult dietary quality [43,44,46,47]. A microsimulation study that directly compared the effects of an increase in SNAP benefits with a targeted subsidy on fruits, vegetables, and milk found that for the cost, targeted subsidies were more than ten times as effective in reducing deficiencies of recommended food groups [47]. One study of Summer EBT observed a small increase in children's fruit and vegetable, whole grain, and dairy intake, but no change in consumption of unhealthful foods and beverages [24,40]. One study showed a reduction in BMI among adults; however, that study assessed the impact of an indirect increase in SNAP benefits resulting from children's enrollment in school (and thus, participation in school meal programs), and may have been confounded by other changes affecting weight that correspond with school enrollment, such as changes in childcare expenses [25].

3.2.2. Provide Financial Incentives for Fruits and Vegetables to Low-Income Households

Nineteen studies examined the impact of supermarket fruit and vegetable subsidies, incentives, vouchers, or prescriptions targeted towards low-income households or individuals [47,49–66]. Results from randomized trials and natural experiments consistently demonstrate increases in household fruit and vegetable purchases or adult fruit and vegetable intake when incentives are targeted towards SNAP participants [50–58]; yet, few studies have been conducted with children [52]. Studies assessing substitution found little evidence that fruit and vegetable incentives changed unhealthful food intake or expenditures [51–53,59]. Intervention effects, however, may not be sustained after the financial incentive ends [54,57]. Although incentive programs in supermarkets would have high start-up costs if implemented nationally, they are expected to be cost-saving in the long-term, largely due to reductions in type 2 diabetes, heart disease, and stroke [60–63]. Compared to research on SNAP incentives, there are limited data on produce prescription programs, which, to date, have been most frequently implemented in farmers' markets or other limited-service food retail settings [49].

When the design and delivery of incentive programs are considered, the impacts on purchasing and consumption may increase with the size of the incentive. For example, the Healthy Incentives Pilot, which provided a 30% incentive on fruits and vegetables, saw a 26% increase (equivalent to approximately $\frac{1}{4}$ serving per day) in consumption among adults participating in SNAP, while the Shop Five for ME study, which provided a 50% incentive, found a 54% increase in fruit and vegetable purchases among SNAP households [52,53]. Additionally, incentives delivered as same-day discounts versus future rebates, administered electronically versus as paper coupons or vouchers, and offered without a minimum purchase requirement may increase uptake by lower-income households [52,55–57]. Frequent engagement with participating households and store staff about how the incentives work, which items qualify, and where they can be used may also be important for increasing utilization [49,52,56,58]. Complementary interventions focused on changing policies or environments to reduce unhealthy food purchases appear more effective in improving total diet quality at the population level than nutrition or cooking education, which tend to have low participation [51,52,59,61,63].

3.2.3. Tax Sweetened Beverages

Forty-eight studies evaluated the impact of sweetened beverage excise taxes on a variety of behavioral, economic, and health outcomes in the U.S [5,60,63–65,67–109]. Evidence from real-world natural experiments shows that these taxes increase retail prices, although pass-through (the proportion of the tax that is passed on to the consumer) varies by city, store type, and beverage type and size [70,71,73,77,98,100]. Excise taxes reduce sales of taxed beverages, but the magnitude of the reduction is highly variable across cities [68,98,100,101]. For example, a $0.01 per ounce tax on calorically sweetened beverages in Berkeley, California was associated with a 9.6% decline in sugary drink sales volume in Berkeley supermarkets after one year [100]. In a natural experiment, a $0.015 per ounce tax on calorically and non-calorically sweetened beverages in Philadelphia, Pennsylvania was associated with a 38% reduction in taxed beverage volume sales after accounting for people who avoided the tax by purchasing sweetened beverages outside city limits [98]. Differences across studies may be due to baseline purchasing habits or income of the population, size of the tax, types of beverages included in the tax, the proportion of the population able to easily avoid the tax (i.e., by shopping in a bordering city), or tax salience.

There are less consistent data on changes in beverage consumption, total diet, or health outcomes, particularly among children. Evidence on dietary intake is mixed, possibly due to measurement error in dietary assessment tools and inadequate sample sizes [69,78,90,100,108]. For example, one study found a statistically significant reduction in sales of sugary drinks and increase in sales of untaxed beverages, but no statistically significant change in adult beverage intake one year after the Berkeley tax [100]. Another study one year after a Philadelphia tax found no changes in children's beverage intake overall, but significant reductions in sugary drink intake among children who were high consumers prior to the tax [71]. There are limited quantitative data on the long-term (>1 year) effects of sweetened beverage taxes; one study of the earliest tax in Berkeley found an average reduction in sugary drink consumption (−0.55 times/day) and increased water consumption (+1.02 times/day) among adults 3 years after the tax [90]. Modeling studies with varying assumptions consistently show taxes improve long-term health outcomes related to obesity, cardiovascular disease, and diabetes among adults, and reduce childhood obesity [5,60,63–65,84,87,91,93,94,96,99,103,104]. Several of these studies suggest a tax on calories or sugar in beverages may better target health harms and encourage industry reformulation, but these taxation strategies have not yet been implemented in the U.S [85,86,106,109].

Economic research shows taxes are highly cost-saving from a public health and societal perspective, but may be costly to industry [104], with some studies documenting reduced supermarket combined sales [98], reduced sugar producer revenues [76,104], and increased cross-border shopping in cities with a tax (which may not be detrimental to supermarkets if shoppers visit the same chain in a different city) [69,70,98,100]. Although the food and beverage industries frequently voice concerns over job loss resulting from taxation, no job loss in these industries within the first year of a tax has been documented [89,97]. Strong and consistent evidence shows that beverage taxes raise revenue for city programs, such as parks and early childhood education, and these investments may affect social determinants of health [76,88]. For example, a simulation of Philadelphia's tax found that investments in quality pre-kindergarten would further reduce sugary beverage consumption among young children by 8% [88].

3.2.4. Revise Composition and Quantities of Foods Provided through the USDA Special Supplemental Nutrition Program for Women, Infants and Children (WIC)

Forty-four studies assessed the association between the 2009 WIC food package revisions and availability of foods and beverages in supermarkets; purchases, redemptions, or dietary intake among WIC participants; obesity in early childhood; perinatal and birth outcomes; or outcomes related to breastfeeding [110–153]. There is consistent evidence of an association between the WIC food package revisions and improvements in household food purchases and dietary intake among both adults and children [111,114–116,119,121,135–140,145,147–149,151]. Specifically, revisions to the food package are associated with improvements in total diet quality, increases in fruit, vegetables, whole grains, dietary fiber, and low-fat dairy, and reductions in full-fat dairy, saturated fat, and juice (with no evidence of complete substitution to other sugary drinks). The cash-value voucher, in particular, increased the perceived value of the program for many participants, although voucher redemption varied across communities and may be limited in some areas by poor access to fresh fruits and vegetables or negative store experiences [112,113,117,123,128,131,132,146]. Impacts of the revisions on breastfeeding are mixed, with some studies showing increases in breastfeeding initiation [129,153], others showing no effect [118], and none finding a relationship with breastfeeding at six months [129,153]. Recent research using interrupted time series or controlled quasi-experimental designs show improvements in maternal and child health outcomes resulting from the food package changes, including reductions in infant and young child obesity [125–127,130], improvements in infant birth weight outcomes (low birth weight, small for gestational age, and large for gestational age) [120], and reductions in maternal weight gain and preeclampsia [120].

With regard to the retail food environment, several studies have documented changes in WIC food availability, variety, quality, or pricing after implementation of the food package revisions and minimum stocking requirements [133,134,141–144,152]. While outcomes have generally been positive for small and medium-sized stores (i.e., greater availability and lower prices of healthful foods), results in supermarkets and mass merchandisers are mixed, likely due to the wide variety of food options offered in these stores at baseline. It is important to note that, in addition to the federal requirements, states have the authority to establish stronger stocking requirements for authorized retailers and there is substantial variation in regulatory guidance across states [142]. Variation in minimum stocking standards, as well as other flexibilities in how WIC programs are administered at the state and local levels, may partially explain observed differences in program impacts across localities; however, this has not been well studied [130].

3.3. Incentives and Rules to Create a Healthy Retail Environment

3.3.1. Provide Financial Assistance to Supermarkets to Locate in Underserved Areas

Twenty-two studies assessed the impacts of new supermarkets locating in underserved areas. Though many community residents support the introduction of a new supermarket [154], studies, including many using controlled, quasi-experimental designs, show low adoption of the new supermarket [155–157] and little or no improvement in body mass indices [155,158–162], household food purchases [156,157,163,164], or dietary intake [155–160,165] attributable to the new store. Similarly, modeling studies show these interventions are less cost-effective for supporting the introduction of new stores and increasing shopping at supermarkets than policies that increase SNAP benefits or coverage [38,166]. However, distance to the store, health and economic characteristics of the community, and baseline shopping habits within the population, may be important effect modifiers [167,168]. Additionally, supermarkets may positively impact health independent of effects on diet. One longitudinal natural experiment showed no improvement in dietary intake, but reductions in SNAP participation, food insecurity, and diagnoses of high cholesterol and arthritis one year after the opening of a new store [169]; however, the mechanism through which these positive health effects occurred is unclear. Several studies have suggested that investments in healthy retail may positively impact health by improving economic opportunity, social cohesion, or safety, but these mechanisms have not been studied [168,170,171].

3.3.2. Allow Payment for Online Grocery Purchases with SNAP

No research has studied the effects of online grocery shopping on the diets of SNAP participants, but several recent studies provide insight on the availability and uptake of online SNAP purchases [172–175]. Three studies have shown that, while online grocery can address transportation barriers and food availability, perceptions related to higher food costs online, lack of control over food quality, and distrust of the online shopping process may prevent SNAP participants from utilizing these services [173–175]. One attempted trial was unable to recruit enough SNAP participants to make online grocery purchases, mainly due to participants' perceived lack of control over the quality of food selected [174]. Additionally, a recent study found that online grocery delivery services disproportionately serve urban areas; services are rarely available in rural areas [172]. It will be important to continue to monitor equitable access to online grocery shopping and delivery over the course of the COVID-19 pandemic, particularly in communities and sub-populations at the highest risk of infection.

4. Discussion

This integrative review aimed to identify governmental policies enacted in the U.S. to promote healthy choices in supermarkets and to synthesize the academic literature on these policies' effects. We identified 147 papers in seven policy areas: calorie labeling, SNAP benefit increases, financial incentives to purchase fruit and vegetables, sweetened beverage taxes, revisions to the WIC food package, financial assistance for supermarkets to locate in underserved areas, and allowing online purchases with SNAP. The majority of identified papers were related to sweetened beverage taxes (33%), followed by revisions to the WIC food package (30%), and financial incentives for supermarkets (15%); few studies assessed calorie labeling of prepared foods in supermarkets (2%) or online SNAP (3%). Most studies leveraged natural experiments to evaluate policy effects, utilizing controlled, quasi-experimental study designs, microsimulation or agent-based modeling, longitudinal approaches, and interrupted time series methods; very few studies employed experimental, qualitative, or mixed methods approaches. With regard to population, many studies were conducted among adults, except in the case of WIC food package revisions, in which studies of young children were more common. Studies frequently used national data or data collected in Northeastern or Western U.S. cities.; far fewer studies were set in the Southern or Midwestern U.S. or in rural areas.

When effects were compared across policy action, we found consistent evidence, including from real-world randomized trials and natural experiments, of an association between economic tools to address food affordability and dietary behaviors. Specifically, sweetened beverage taxes were associated with increased prices and decreased purchases of taxed beverages, revisions to the WIC food package were associated with improvements in total diet quality and maternal/child health outcomes, and fruit and vegetable incentives increased purchases and consumption of discounted foods. In modeling studies, all three policies reduced the incidence of cardiometabolic diseases and were cost-effective in the long-term, but those restricting or discouraging consumption of unhealthful foods (i.e., taxes, WIC revisions) showed greater gains than those solely encouraging consumption of healthful foods (i.e., incentives). When incentives were paired with restrictions or taxes on unhealthful purchases, however, their combined effects on dietary behaviors were greater than those of any single policy action. This highlights the importance of multiple, synergistic policy interventions delivered together.

In contrast to the economic levers described above, financial assistance for supermarkets to open in underserved neighborhoods and increases in the SNAP benefit amount had little effect on diet, but reduced food insecurity. Food insecurity is associated with a wide range of negative outcomes, including increased risk of obesity and cardiometabolic diseases [176], poor mental health [177], and poor early childhood development [178]. Thus, these policy interventions could improve long-term health by reducing food insecurity, but these mechanisms have not yet been studied. Longitudinal natural experiments are needed to understand the role of supermarkets in neighborhood revitalization and the complex relationship between economic development strategies and improved health of neighborhood residents.

This review exposed several gaps in the literature that could be addressed in future research. First, research on calorie labeling of prepared foods in supermarkets and online SNAP is nascent and could be examined using natural experiments or interrupted time series designs. Second, very little research has been conducted in rural areas or in the Southern or Midwestern U.S.—regions with a disproportionately high prevalence of obesity and related health conditions [179]. Similarly, few studies assessed policy impacts on racial or socioeconomic disparities. While some policies may not substantially improve average dietary intake, they may contribute to improving equity. Third, although this review sought to include a wide range of outcomes, most studies evaluated policy effects on food security, household purchases, dietary intake, or obesity. Other important health-related outcomes, such as changes to social norms, parental feeding practices, and modeling of healthful behaviors, are needed and could be assessed using qualitative or mixed methods. Fourth, very few studies examined outcomes of importance to retailers, such as customer loyalty or sales revenue, which could help foster retail partnerships and industry buy-in. Fifth, policy implementation was rarely addressed. Implementation of federal policies often varies at the state level, and state and local policies with similar goals often differ in scope. This variation in implementation could explain variation in outcomes across settings, but it has not been quantitatively or qualitatively assessed. Similarly, process outcomes, such as policy adoption, acceptability, or fidelity, were infrequently measured and could help explain null effects. Lastly, many quasi-experimental studies were limited by small sample sizes and crude dietary assessment tools, which may have limited investigators' abilities to detect small policy effects. Investigators should carefully consider required sample sizes and appropriate dietary assessment methods to avoid false null findings, which can be detrimental to policy and advocacy efforts.

Strengths and Limitations

This review has several limitations and strengths that should be considered. In line with the project aims, a large amount of literature was reviewed and, thus, strength and quality of evidence was not quantitatively assessed but rather qualitatively synthesized. As a means to limit included studies to the highest quality papers, non-academic, non-peer reviewed sources were not included. This decision likely led to exclusion of some important evidence, such as reports commissioned by the USDA or other agencies or organizations. It also excludes industry reports, which may be more likely to assess outcomes relevant to retailers. We did not include food formulation, front-of-pack, or back-of-pack labeling policies in this review, although such policies could theoretically influence the types of products stocked or how they are priced or promoted within the store. Strengths of the study include extraction of relevant policies from five policy databases, comprehensive search strings and database searches across the psychology, economics, business, marketing, policy, and public health literature, inclusion of a wide range of effects on individuals, retailers, and community health, and narrative comparison of effects across seven distinct policy actions.

5. Conclusions

Governmental policies, particularly sweetened beverage taxes, revisions to the WIC food package, and financial incentives for fruits and vegetables, are associated with improvements in dietary behaviors. Providing financial incentives to supermarkets to open in underserved areas and increases in SNAP benefits are not associated with changes in food purchasing or diet quality but may improve food security. More research is needed to understand the effects of calorie labeling in supermarkets and allowing online purchases with SNAP.

Author Contributions: Conceptualization, A.J.M., A.P.; Methodology, A.J.M., A.G., C.A.R.; Formal analysis, A.J.M., Y.G., S.C.; Investigation, S.C. and Y.G.; Data curation, S.C. and Y.G.; Writing—original draft preparation, A.J.M.; Writing—review and editing, A.J.M., Y.G., S.C., A.G., A.P., C.A.R.; Visualization, A.J.M.; Supervision, A.J.M., A.P., A.G., C.A.R.; Project administration, A.J.M.; Funding acquisition, A.P., A.J.M. All authors have read and agreed to the published version of the manuscript.

Funding: This research was supported by the Johns Hopkins Center for a Livable Future. Publication fees were supported by Healthy Eating Research, a national program of the Robert Wood Johnson Foundation.

Acknowledgments: A version of this work was presented at the January 2020 Healthy Retail Research Convening in Washington, D.C. The authors would like to thank the meeting attendees for their constructive feedback, and Donna Hesson for her assistance in developing the search strategy for this paper.

Conflicts of Interest: The authors declare no conflict of interest. The funders had no role in the design of the study; in the collection, analyses, or interpretation of data; in the writing of the manuscript, or in the decision to publish the results.

Appendix A. Search Terms

Search #1

Terms related to supermarket
(grocer* OR supermarket OR store OR Retail* OR outlet OR e-commerce OR mercado)
AND
Terms related to food and beverage
food OR foods OR beverage* OR fruit OR fruits OR vegetable* OR snack* OR drink OR drinks OR lunch OR dinner* OR breakfast OR meat OR poultry OR beef OR chicken OR fish OR milk OR cheese OR yogurt OR juice OR soda OR grain OR grains OR meal OR bean OR beans OR nut OR nuts OR candy OR sweets OR cookies OR chips OR "ice cream" OR sugar OR salt OR sugar-sweetened OR "sugar sweetened" OR sweet OR nutrition* OR calorie OR calories
AND
Terms related to policy
policy OR policies OR Law OR laws OR regulat* OR ordinance* OR statute* OR tax OR taxes OR taxation OR incentive* OR "healthy food financing" OR subsid* OR "menu labeling" OR "calorie labeling" OR WIC OR "supplemental nutrition" OR "food stamps" OR access OR rule OR rules OR "retail expansion" OR "community development" OR "food trust" OR "food desert" OR loan OR loans OR "healthy food business" OR "healthy neighborhood" OR "federal nutrition program" OR "fresh food fund" OR "grocery financing" OR zoning OR "minimum stocking" OR "staple food" OR "excess food" OR "food waste" OR "grocery store development program" OR "closer to my grocer" OR license OR licensing OR permit OR permitting OR "Baton Rouge" OR frameworks OR "grocery access" OR "fresh food financing" OR "supermarket access" OR "healthy food center" OR "neighborhood development" OR "healthy families" OR "fresh food retailer"

Search #2

Terms related to beverage taxes
("sweetened beverage*" OR "sugary drink*" OR "sugary beverage*") AND (tax OR taxes OR taxation)

Search #3
Terms related to SNAP benefit increases
(ARRA OR (benefit AND increase)) AND "Supplemental Nutrition Assistance Program"
Search #4
Terms related to WIC food package revisions
((WIC AND (fruit* OR vegetable*) AND voucher)
OR
(((WIC OR "Special Supplemental Nutrition Program for Women, Infants, and Children") AND ("food package OR revisions))) AND ("2014/04"[Date–Publication]: "3000"[Date-Publication]))
Search #5
Terms related to the online purchasing pilot
"online grocery" OR "online purchas* pilot" OR (online AND shopping AND "Supplemental Nutrition Assistance Program")
Search #6
Terms related to produce prescription programs
((fruit OR vegetable* OR produce) AND (prescription OR rx)) AND (supermarket OR grocer*)

References

1. Afshin, A.; Sur, P.J.; Fay, K.A.; Cornaby, L.; Ferrara, G.; Salama, J.S.; Mullany, E.C.; Abate, K.H.; Abbafati, C.; Abebe, Z. Health effects of dietary risks in 195 countries, 1990–2017: A systematic analysis for the Global Burden of Disease Study 2017. *Lancet* **2019**, *393*, 1958–1972. [CrossRef]
2. Jardim, T.V.; Mozaffarian, D.; Abrahams-Gessel, S.; Sy, S.; Lee, Y.; Liu, J.; Huang, Y.; Rehm, C.; Wilde, P.; Micha, R. Cardiometabolic disease costs associated with suboptimal diet in the United States: A cost analysis based on a microsimulation model. *PLoS Med.* **2019**, *16*, e1002981. [CrossRef] [PubMed]
3. Hoffman, J.S.; Salerno, J.; Moss, A.; Dunne, B.; Fineberg, H.V.; Brownell, K.D. *The Weight of the Nation: Surprising Lessons About Diets, Food, and Fat from the Extraordinary Series from HBO Documentary Series*; St. Martin's Press: New York, NY, USA, 2012.
4. Food-PRICE: Food Policy Review and Intervention Cost-Effectiveness. Available online: https://www.food-price.org/ (accessed on 28 July 2020).
5. Gortmaker, S.L.; Long, M.W.; Resch, S.C.; Ward, Z.J.; Cradock, A.L.; Barrett, J.L.; Wright, D.R.; Sonneville, K.R.; Giles, C.M.; Carter, R.C. Cost effectiveness of childhood obesity interventions: Evidence and methods for CHOICES. *Am. J. Prev. Med.* **2015**, *49*, 102–111. [CrossRef] [PubMed]
6. Mancino, L.; Guthrie, J.; Ver Ploeg, M.; Lin, B.-H. *Nutritional Quality of Foods Acquired by Americans: Findings from USDA's National Household Food Acquisition and Purchase Survey*; United States Department of Agriculture, Economic Research Service: Washington, DC, USA, 2018.
7. Ver Ploeg, M.; Mancino, L.; Todd, J.E.; Clay, D.M.; Scharadin, B. *Where Do Americans Usually Shop for Food and How Do They Travel to Get There? Initial Findings from the National Household Food Acquisition and Purchase Survey*; United States Department of Agriculture, Economic Research Service: Washington, DC, USA, 2015.
8. Glanz, K.; Bader, M.D.; Iyer, S. Retail grocery store marketing strategies and obesity: An integrative review. *Am. J. Prev. Med.* **2012**, *42*, 503–512. [CrossRef]
9. Cohen, D.A.; Bogart, L.; Castro, G.; Rossi, A.D.; Williamson, S.; Han, B. Beverage marketing in retail outlets and The Balance Calories Initiative. *Prev. Med.* **2018**, *115*, 1–7. [CrossRef]
10. Shan, Z.; Rehm, C.D.; Rogers, G.; Ruan, M.; Wang, D.D.; Hu, F.B.; Mozaffarian, D.; Zhang, F.F.; Bhupathiraju, S.N. Trends in dietary carbohydrate, protein, and fat intake and diet quality among US adults, 1999–2016. *JAMA* **2019**, *322*, 1178–1187. [CrossRef]
11. An FTC Staff Study. *Slotting Allowances in the Retail Grocery Industry: Selected Case Studies in Five Product Categories*; Federal Trade Commission: Washington, DC, USA, 2003.
12. Rivlin, G. *Rigged Supermarket Shelves for Sale*; Center for Science in the Public Interest: Washington, DC, USA, 2016.
13. Moher, D.; Liberati, A.; Tetzlaff, J.; Altman, D.G.; Group, P. Preferred reporting items for systematic reviews and meta-analyses: The PRISMA statement. *PLoS Med.* **2009**, *6*, e1000097. [CrossRef]
14. World Cancer Research Fund. *NOURISHING Database*; World Cancer Research Fund International: London, UK, 2018.

15. World Health Organization. Global database on the Implementation of Nutrition Action (GINA). In *World Health Organization*; World Health Organization: Geneva, Switzerland, 2012.
16. Healthy Food Access Portal. Healthy Food Financing Funds. Available online: https://extranet.who.int/nutrition/gina/en/home/ (accessed on 28 July 2020).
17. Growing Food Connections, Briefs. *Growing Food Connections*; Metropolitan Universities: Towson, MD, USA, 2017; p. 1.
18. Healthy Food Policy Project. Available online: https://healthyfoodpolicyproject.org/ (accessed on 11 October 2020).
19. Food and Drug Administration. Menu Labeling Requirements. Available online: https://www.fda.gov/food/food-labeling-nutrition/menu-labeling-requirements (accessed on 28 July 2020).
20. Food and Drug Administration. Menu Labeling Social Media Toolkit for Consumer Outreach. Available online: https://www.fda.gov/food/nutrition-education-resources-materials/menu-labeling-social-media-toolkit-consumer-outreach (accessed on 28 July 2020).
21. *Supplemental Nutrition Assistance Program Participation and Costs*; United States Department of Agriculture, Food and Nutrition Services: Washington, DC, USA, 2020.
22. Center on Budget and Policy Priorities. Chart Book: SNAP Helps Struggling Families Put Food on the Table. Available online: https://www.cbpp.org/sites/default/files/atoms/files/3-13-12fa-chartbook.pdf (accessed on 28 July 2020).
23. Center on Budget and Policy Priorities. Policy Basics: The Supplemental Nutrition Assistance Program (SNAP). Available online: https://www.cbpp.org/research/food-assistance/policy-basics-the-supplemental-nutrition-assistance-program-snap (accessed on 8 October 2020).
24. Gordon, A.R.; Briefel, R.R.; Collins, A.M.; Rowe, G.M.; Klerman, J.A. Delivering summer electronic benefit transfers for children through the supplemental nutrition assistance program or the special supplemental nutrition program for women, infants, and children: Benefit use and impacts on food security and foods consumed. *J. Acad. Nutr. Diet.* **2017**, *117*, 367–375. [CrossRef] [PubMed]
25. Almada, L.N.; Tchernis, R. Measuring effects of SNAP on obesity at the intensive margin. *Econ. Hum. Biol.* **2018**, *31*, 150–163. [CrossRef]
26. United States Department of Agriculture. Local and Regional Foods. Available online: https://www.ers.usda.gov/agriculture-improvement-act-of-2018-highlights-and-implications/local-and-regional-foods/ (accessed on 28 July 2020).
27. Healthy Food America. TAXING SUGARY DRINKS. Available online: http://www.healthyfoodamerica.org/taxing_sugary_drinks#:~{}:text=The%20evidence%20of%20harm%20from,diet%20drinks%20in%20beverage%20taxes (accessed on 28 July 2020).
28. Institute of Medicine. *WIC Food Packages: Time for a Change*; The National Academies Press: Washington, DC, USA, 2006.
29. *Dietary Guidelines for Americans*; United States Department of Health and Human Services, United States Department of Agriculture: Washington, DC, USA, 2005.
30. Kleinmann, R. *Pediatric Nutrition Handbook*; American Academy of Pediatrics: Elk Grove Village, IL, USA, 2004.
31. United States Department of Agriculture. Final Rule: Revisions in the WIC Food Packages. Available online: https://www.fns.usda.gov/wic/fr-030414 (accessed on 28 July 2020).
32. The Food Trust. Special Report: HFFI Impacts. Available online: http://thefoodtrust.org/administrative/hffi-impacts (accessed on 28 July 2020).
33. Lange, S.J.; Moore, L.V.; Galuska, D.A. Local government retail incentives for healthier food retailers in the USA, 2014. *Public Health Nutr.* **2019**, *22*, 2521–2529. [CrossRef] [PubMed]
34. United States Department of Agriculture. FNS Launches the Online Purchasing Pilot. Available online: https://www.fns.usda.gov/snap/online-purchasing-pilot (accessed on 28 July 2020).
35. Bachman, J.L.; Arigo, D. Reported Influences on Restaurant-Type Food Selection Decision Making in a Grocery Store Chain. *J. Nutr. Educ. Behav.* **2018**, *50*, 555–563. [CrossRef] [PubMed]
36. Cleveland, L.P.; Simon, D.; Block, J.P. Compliance in 2017 with Federal Calorie Labeling in 90 Chain Restaurants and 10 Retail Food Outlets Prior to Required Implementation. *Am. J. Public Health* **2018**, *108*, 1099–1102. [CrossRef]

37. Nianogo, R.A.; Kuo, T.; Smith, L.V.; Arah, O.A. Associations between self-perception of weight, food choice intentions, and consumer response to calorie information: A retrospective investigation of public health center clients in Los Angeles County before the implementation of menu-labeling regulation. *BMC Public Health* **2016**, *16*, 8. [CrossRef] [PubMed]
38. Andrews, M.; Bhatta, R.; Ploeg, M.V. An Alternative to Developing Stores in Food Deserts: Can Changes in SNAP Benefits Make a Difference? *Appl. Econ. Perspect. Policy* **2013**, *35*, 150–170. [CrossRef]
39. Beatty, T.K.M.; Tuttle, C.J. Expenditure Response to Increases in In-Kind Transfers: Evidence from the Supplemental Nutrition Assistance Program. *Am. J. Agric. Econ.* **2015**, *97*, 390–404. [CrossRef]
40. Collins, A.M.; Klerman, J.A. Improving Nutrition by Increasing Supplemental Nutrition Assistance Program Benefits. *Am. J. Prev. Med.* **2017**, *52*, S179–S185. [CrossRef]
41. Jiyoon, K. Do SNAP participants expand non-food spending when they receive more SNAP benefits?—Evidence from the 2009 SNAP benefits increase. *Food Policy* **2016**, *65*, 9–20. [CrossRef]
42. Cheng, X.H.; Jo, Y.; Kim, J. Heterogeneous Impact of Supplemental Nutrition Assistance Program Benefit Changes on Food Security by Local Prices. *Am. J. Prev. Med.* **2019**. [CrossRef]
43. McClain, A.C.; Tucker, K.L.; Falcon, L.M.; Mattei, J. Food insecurity and dietary intake by Supplemental Nutrition Assistance Program participation status among mainland US Puerto Rican adults after the 2009 American Recovery and Reinvestment Act. *Public Health Nutr.* **2019**, *22*, 2989–2998. [CrossRef]
44. Todd, J.E. Revisiting the Supplemental Nutrition Assistance Program Cycle of Food Intake: Investigating Heterogeneity, Diet Quality, and a Large Boost in Benefit Amounts. *Appl. Econ. Perspect. Policy* **2015**, *37*, 437–458. [CrossRef]
45. Todd, J.E.; Gregory, C. Changes in Supplemental Nutrition Assistance Program real benefits and daily caloric intake among adults. *Food Policy* **2018**, *79*, 111–120. [CrossRef]
46. Waehrer, G.; Deb, P.; Decker, S.L. Did the 2009 American Recovery and Reinvestment Act affect dietary intake of low-income individuals? *Econ. Hum. Biol.* **2015**, *19*, 170–183. [CrossRef] [PubMed]
47. Lin, B.-H.; Yen, S.T.; Dong, D.; Smallwood, D.M. Economic Incentives for Dietary Improvement among Food Stamp Recipients. *Contemp. Econ. Policy* **2010**, *28*, 524–536. [CrossRef]
48. Morrissey, T.W.; Miller, D.P. Supplemental Nutrition Assistance Program Participation Improves Children's Health Care Use: An Analysis of the American Recovery and Reinvestment Act's Natural Experiment. *Acad. Pediatr.* **2019**. [CrossRef] [PubMed]
49. Marcinkevage, J.; Auvinen, A.; Nambuthiri, S. Washington state's fruit and vegetable prescription program: Improving affordability of healthy foods for low-income patients. *Prev. Chronic Dis.* **2019**. [CrossRef]
50. Grindal, T.; Wilde, P.; Schwartz, G.; Klerman, J.; Bartlett, S.; Berman, D. Does food retail access moderate the impact of fruit and vegetable incentives for SNAP participants? Evidence from western Massachusetts. *Food Policy* **2016**, *61*, 59–69. [CrossRef]
51. Harnack, L.; Oakes, J.M.; Elbel, B.; Beatty, T.; Rydell, S.; French, S. Effects of Subsidies and Prohibitions on Nutrition in a Food Benefit Program A Randomized Clinical Trial. *JAMA Intern. Med.* **2016**, *176*, 1610–1618. [CrossRef]
52. Moran, A.; Thorndike, A.; Franckle, R.; Boulos, R.; Doran, H.; Fulay, A.; Greene, J.; Blue, D.; Block, J.P.; Rimm, E.B.; et al. Financial Incentives Increase Purchases Of Fruit And Vegetables Among Lower-Income Households With Children. *Health Aff.* **2019**, *38*, 1557–1566. [CrossRef]
53. Olsho, L.E.W.; Klerman, J.A.; Wilde, P.E.; Bartlett, S. Financial incentives increase fruit and vegetable intake among Supplemental Nutrition Assistance Program participants: A randomized controlled trial of the USDA Healthy Incentives Pilot. *Am. J. Clin. Nutr.* **2016**, *104*, 423–435. [CrossRef]
54. Phipps, E.J.; Braitman, L.E.; Stites, S.D.; Singletary, S.B.; Wallace, S.L.; Hunt, L.; Axelrod, S.; Glanz, K.; Uplinger, N. Impact of a Rewards-Based Incentive Program on Promoting Fruit and Vegetable Purchases. *Am. J. Public Health* **2015**, *105*, 166–172. [CrossRef]
55. Phipps, E.J.; Braitman, L.E.; Stites, S.D.; Wallace, S.L.; Singletary, S.B.; Hunt, L.H. The Use of Financial Incentives to Increase Fresh Fruit and Vegetable Purchases in Lower-Income Households: Results of a Pilot Study. *J. Health Care Poor Underserved* **2013**, *24*, 864–874. [CrossRef] [PubMed]
56. Polacsek, M.; Moran, A.; Thorndike, A.N.; Boulos, R.; Franckle, R.L.; Greene, J.C.; Blue, D.J.; Block, J.P.; Rimm, E.B. A Supermarket Double-Dollar Incentive Program Increases Purchases of Fresh Fruits and Vegetables Among Low-Income Families With Children: The Healthy Double Study. *J. Nutr. Educ. Behav.* **2018**, *50*, 217–228. [CrossRef] [PubMed]

57. Steele-Adjognon, M.; Weatherspoon, D. Double Up Food Bucks program effects on SNAP recipients' fruit and vegetable purchases. *BMC Public Health* **2017**, *17*, 7. [CrossRef] [PubMed]
58. Wilde, P.; Klerman, J.A.; Olsho, L.E.W.; Bartlett, S. Explaining the Impact of USDA's Healthy Incentives Pilot on Different Spending Outcomes. *Appl. Econ. Perspect. Policy* **2016**, *38*, 655–672. [CrossRef]
59. French, S.A.; Rydell, S.A.; Mitchell, N.R.; Oakes, J.M.; Elbel, B.; Harnack, L. Financial incentives and purchase restrictions in a food benefit program affect the types of foods and beverages purchased: Results from a randomized trial. *Int. J. Behav. Nutr. Phys. Act.* **2017**, *14*, 10. [CrossRef]
60. Basu, S.; Seligman, H.; Bhattacharya, J. Nutritional policy changes in the supplemental nutrition assistance program: A microsimulation and cost-effectiveness analysis. *Med Decis. Mak.* **2013**, *33*, 937–948. [CrossRef]
61. Mozaffarian, D.; Liu, J.; Sy, S.; Huang, Y.; Rehm, C.; Lee, Y.; Wilde, P.; Abrahams-Gessel, S.; Veiga Jardim, T.d.S.; Gaziano, T.; et al. Cost-effectiveness of financial incentives and disincentives for improving food purchases and health through the US Supplemental Nutrition Assistance Program (SNAP): A microsimulation study. *PLoS Med.* **2018**, *15*. [CrossRef]
62. Choi, S.E.; Seligman, H.; Basu, S. Cost effectiveness of subsidizing fruit and vegetable purchases through the Supplemental Nutrition Assistance Program. *Am. J. Prev. Med.* **2017**, *52*, e147–e155. [CrossRef]
63. Penalvo, J.L.; Cudhea, F.; Micha, R.; Rehm, C.D.; Afshin, A.; Whitsel, L.; Wilde, P.; Gaziano, T.; Pearson-Stuttard, J.; O'Flaherty, M.; et al. The potential impact of food taxes and subsidies on cardiovascular disease and diabetes burden and disparities in the United States. *BMC Med.* **2017**, *15*. [CrossRef]
64. Pearson-Stuttard, J.; Bandosz, P.; Rehm, C.D.; Penalvo, J.; Whitsel, L.; Gaziano, T.; Conrad, Z.; Wilde, P.; Micha, R.; Lloyd-Williams, F.; et al. Reducing US Cardiovascular Disease Disparities Through Dietary Policy. *Circulation* **2017**, *135*. [CrossRef]
65. Wilde, P.E.; Conrad, Z.; Rehm, C.D.; Pomeranz, J.L.; Penalvo, J.L.; Cudhea, F.; Pearson-Stuttard, J.; O'Flaherty, M.; Micha, R.; Mozaffarian, D. Reductions in national cardiometabolic mortality achievable by food price changes according to Supplemental Nutrition Assistance Program (SNAP) eligibility and participation. *J. Epidemiol. Community Health* **2018**, *72*, 817–824. [CrossRef] [PubMed]
66. Klerman, J.A.; Bartlett, S.; Wilde, P.; Olsho, L. The short-run impact of the healthy incentives pilot program on fruit and vegetable intake. *Am. J. Agric. Econ.* **2014**, *96*, 1372–1382. [CrossRef]
67. Andreyeva, T.; Chaloupka, F.J.; Brownell, K.D. Estimating the potential of taxes on sugar-sweetened beverages to reduce consumption and generate revenue. *Prev. Med. Int. J. Devoted Pract. Theory* **2011**, *52*, 413–416. [CrossRef] [PubMed]
68. Baskin, E.; Coary, S.P. Implications of the Philadelphia beverage tax on sales and beverage substitution for a major grocery retailer chain. *J. Int. Food Agribus. Mark.* **2019**, *31*, 293–307. [CrossRef]
69. Cawley, J.; Frisvold, D.; Hill, A.; Jones, D. The impact of the Philadelphia beverage tax on purchases and consumption by adults and children. *J. Health Econ.* **2019**, *67*, 16. [CrossRef]
70. Cawley, J.; Frisvold, D.E. The Pass-Through of Taxes on Sugar-Sweetened Beverages to Retail Prices: The Case of Berkeley, California. *J. Policy Anal. Manag.* **2017**, *36*, 303–326. [CrossRef]
71. Cawley, J.; Willage, B.; Frisvold, D. Pass-through of a tax on sugar-sweetened beverages at the Philadelphia International Airport. *JAMA* **2018**, *319*, 305–306. [CrossRef] [PubMed]
72. Chen, Z.; Finkelstein, E.A.; Nonnemaker, J.M.; Karns, S.A.; Todd, J.E. Predicting the effects of sugar-sweetened beverage taxes on food and beverage demand in a large demand system. *Am. J. Agric. Econ.* **2014**, *96*, 1–25.
73. Coary, S.P.; Baskin, E. Sweetened beverages excise tax pass-through rates: A case study in Philadelphia. *J. Int. Food Agribus. Mark.* **2018**, *30*, 382–391. [CrossRef]
74. Debnam, J. Selection Effects and Heterogeneous Demand Responses to the Berkeley Soda Tax Vote. *Am. J. Agric. Econ.* **2017**, *99*, 1172–1187. [CrossRef]
75. Dharmasena, S.; Capps, O., Jr. Intended and unintended consequences of a proposed national tax on sugar-sweetened beverages to combat the U.S. obesity problem. *Health Econ.* **2012**, *21*, 669–694. [CrossRef] [PubMed]
76. Dharmasena, S.; Davis, G.C.; Capps, O., Jr. Partial versus General Equilibrium Calorie and Revenue Effects Associated with a Sugar-Sweetened Beverage Tax. *J. Agric. Resour. Econ.* **2014**, *39*, 157–173.
77. Falbe, J.; Rojas, N.; Grummon, A.H.; Madsen, K.A. Higher Retail Prices of Sugar-Sweetened Beverages 3 Months After Implementation of an Excise Tax in Berkeley, California. *Am. J. Public Health* **2015**, *105*, 2194–2201. [CrossRef]

78. Falbe, J.; Thompson, H.R.; Becker, C.M.; Rojas, N.; McCulloch, C.E.; Madsen, K.A. Impact of the Berkeley excise tax on sugar-sweetened beverage consumption. *Am. J. Public Health* **2016**, *106*, 1865–1871. [CrossRef]
79. Finkelstein, E.A.; Zhen, C.; Bilger, M.; Nonnemaker, J.; Farooqui, A.M.; Todd, J.E. Implications of a sugar-sweetened beverage (SSB) tax when substitutions to non-beverage items are considered. *J. Health Econ.* **2013**, *32*, 219–239. [CrossRef] [PubMed]
80. Finkelstein, E.A.; Zhen, C.; Nonnemaker, J.; Todd, J.E. Impact of targeted beverage taxes on higher- and lower-income households. *Arch Intern Med* **2010**, *170*, 2028–2034. [CrossRef]
81. Fletcher, J.M.; Frisvold, D.E.; Tefft, N. Non-linear effects of soda taxes on consumption and weight outcomes. *Health Econ.* **2015**, *24*, 566–582. [CrossRef] [PubMed]
82. Ford, C.N.; Ng, S.W.; Popkin, B.M. Targeted Beverage Taxes Influence Food and Beverage Purchases among Households with Preschool Children. *J. Nutr.* **2015**, *145*, 1835–1843. [CrossRef] [PubMed]
83. Ford, C.N.; Poti, J.M.; Ng, S.W.; Popkin, B.M. SSB taxes and diet quality in US preschoolers: Estimated changes in the 2010 Healthy Eating Index. *Pediatr. Obes.* **2017**, *12*, 146–154. [CrossRef] [PubMed]
84. Gortmaker, S.L.; Wang, Y.C.; Long, M.W.; Giles, C.M.; Ward, Z.J.; Barrett, J.L.; Kenney, E.L.; Sonneville, K.R.; Afzal, A.S.; Resch, S.C.; et al. Three Interventions That Reduce Childhood Obesity Are Projected To Save More Than They Cost To Implement. *Health Aff. (Proj. Hope)* **2015**, *34*, 1932–1939. [CrossRef] [PubMed]
85. Harding, M.; Lovenheim, M. The effect of prices on nutrition: Comparing the impact of product- and nutrient-specific taxes. *J. Health Econ.* **2017**, *53*, 53–71. [CrossRef] [PubMed]
86. Jithitikulchai, T.; Andreyeva, T. Sugar-Sweetened Beverage Demand and Tax Simulation for Federal Food Assistance Participants: A Case of Two New England States. *Appl. Health Econ. Health Policy* **2018**, *16*, 549–558. [CrossRef] [PubMed]
87. Kristensen, A.H.; Flottemesch, T.J.; Maciosek, M.V.; Jenson, J.; Barclay, G.; Ashe, M.; Sanchez, E.J.; Story, M.; Teutsch, S.M.; Brownson, R.C. Reducing childhood obesity through U.S. federal policy: A microsimulation analysis. *Am. J. Prev. Med.* **2014**, *47*, 604–612. [CrossRef] [PubMed]
88. Langellier, B.A.; Lê-Scherban, F.; Purtle, J. Funding quality pre-kindergarten slots with Philadelphia's new 'sugary drink tax': Simulating effects of using an excise tax to address a social determinant of health. *Public Health Nutr.* **2017**, *20*, 2450–2458. [CrossRef] [PubMed]
89. Lawman, H.G.; Bleich, S.N.; Yana, J.L.; LeVasseur, M.T.; Mitra, N.; Roberto, C.A. Unemployment claims in Philadelphia one year after implementation of the sweetened beverage tax. *PLoS ONE* **2019**, *14*, e0213218. [CrossRef] [PubMed]
90. Lee, M.M.; Falbe, J.; Schillinger, D.; Basu, S.; McCulloch, C.E.; Madsen, K.A. Sugar-Sweetened Beverage Consumption 3 Years After the Berkeley, California, Sugar-Sweetened Beverage Tax. *Am. J. Public Health* **2019**, *109*, 637–639. [CrossRef] [PubMed]
91. Lin, B.H.; Smith, T.A.; Lee, J.Y.; Hall, K.D. Measuring weight outcomes for obesity intervention strategies: The case of a sugar-sweetened beverage tax. *Econ. Hum. Biol.* **2011**, *9*, 329–341. [CrossRef]
92. Liu, S.; Osgood, N.; Gao, Q.; Xue, H.; Wang, Y. Systems simulation model for assessing the sustainability and synergistic impacts of sugar-sweetened beverages tax and revenue recycling on childhood obesity prevention. *J. Oper. Res. Soc.* **2016**, *67*, 708–721. [CrossRef]
93. Long, M.W.; Gortmaker, S.L.; Ward, Z.J.; Resch, S.C.; Moodie, M.L.; Sacks, G.; Swinburn, B.A.; Carter, R.C.; Wang, Y.C. Cost effectiveness of a sugar-sweetened beverage excise tax in the US. *Am. J. Prev. Med.* **2015**, *49*, 112–123. [CrossRef]
94. Long, M.W.; Polacsek, M.; Bruno, P.; Giles, C.M.; Ward, Z.J.; Cradock, A.L.; Gortmaker, S.L. Cost-Effectiveness Analysis and Stakeholder Evaluation of 2 Obesity Prevention Policies in Maine, US. *J. Nutr. Educ. Behav.* **2019**, *51*, 1177–1187. [CrossRef]
95. Lusk, J.L.; Schroeter, C. When do fat taxes increase consumer welfare? *Health Econ.* **2012**, *21*, 1367–1374. [CrossRef] [PubMed]
96. Mekonnen, T.A.; Odden, M.C.; Coxson, P.G.; Guzman, D.; Lightwood, J.; Wang, Y.C.; Bibbins-Domingo, K. Health benefits of reducing sugar-sweetened beverage intake in high risk populations of California: Results from the cardiovascular disease (CVD) policy model. *PLoS ONE* **2013**, *8*, e81723. [CrossRef] [PubMed]

97. Powell, L.M.; Wada, R.; Persky, J.J.; Chaloupka, F.J. Employment Impact of Sugar-Sweetened Beverage Taxes. *Am. J. Public Health* **2014**, *104*, 672–677. [CrossRef] [PubMed]
98. Roberto, C.A.; Lawman, H.G.; LeVasseur, M.T.; Mitra, N.; Peterhans, A.; Herring, B.; Bleich, S.N. Association of a Beverage Tax on Sugar-Sweetened and Artificially Sweetened Beverages With Changes in Beverage Prices and Sales at Chain Retailers in a Large Urban Setting. *JAMA* **2019**, *321*, 1799–1810. [CrossRef]
99. Ruff, R.R.; Zhen, C. Estimating the effects of a calorie-based sugar-sweetened beverage tax on weight and obesity in New York City adults using dynamic loss models. *Ann. Epidemiol.* **2015**, *25*, 350–357. [CrossRef]
100. Silver, L.D.; Ng, S.W.; Ryan-Ibarra, S.; Taillie, L.S.; Induni, M.; Miles, D.R.; Poti, J.M.; Popkin, B.M. Changes in prices, sales, consumer spending, and beverage consumption one year after a tax on sugar-sweetened beverages in Berkeley, California, US: A before-and-after study. *PLoS Med.* **2017**, *14*, 19. [CrossRef]
101. Taylor, R.L.; Kaplan, S.; Villas-Boas, S.B.; Jung, K. Soda wars: The effect of a soda tax election on university beverage sales. *Econ. Inq.* **2019**, *57*, 1480–1496. [CrossRef]
102. Wang, E.Y. The impact of soda taxes on consumer welfare: Implications of storability and taste heterogeneity. *Rand J. Econ.* **2015**, *46*, 409–441. [CrossRef]
103. Wang, Y.C.; Coxson, P.; Shen, Y.-M.; Goldman, L.; Bibbins-Domingo, K. A Penny-Per-Ounce Tax On Sugar-Sweetened Beverages Would Cut Health And Cost Burdens Of Diabetes. *Health Aff.* **2012**, *31*, 199–207. [CrossRef]
104. Wilde, P.; Huang, Y.; Sy, S.; Abrahams-Gessel, S.; Jardim, T.V.; Paarlberg, R.; Mozaffarian, D.; Micha, R.; Gaziano, T. Cost-Effectiveness of a US National Sugar-Sweetened Beverage Tax With a Multistakeholder Approach: Who Pays and Who Benefits. *Am. J. Public Health* **2019**, *109*, 276–284. [CrossRef]
105. Zeiss, J.; Carlson, L.; Ball, A.D. Uncalculated first-party externalities given a beverage tax. *Soc. Sci. Q.* **2019**, *100*, 736–748. [CrossRef]
106. Zhen, C.; Brissette, I.F.; Ruff, R.R. By Ounce or by Calorie: The Differential Effects of Alternative Sugar-Sweetened Beverage Tax Strategies. *Am. J. Agric. Econ.* **2014**, *96*, 1070–1083. [CrossRef] [PubMed]
107. Zheng, H.; Huang, L.; Ross, W., Jr. Reducing Obesity by Taxing Soft Drinks: Tax Salience and Firms' Strategic Responses. *J. Public Policy Mark.* **2019**, *38*, 297–315. [CrossRef]
108. Zhong, Y.; Auchincloss, A.H.; Lee, B.K.; Kanter, G.P. The Short-Term Impacts of the Philadelphia Beverage Tax on Beverage Consumption. *Am. J. Prev. Med.* **2018**, *55*, 26–34. [CrossRef] [PubMed]
109. Grummon, A.H.; Lockwood, B.B.; Taubinsky, D.; Allcott, H. Designing better sugary drink taxes. *Science* **2019**, *365*, 989–990. [CrossRef] [PubMed]
110. Vercammen, K.A.; Moran, A.J.; Zatz, L.Y.; Rimm, E.B. 100% Juice, Fruit, and Vegetable Intake Among Children in the Special Supplemental Nutrition Program for Women, Infants, and Children and Nonparticipants. *Am. J. Prev. Med.* **2018**, *55*, e11–e18. [CrossRef]
111. Meiqari, L.; Torre, L.; Gazmararian, J.A. Exploring the Impact of the New WIC Food Package on Low-Fat Milk Consumption Among WIC Recipients: A Pilot Study. *J. Health Care Poor Underserved* **2015**, *26*, 712–725. [CrossRef]
112. Ritchie, L.D.; Whaley, S.E.; Crocker, N.J. Satisfaction of California WIC participants with food package changes. *J. Nutr. Educ. Behav.* **2014**, *46*, S71–S78. [CrossRef]
113. McLaury, K.C.; Jernigan, V.B.B.; Johnson, D.B.; Buchwald, D.; Duncan, G.E. Variation in WIC Cash-Value Voucher Redemption Among American Indian Reservation Communities in Washington State. *J. Hunger Environ. Nutr.* **2016**, *11*, 254–262. [CrossRef]
114. Tester, J.M.; Leung, C.W.; Crawford, P.B. Revised WIC Food Package and Children's Diet Quality. *Pediatrics* **2016**, *137*. [CrossRef]
115. Ng, S.W.; Hollingsworth, B.A.; Busey, E.A.; Wandell, J.L.; Miles, D.R.; Poti, J.M. Federal Nutrition Program Revisions Impact Low-income Households' Food Purchases. *Am. J. Prev. Med.* **2018**, *54*, 403–412. [CrossRef] [PubMed]
116. Kong, A.; Odoms-Young, A.M.; Schiffer, L.A.; Kim, Y.; Berbaum, M.L.; Porter, S.J.; Blumstein, L.B.; Bess, S.L.; Fitzgibbon, M.L. The 18-month impact of special supplemental nutrition program for women, infants, and children food package revisions on diets of recipient families. *Am. J. Prev. Med.* **2014**, *46*, 543–551. [CrossRef] [PubMed]
117. Kim, L.P.; Whaley, S.E.; Gradziel, P.H.; Crocker, N.J.; Ritchie, L.D.; Harrison, G.G. Mothers prefer fresh fruits and vegetables over jarred baby fruits and vegetables in the new special supplemental nutrition program for women, infants, and children food package. *J. Nutr. Educ. Behav.* **2013**, *45*, 723–727. [CrossRef] [PubMed]

118. Joyce, T.; Reeder, J. Changes in breastfeeding among WIC participants following implementation of the new food package. *Matern. Child Health J.* **2015**, *19*, 868–876. [CrossRef]
119. Hamner, H.C.; Paolicelli, C.; Casavale, K.O.; Haake, M.; Bartholomew, A. Food and Beverage Intake From 12 to 23 Months by WIC Status. *Pediatrics* **2019**, *143*. [CrossRef]
120. Hamad, R.; Collin, D.F.; Baer, R.J.; Jelliffe-Pawlowski, L.L. Association of Revised WIC Food Package With Perinatal and Birth Outcomes: A Quasi-Experimental Study. *JAMA Pediatr.* **2019**. [CrossRef]
121. Hamad, R.; Batra, A.; Karasek, D.; LeWinn, K.Z.; Bush, N.R.; Davis, R.L.; Tylavsky, F.A. The Impact of the Revised WIC Food Package on Maternal Nutrition During Pregnancy and Postpartum. *Am. J. Epidemiol.* **2019**, *188*, 1493–1502. [CrossRef]
122. Au, L.E.; Paolicelli, C.; Gurzo, K.; Ritchie, L.D.; Weinfield, N.S.; Plank, K.R.; Whaley, S.E. Contribution of WIC-Eligible Foods to the Overall Diet of 13- and 24-Month-Old Toddlers in the WIC Infant and Toddler Feeding Practices Study-2. *J. Acad. Nutr. Diet.* **2019**, *119*, 435–448. [CrossRef]
123. Bertmann, F.M.; Barroso, C.; Ohri-Vachaspati, P.; Hampl, J.S.; Sell, K.; Wharton, C.M. Women, infants, and children cash value voucher (CVV) use in Arizona: A qualitative exploration of barriers and strategies related to fruit and vegetable purchases. *J. Nutr. Educ. Behav.* **2014**, *46*, S53–S58. [CrossRef]
124. Cakir, M.; Beatty, T.K.M.; Boland, M.A.; Park, T.A.; Snyder, S.; Wang, Y. Spatial and Temporal Variation in the Value of the Women, Infants, and Children Program's Fruit and Vegetable Voucher. *Am. J. Agric. Econ.* **2018**, *100*, 691–706. [CrossRef]
125. Chaparro, M.P.; Anderson, C.E.; Crespi, C.M.; Whaley, S.E.; Wang, M.C. The effect of the 2009 WIC food package change on childhood obesity varies by gender and initial weight status in Los Angeles County. *Pediatr. Obes.* **2019**, *14*, e12526. [CrossRef] [PubMed]
126. Chaparro, M.P.; Crespi, C.M.; Anderson, C.E.; Wang, M.C.; Whaley, S.E. The 2009 Special Supplemental Nutrition Program for Women, Infants, and Children (WIC) food package change and children's growth trajectories and obesity in Los Angeles County. *Am. J. Clin. Nutr.* **2019**, *109*, 1414–1421. [CrossRef] [PubMed]
127. Chaparro, M.P.; Wang, M.C.; Anderson, C.E.; Crespi, C.M.; Whaley, S.E. The Association between the 2009 WIC Food Package Change and Early Childhood Obesity Risk Varies by Type of Infant Package Received. *J. Acad. Nutr. Diet.* **2019**. [CrossRef] [PubMed]
128. Ishdorj, A.; Capps, O., Jr. The effect of revised wic food packages on native American children. *Am. J. Agric. Econ.* **2013**, *95*, 1266–1272. [CrossRef]
129. Li, K.; Wen, M.; Reynolds, M.; Zhang, Q. WIC Participation and Breastfeeding after the 2009 WIC Revision: A Propensity Score Approach. *Int. J. Environ. Res. Public Health* **2019**, *16*, 2645. [CrossRef]
130. Daepp, M.I.G.; Gortmaker, S.L.; Wang, Y.C.; Long, M.W.; Kenney, E.L. WIC Food Package Changes: Trends in Childhood Obesity Prevalence. *Pediatrics* **2019**, *143*. [CrossRef]
131. Singleton, C.R.; Opoku-Agyeman, W.; Affuso, E.; Baskin, M.L.; Levitan, E.B.; Sen, B.; Affuso, O. WIC Cash Value Voucher Redemption Behavior in Jefferson County, Alabama, and Its Association With Fruit and Vegetable Consumption. *Am. J. Health Promot.* **2018**, *32*, 325–333. [CrossRef]
132. Solomon, C.A.; Batada, A.; Zillante, A.; Kennedy, A.; Hudak, K.M.; Racine, E.F. Food cost is the least of my worries: A qualitative study exploring food and beverage purchasing decisions among parents enrolled in the WIC program. *J. Hunger Environ. Nutr.* **2018**, *13*, 497–506. [CrossRef]
133. Zenk, S.N.; Odoms-Young, A.; Powell, L.M.; Campbell, R.T.; Block, D.; Chavez, N.; Krauss, R.C.; Strode, S.; Armbruster, J. Fruit and Vegetable Availability and Selection Federal Food Package Revisions, 2009. *Am. J. Prev. Med.* **2012**, *43*, 423–428. [CrossRef]
134. Zenk, S.N.; Powell, L.M.; Odoms-Young, A.M.; Krauss, R.; Fitzgibbon, M.L.; Block, D.; Campbell, R.T. Impact of the Revised Special Supplemental Nutrition Program for Women, Infants, and Children (WIC) Food Package Policy on Fruit and Vegetable Prices. *J. Acad. Nutr. Diet.* **2014**, *114*, 288–296. [CrossRef]
135. Andreyeva, T.; Luedicke, J. Federal Food Package Revisions Effects on Purchases of Whole-Grain Products. *Am. J. Prev. Med.* **2013**, *45*, 422–429. [CrossRef] [PubMed]
136. Andreyeva, T.; Luedicke, J. Incentivizing fruit and vegetable purchases among participants in the Special Supplemental Nutrition Program for Women, Infants, and Children. *Public Health Nutr.* **2015**, *18*, 33–41. [CrossRef] [PubMed]
137. Andreyeva, T.; Luedicke, J.; Henderson, K.E.; Schwartz, M.B. The Positive Effects of the Revised Milk and Cheese Allowances in the Special Supplemental Nutrition Program for Women, Infants, and Children. *J. Acad. Nutr. Diet.* **2014**, *114*, 622–630. [CrossRef]

138. Andreyeva, T.; Luedicke, J.; Tripp, A.S.; Henderson, K.E. Effects of Reduced Juice Allowances in Food Packages for the Women, Infants, and Children Program. *Pediatrics* **2013**, *131*, 919–927. [CrossRef] [PubMed]
139. Andreyeva, T.; Tripp, A.S. The healthfulness of food and beverage purchases after the federal food package revisions: The case of two New England states. *Prev. Med.* **2016**, *91*, 204–210. [CrossRef]
140. Herman, D.R.; Harrison, G.G.; Afifi, A.A.; Jenks, E. Effect of a targeted subsidy on intake of fruits and vegetables among low-income women in the special supplemental nutrition program for women, infants, and children. *Am. J. Public Health* **2008**, *98*, 98–105. [CrossRef]
141. Hillier, A.; McLaughlin, J.; Cannuscio, C.C.; Chilton, M.; Krasny, S.; Karpyn, A. The Impact of WIC Food Package Changes on Access to Healthful Food in 2 Low-Income Urban Neighborhoods. *J. Nutr. Educ. Behav.* **2012**, *44*, 210–216. [CrossRef]
142. Pelletier, J.E.; Schreiber, L.R.N.; Laska, M.N. Minimum Stocking Requirements for Retailers in the Special Supplemental Nutrition Program for Women, Infants, and Children: Disparities Across US States. *Am. J. Public Health* **2017**, *107*, 1171–1174. [CrossRef]
143. Lu, W.H.; McKyer, E.L.J.; Dowdy, D.; Evans, A.; Ory, M.; Hoelscher, D.M.; Wang, S.J.; Miao, J.G. Evaluating the Influence of the Revised Special Supplemental Nutrition Program for Women, Infants, and Children (WIC) Food Allocation Package on Healthy Food Availability, Accessibility, and Affordability in Texas. *J. Acad. Nutr. Diet.* **2016**, *116*, 292–301. [CrossRef]
144. O'Malley, K.; Luckett, B.G.; Dunaway, L.F.; Bodor, J.N.; Rose, D. Use of a new availability index to evaluate the effect of policy changes to the Special Supplemental Nutrition Program for Women, Infants, and Children (WIC) on the food environment in New Orleans. *Public Health Nutr.* **2015**, *18*, 25–32. [CrossRef]
145. Herman, D.R.; Harrison, G.G.; Jenks, E. Choices made by low-income women provided with an economic supplement for fresh fruit and vegetable purchase. *J. Am. Diet. Assoc.* **2006**, *106*, 740–744. [CrossRef] [PubMed]
146. Okeke, J.O.; Ekanayake, R.M.; Santorelli, M.L. Effects of a 2014 Statewide Policy Change on Cash-Value Voucher Redemptions for Fruits/Vegetables Among Participants in the Supplemental Nutrition Program for Women, Infants, and Children (WIC). *Matern. Child Health J.* **2017**, *21*, 1874–1879. [CrossRef] [PubMed]
147. Zimmer, M.C.; Vernarelli, J.A. Changes in nutrient and food group intakes among children and women participating in the Special Supplemental Nutrition Program for Women, Infants, and Children: Findings from the 2005-2008 and 2011-2014 National Health and Nutrition Examination Surveys. *Public Health Nutr.* **2019**, *22*, 3309–3314. [CrossRef] [PubMed]
148. Oh, M.; Jensen, H.H.; Rahkovsky, I. Did revisions to the WIC program affect household expenditures on whole grains? *Appl. Econ. Perspect. Policy* **2016**, ppw020. [CrossRef]
149. Chiasson, M.A.; Findley, S.; Sekhobo, J.; Scheinmann, R.; Edmunds, L.; Faly, A.; McLeod, N. Changing WIC changes what children eat. *Obesity* **2013**, *21*, 1423–1429. [CrossRef]
150. Morshed, A.B.; Davis, S.M.; Greig, E.A.; Myers, O.B.; Cruz, T.H. Effect of WIC food package changes on dietary intake of preschool children in New Mexico. *Health Behav. Policy Rev.* **2015**, *2*, 3–12. [CrossRef]
151. Whaley, S.E.; Ritchie, L.D.; Spector, P.; Gomez, J. Revised WIC food package improves diets of WIC families. *J. Nutr. Educ. Behav.* **2012**, *44*, 204–209. [CrossRef] [PubMed]
152. Cobb, L.K.; Anderson, C.A.M.; Appel, L.; Jones-Smith, J.; Bilal, U.; Gittelsohn, J.; Franco, M. Baltimore City Stores Increased The Availability Of Healthy Food After WIC Policy Change. *Health Aff.* **2015**, *34*, 1849–1857. [CrossRef]
153. Langellier, B.A.; Chaparro, M.P.; Wang, M.C.; Koleilat, M.; Whaley, S.E. The new food package and breastfeeding outcomes among women, infants, and children participants in Los Angeles County. *Am. J. Public Health* **2014**, *104*, S112–S118. [CrossRef]
154. Evans, A.; Banks, K.; Jennings, R.; Nehme, E.; Nemec, C.; Sharma, S.; Hussaini, A.; Yaroch, A. Increasing access to healthful foods: A qualitative study with residents of low-income communities. *Int. J. Behav. Nutr. Phys. Act.* **2015**, *12* (Suppl. 1), S5. [CrossRef]
155. Cummins, S.; Flint, E.; Matthews, S.A. New Neighborhood Grocery Store Increased Awareness Of Food Access But Did Not Alter Dietary Habits Or Obesity. *Health Aff.* **2014**, *33*, 283–291. [CrossRef] [PubMed]
156. Elbel, B.; Mijanovich, T.; Kiszko, K.; Abrams, C.; Cantor, J.; Dixon, L.B. The Introduction of a Supermarket via Tax-Credits in a Low-Income Area: The Influence on Purchasing and Consumption. *Am. J. Health Promot.* **2017**, *31*, 59–66. [CrossRef] [PubMed]

157. Elbel, B.; Moran, A.; Dixon, L.B.; Kiszko, K.; Cantor, J.; Abrams, C.; Mijanovich, T. Assessment of a government-subsidized supermarket in a high-need area on household food availability and children's dietary intakes. *Public Health Nutr.* **2015**, *18*, 2881–2890. [CrossRef] [PubMed]
158. Dubowitz, T.; Ghosh-Dastidar, M.; Cohen, D.A.; Beckman, R.; Steiner, E.D.; Hunter, G.P.; Flórez, K.R.; Huang, C.; Vaughan, C.A.; Sloan, J.C. Changes in diet after introduction of a full service supermarket in a food desert. *Health Aff. (Proj. Hope)* **2015**, *34*, 1858. [CrossRef]
159. Dubowitz, T.; Ghosh-Dastidar, M.; Cohen, D.A.; Beckman, R.; Steiner, E.D.; Hunter, G.P.; Florez, K.R.; Huang, C.; Vaughan, C.A.; Sloan, J.C.; et al. Diet And Perceptions Change With Supermarket Introduction In A Food Desert, But Not Because Of Supermarket Use. *Health Aff.* **2015**, *34*, 1858–1868. [CrossRef]
160. Pitts, S.B.J.; Wu, Q.; McGuirt, J.T.; Sharpe, P.A.; Rafferty, A.P. Impact on Dietary Choices After Discount Supermarket Opens in Low-Income Community. *J. Nutr. Educ. Behav.* **2018**, *50*, 729–735. [CrossRef]
161. Zeng, D.; Thomsen, M.R.; Nayga, R.M.; Bennett, J.L. Supermarket access and childhood bodyweight: Evidence from store openings and closings. *Econ. Hum. Biol.* **2019**, *33*, 78–88. [CrossRef]
162. Zhang, Y.T.; Laraia, B.A.; Mujahid, M.S.; Blanchard, S.D.; Warton, E.M.; Moffet, H.H.; Karter, A.J. Is a reduction in distance to nearest supermarket associated with BMI change among type 2 diabetes patients? *Health Place* **2016**, *40*, 15–20. [CrossRef]
163. Freedman, M.; Kuhns, A. Supply-side subsidies to improve food access and dietary outcomes: Evidence from the New Markets Tax Credit. *Urban Stud.* **2018**, *55*, 3234–3251. [CrossRef]
164. Ulrich, V.; RD, A.H.; MSW PHD, K.I.D. The impact of a new nonprofit supermarket within an urban food desert on household food shopping. *Med. Res. Arch.* **2015**. [CrossRef]
165. Wang, M.C.; MacLeod, K.E.; Steadman, C.; Williams, L.; Bowie, S.L.; Herd, D.; Luluquisen, M.; Woo, M. Is the Opening of a Neighborhood Full-Service Grocery Store Followed by a Change in the Food Behavior of Residents? *J. Hunger Environ. Nutr.* **2007**, *2*, 3–18. [CrossRef]
166. Cleary, R.; Bonanno, A.; Chenarides, L.; Goetz, S.J. Store profitability and public policies to improve food access in non-metro US counties. *Food Policy* **2018**, *75*, 158–170. [CrossRef]
167. Chen, S.E.; Florax, R. Zoning for Health: The Obesity Epidemic and Opportunities for Local Policy Intervention. *J. Nutr.* **2010**, *140*, 1181–1184. [CrossRef] [PubMed]
168. Rogus, S.; Athens, J.; Cantor, J.; Elbel, B. Measuring Micro-Level Effects of a New Supermarket: Do Residents Within 0.5 Mile Have Improved Dietary Behaviors? *J. Acad. Nutr. Diet.* **2018**, *118*, 1037–1046. [CrossRef] [PubMed]
169. Richardson, A.S.; Ghosh-Dastidar, M.; Beckman, R.; Florez, K.R.; DeSantis, A.; Collins, R.L.; Dubowitz, T. Can the introduction of a full-service supermarket in a food desert improve residents' economic status and health? *Ann. Epidemiol.* **2017**, *27*, 771–776. [CrossRef]
170. Chrisinger, B. A Mixed-Method Assessment of a New Supermarket in a Food Desert: Contributions to Everyday Life and Health. *J. Urban Health Bull. N. Y. Acad. Med.* **2016**, *93*, 425–437. [CrossRef]
171. Giang, T.; Karpyn, A.; Laurison, H.B.; Hillier, A.; Perry, R.D. Closing the grocery gap in underserved communities: The creation of the Pennsylvania fresh food financing initiative. *J. Public Health Manag. Pract.* **2008**, *14*, 272–279. [CrossRef]
172. Brandt, E.J.; Silvestri, D.M.; Mande, J.R.; Holland, M.L.; Ross, J.S. Availability of Grocery Delivery to Food Deserts in States Participating in the Online Purchase Pilot. *JAMA Netw. Open* **2019**, *2*, e1916444. [CrossRef]
173. Lagisetty, P.; Flamm, L.; Rak, S.; Landgraf, J.; Heisler, M.; Forman, J. A multi-stakeholder evaluation of the Baltimore City virtual supermarket program. *BMC Public Health* **2017**, *17*, 9. [CrossRef]
174. Martinez, O.; Tagliaferro, B.; Rodriguez, N.; Athens, J.; Abrams, C.; Elbel, B. EBT Payment for Online Grocery Orders: A Mixed-Methods Study to Understand Its Uptake among SNAP Recipients and the Barriers to and Motivators for Its Use. *J. Nutr. Educ. Behav.* **2018**, *50*, 396–402. [CrossRef]
175. Rogus, S.; Guthrie, J.F.; Niculescu, M.; Mancino, L. Online grocery shopping knowledge, attitudes, and behaviors among SNAP participants. *J. Nutr. Educ. Behav.* **2020**, *52*, 539–545. [CrossRef]
176. Decker, D.; Flynn, M. Food Insecurity and Chronic Disease: Addressing Food Access as a Healthcare Issue. *Rhode Isl. Med J.* **2018**, *101*, 28–30.
177. Arenas, D.J.; Thomas, A.; Wang, J.; DeLisser, H.M. A systematic review and meta-analysis of depression, anxiety, and sleep disorders in US adults with food insecurity. *J. Gen. Intern. Med.* **2019**, 1–9. [CrossRef]

178. de Oliveira, K.H.D.; de Almeida, G.M.; Gubert, M.B.; Moura, A.S.; Spaniol, A.M.; Hernandez, D.C.; Pérez-Escamilla, R.; Buccini, G. Household food insecurity and early childhood development: Systematic review and meta-analysis. *Matern. Child Nutr.* **2020**, e12967. [CrossRef]
179. Trust for America's Health. *The State of Obesity: Better Policies for a Healthier America 2019*; Trust for America's Health: Washington, DC, USA, 2019.

Publisher's Note: MDPI stays neutral with regard to jurisdictional claims in published maps and institutional affiliations.

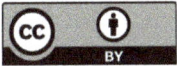

© 2020 by the authors. Licensee MDPI, Basel, Switzerland. This article is an open access article distributed under the terms and conditions of the Creative Commons Attribution (CC BY) license (http://creativecommons.org/licenses/by/4.0/).

Review

Influence of Food and Beverage Companies on Retailer Marketing Strategies and Consumer Behavior

Amelie A. Hecht [1,*], Crystal L. Perez [1], Michele Polacsek [2], Anne N. Thorndike [3], Rebecca L. Franckle [4] and Alyssa J. Moran [1]

1. Department of Health Policy and Management, Johns Hopkins Bloomberg School of Public Health, Baltimore, MD 21205, USA; CPerez20@jhu.edu (C.L.P.); AMoran10@jhu.edu (A.J.M.)
2. Westbrook College of Health Professions, University of New England, Portland, ME 04103, USA; mpolacsek@une.edu
3. Department of Medicine, Massachusetts General Hospital and Harvard Medical School, Boston, MA 02114, USA; athorndike@mgh.harvard.edu
4. Program in Global Public Health and the Common Good, Department of Biology, Boston College, Chestnut Hill, MA 02467, USA; franckle@bc.edu
* Correspondence: AHecht3@jhu.edu

Received: 11 September 2020; Accepted: 3 October 2020; Published: 10 October 2020

Abstract: The retail food environment plays an important role in shaping dietary habits that contribute to obesity and other chronic diseases. Food and beverage manufacturers use trade promotion—incentives paid to retailers—to influence how products are placed, priced, and promoted in stores. This review aims to: (1) catalogue trade promotion practices that manufacturers use to influence retailer marketing strategies, and (2) describe how these retailer marketing strategies affect consumer purchasing behavior and attitudes. Researchers searched five databases, Academic Search Ultimate, Business Source Ultimate, PsycINFO, PubMed, and Web of Science, to identify literature from industry and academic sources published in English through November 2019. Twenty articles describing manufacturer trade promotion practices were synthesized and provided insight into four types of trade promotion practices: category management, slotting allowances, price discounts, and cooperative advertising. Fifty-four articles describing the impact of retailer marketing on consumers were synthesized and graded for quality of evidence. While comparison across studies is challenging, findings suggest that retailer marketing strategies, such as price promotions and prominent placement, lead to increased sales. Results can guide efforts by policymakers, public health practitioners, and food retailers to design retail environments that improve healthy eating while maintaining retailer financial interests. Additional research should measure the impact of retailer marketing strategies on consumer diet quality and retailer outcomes (e.g., return-on-investment).

Keywords: trade promotion; price; promotion; placement; food and beverage; food retailer; grocery; consumer behavior; marketing; chronic disease; choice architecture

1. Introduction

The retail food environment plays a critical role in shaping dietary habits and is an important setting for interventions to improve diet quality and prevent diet-related chronic diseases, including diabetes, obesity, and cardiovascular disease [1]. Evidence suggests that marketing of unhealthy foods and beverages may be more common and effective at driving sales compared to marketing of healthy foods and beverages [2–9]. Low-income and racial and ethnic minority populations are disproportionately targeted by unhealthy food marketing, which may exacerbate disparities in diet quality and diet-related chronic disease [10]. For example, advertisements for low-cost, high-calorie, and low-nutrition foods and beverages appear more often in media watched by African Americans [11]; and retailers increase marketing of sugar-sweetened beverages when Supplemental Nutrition Assistance Program (SNAP) benefits are issued each month [12].

Retail food stores, which include both online and brick-and-mortar retailers (see Appendix A for a list of retail formats), are the primary source of food for many populations in both developed and developing economies [13]. In the US, consumers acquire the majority of their calories from supermarkets and superstores [14]. Considering that consumers make an estimated three-quarters of their purchasing decisions while shopping [15], in-store marketing techniques may play an important role in shaping purchase attitudes and decisions [9,16].

Food and beverage manufacturers use trade promotion practices (TPP), or incentives to retailers, to shape in-store marketing [17]. This paper focuses on how TPP influence three out of the "4Ps" of marketing: price, place (both the channels through which products are sold and where products are placed in stores), and promotion (efforts to engage consumers and communicate product features, such as signs) [18]. The fourth "P" of marketing, "product," is less frequently shaped by TPP, but rather by manufacturers in-house, through efforts such as packaging and product formulation. Similarly, TPP more commonly shapes where items are placed in stores and on shelves (i.e., product placement) rather than the channels through which products are sold. Food and beverage manufacturers allocate about $1 trillion annually to TPP—between 50 and 70% of their marketing budgets and nearly 20% of their total revenue [17,19].

There is growing interest among policymakers, researchers, advocates, and retailers in creating policies and corporate practices that promote healthy food retail. To inform efforts to improve the food retail environment, it is important to understand (1) the types of TPP currently used by food and beverage manufacturers to influence retailer marketing strategies, and (2) how retailer marketing strategies, in turn, affect consumers. The first part of this research question—which types of TPP are used to influence retailers—is understudied, particularly in the public health literature. A 2016 investigative report commissioned by the Center for Science in the Public Interest, which describes TPP but did not use a systematic approach to gather data or survey the literature, served as a launching point for this aim [17].

The second part of this research question—how retailer marketing strategies impact consumers—has been only partially explored in previous reviews. Specifically, three previous reviews have focused on price promotions' impact on consumers; all three concluded that price promotions were associated with consumer behavior [3,9,20]. In a 2012 integrative review, Glanz et al. synthesized literature on the impact of price, placement, and promotion on consumer behavior but limited their search to literature focused on brick-and-mortar grocery stores. They found that all three marketing strategies were associated with increased product liking and purchasing, with some variation in degree of impact by strategy [21]. This review serves as an update to and expansion of the Glanz et al. review, synthesizing literature since 2011 and including other nontraditional retail settings such as online retailers and convenience stores. This review focuses on identifying, where possible, whether and how outcomes differ when healthy versus unhealthy products are marketed. Findings from this study can inform efforts by advocates, policymakers, public health practitioners, and food retailers to design food retail environments that promote healthy eating while maintaining retailer financial interests. This study will also identify gaps in the literature and provide directions for future research.

2. Methods

Two research questions were identified: (1) how do food and beverage manufacturers use TPP to influence retailer marketing strategies; and (2) how do retailer marketing strategies impact consumer purchasing behavior and attitudes? Searches were conducted for peer-reviewed and grey literature (e.g., conference abstracts and proceedings, reports, dissertations) in English. To identify publications from diverse disciplines including public health, business, economics, marketing, and social sciences, the following databases were searched: Academic Search Ultimate, Business Source Ultimate, PsycINFO, PubMed, and Web of Science. Search terms for each research question were developed by the study authors in consultation with industry and academic experts and a research librarian (Appendix B). The selection and analysis of the results were carried out under the Preferred Reporting Items for Systematic Reviews and Meta-Analyses (PRISMA) guidelines [22].

2.1. Research Question 1: Search Strategy and Inclusion Criteria

To answer the first research question, a narrative review was conducted to identify and catalogue types of trade promotion practices used by food and beverage manufacturers to influence retailer marketing strategies (Figure 1). Articles published through November 2019 were included. Article titles and abstracts were independently screened by two authors (AH and CP) for inclusion. Full-text review was completed by the first author (AH). Any questions about study inclusion were resolved through discussion with the second author (CP).

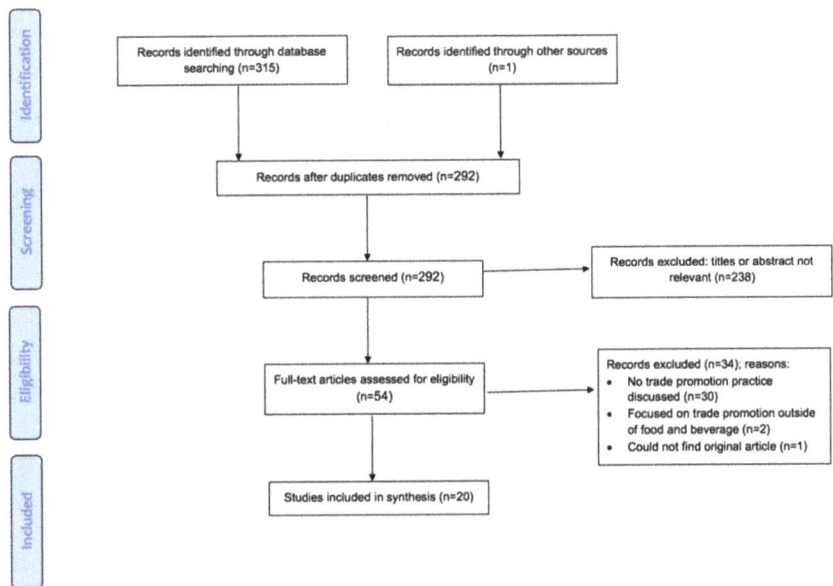

Figure 1. Preferred Reporting Items for Systematic Reviews and Meta-Analyses (PRISMA) Diagram for Research Question 1.

2.2. Research Question 2: Search Strategy and Inclusion Criteria

To answer the second research question, a systematic review was conducted to understand the impact of retailer marketing strategies on consumer behavior and attitudes (Figure 2). Inclusion criteria were that the article must (1) be published between January 2011 and November 2019 (to capture studies published since the Glanz et al. review) and (2) measure the impact of retailer marketing strategies influenced by TPP on consumer purchasing behavior or attitudes. Studies were excluded if they assessed (1) an investigator-driven healthy retail intervention (review by Karpyn et al., forthcoming); (2) retailer or manufacturer practices unrelated to TPP (e.g., product labeling); (3) restaurants, vending machines, cafeterias, or schools, or (4) were not original research (e.g., literature reviews). The excluded literature reviews were incorporated into the background and discussion section of this review. Two authors (AH and CP) independently reviewed titles, abstracts, and full texts for inclusion and met to reconcile differences. Reference lists of included articles were also scanned, and relevant articles included.

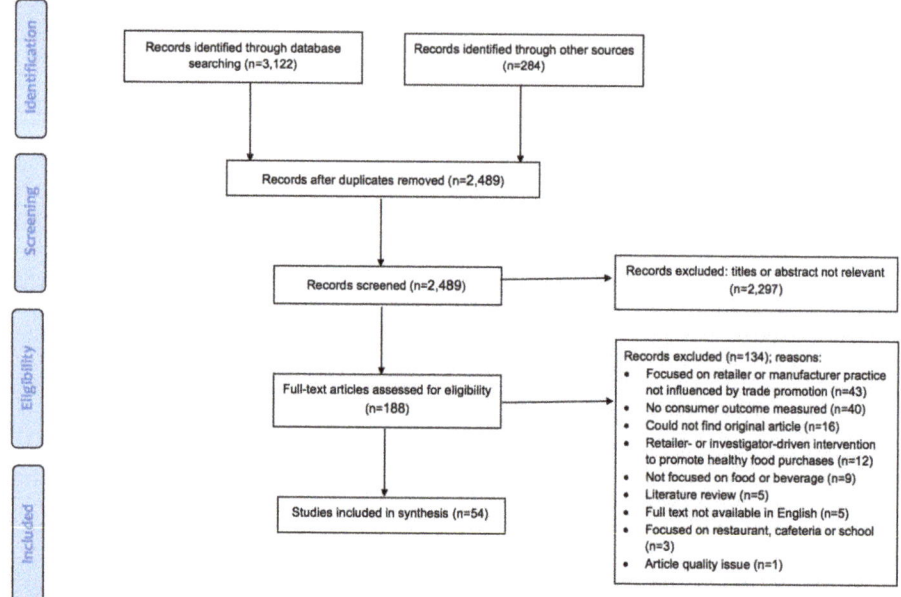

Figure 2. PRISMA Diagram for Research Question 2.

2.3. Quality of Studies

The quality of included studies for the second research question was assessed using the Newcastle–Ottawa quality assessment scale, adapted for cross-sectional studies [23] (Appendix C). The Newcastle–Ottawa scale assigns studies composite quality scores by awarding a certain number of stars out of a total of nine possible stars. Similar to an approach used by Bennett et al., amendments were made to the scale; for articles using aggregate sales data, a "not applicable" option was allowed for categories of "non-respondents" and "controlling for confounding variables" [3]. The denominator (total number of possible stars) was reduced appropriately. Two authors (AH and CP) independently graded the included studies and met to reconcile differences. As described by Takehashi and Hashizume [24], studies that earned fewer than a third of the possible stars were classified as low-quality studies.

3. Results

3.1. Narrative Review of Trade Promotion Practices

Twenty articles were identified that described TPP used by manufacturers to influence retailer marketing strategies [25–44]. Of these, 13 articles were published in the peer-reviewed literature or through conference proceedings and seven articles were published in trade publications. Of peer-reviewed publications, two were in public health or public policy journals and the remainder were in journals focused on retail, economics, or marketing. Thirteen articles focused on the US, six focused on other countries, including Brazil, the United Kingdom (UK), New Zealand, Sweden, Finland, Italy, and Portugal, and one used a global perspective.

Results indicate that manufacturers use four types of TPP to shape retailer marketing strategies: (1) category management, (2) slotting allowances, (3) price discounts, and (4) cooperative advertising (Table 1). These terms may differ across retailers, manufacturers, and countries; for example, in Europe, slotting allowances are also referred to as listing charges [25]. Certain types of TPP may be used more often for some product categories and in some retail formats. For example, slotting allowances are more often used in highly concentrated, processed product categories such as beverages, snacks, and candy [32]. In smaller stores, such as convenience and corner stores, more informal incentive-based agreements between suppliers and retailers are common [36].

Table 1. Definitions of trade promotion practices.

Trade Promotion Practice (n)	Definition
Category management (11)	Collaboration between retailers and manufacturers to make decisions regarding product assortment, supply, pricing, and promotion for entire categories
Slotting allowances (7)	Lump-sum fees paid by manufacturers to retailers in exchange for access to the consumer market (e.g., shelf space, prominent placement)
Price discounts (4)	Fixed discounts (merchandise is sold at a set discount for a specified period) or performance-based discounts (discounts are tied to a measure of performance such as units sold or displayed)
Cooperative advertising (1)	Cost-sharing between retailers and manufacturers to create and distribute promotional materials

Note: some articles discussed multiple trade promotion practices, so ns sum to greater than the total number of included articles.

3.1.1. Category Management

Eleven articles focused on category management [27,28,31,34,35,37–39,41,43,44]. Category management is the collaboration between manufacturers and retailers to make decisions regarding product assortment, space allocation, pricing, and in-store promotion for entire product categories. Categories (e.g., ice cream, yogurt) are treated as strategic business units to ensure maximum efficiency and boost sales for the whole category, rather than for individual brands [27]. Category management typically uses a shopper-centric and research-based approach to promote consumer satisfaction and loyalty [39,41,44].

A leading manufacturer in a category often serves as the "category captain," overseeing category management and customizing plans on a store-by-store basis. Such an arrangement is often considered beneficial for both retailers and manufacturers: it allows retailers to concentrate on other aspects of their business, and manufacturers to focus on increasing category market share and profitability [28]. While some retailers have safeguards in place to ensure category captains are not unfairly advantaged, critics contend that because category captains have influence over which brands and products within a category are stocked and promoted, category captains may be able to exclude competitors [28,43].

3.1.2. Slotting Allowances

Seven articles focused on slotting allowances, or lump-sum fees paid by manufacturers to retailers in exchange for access to the consumer market (i.e., shelf space) [25,29,32,33,36,40,42]. These include slotting fees to introduce a new product onto shelves, pay-to-stay fees to maintain shelf position, floor fees to make sales presentations and offer in-store samples, and display fees, which may cover premium placement, display materials (e.g., wire racks, prefabricated displays), and promotional signage. Theoretical explanations for why slotting allowances have become widely used include a market power explanation (i.e., slotting allowances reflect growing power among retailers who control access to the market) and an efficient market explanation (i.e., slotting allowances enable efficient allocation of scarce shelf space) [25]. According to the efficient market rationale, slotting allowances help retailers defray the costs and risks associated with new product introductions in light of an estimated 70% failure rate for new products [45]. Evidence suggests that slotting allowances in the US alone total between $6 billion and $18 billion per year [25,46]. Nationwide introduction of a new product in the US can cost up to $1–2 million in slotting fees [45]. In countries with more independent retailers, slotting allowances are less common.

3.1.3. Price Discounts

Four articles discussed price discounts that manufacturers provide to retailers to incentivize retailers to stock, display, or provide promotional discounts for their products [26,33,36,47]. Manufacturer discounts may be fixed or performance-based [47]. Fixed discounts are price reductions offered to the retailer on a per unit or per case basis, often at the time of billing, for a limited period of time. Performance-based discounts are tied to a measure of retailer performance such as number of units sold, displayed, or offered on price promotion. Discounts may be passed on to the consumer in the form of temporary price reductions (TPR) or coupons, affecting final sale prices [33,47]. Manufacturers may also provide retailers products for free to encourage retailers to stock new products or provide customer discounts, giveaways, or in-store samples [26,36].

3.1.4. Cooperative Advertising

One article focused on cooperative advertising. Cooperative advertising is the collaboration between manufacturers and retailers to create and distribute local promotional materials such as newspaper inserts or direct mail flyers [42]. A cooperative advertising agreement may be initiated by either a retailer or manufacturer. Typically, the manufacturer will design the promotional materials, providing product images and templates, and the manufacturer and retailer will share the cost of printing and distribution.

3.2. Literature Review of Impacts of Retailer Marketing Strategies on Consumers

Fifty-four articles that describe the impact of retailer marketing strategies on consumer behavior or attitudes were identified (Table 2). These included peer-reviewed literature ($n = 44$), dissertations ($n = 4$), conference proceedings ($n = 3$), reports from government or industry ($n = 2$), and trade publications ($n = 1$). Studies occurred in the US ($n = 17$), UK ($n = 11$), other European countries ($n = 8$), Asian and Middle Eastern countries ($n = 8$), Australia or New Zealand ($n = 6$), Canada ($n = 1$), and Egypt ($n = 1$); two articles did not specify location. Articles focused on a range of retail formats, including supermarket/grocery stores ($n = 43$); convenience/corner stores ($n = 9$); online retailers ($n = 4$); dollar stores ($n = 1$); other (e.g., organic markets, liquor stores, pharmacies, $n = 9$); and four articles did not specify the retail format assessed. Ten articles evaluated multiple retail formats. Data sources used varied widely; scanner or panel data was the most commonly used data source (e.g., Kantar Worldpanel data) ($n = 26$), followed by customer survey ($n = 21$), direct observation ($n = 9$), customer interviews or focus groups ($n = 8$), marketing data from the manufacturer or retailer ($n = 5$), retailer loyalty card data ($n = 4$), and other data sources (e.g., customer diaries, eye scanner, store audits, bag checks, $n = 6$); one article did not specify the data source used. Nearly one third ($n = 17$) used multiple data sources. No articles declared conflicts of interest.

TPP influence three categories of retailer marketing strategies: how products are priced, placed, and promoted. Results below are organized according to these three domains. Notably, comparison across studies is challenging given they focus on different products, use different study designs, and employ different outcome measures. The two final sections of the results describe findings from studies that compare outcomes across two or more retailer marketing strategies and compare the impact of marketing of healthy versus unhealthy products.

3.2.1. Pricing

Retailers employ a variety of price promotion strategies, including coupons, bundle deals (e.g., buy-one-get-one, 2-for-1), and TPR (also called rollbacks). In the US and the UK, an estimated 40% and 34% of all purchases are price promoted, respectively [6,48]. Estimates indicate that between 24% [49] and 67% [4] of unhealthy foods and beverages are purchased while price promoted, though prevalence of promotions differ across retailer formats and neighborhood [4]. A review of price promotions among Scottish retailers found that TPR are the most prevalent form of price promotion, accounting for 74%

of promotions, followed by bundle deals, which represent 23% of promotions [9]. Price promotions are offered more frequently for unhealthy compared to healthy products [2,3,5,7–9,20,50,51].

Thirty-two articles focused on price promotions. Eight presented results separately for coupons, seven presented results separately for TPR, and the remainder did not specify the type of price promotion assessed or assessed multiple types of price promotion and did not present results separately.

Coupons

Coupons may be distributed by retailers or manufacturers. In 2017, 302 billion coupons for consumer packaged goods were distributed in the US [52]. Six studies evaluated coupons and reported coupons were associated with increases in overall purchase volume, impulse purchase volume, brand choice, and product trialing (first-time purchase), but not brand loyalty [53–58]. Two studies assessed customized coupons, which target consumer groups based on demographic characteristics or past shopping behavior, and found they were associated with increased purchasing of targeted products [54,56]. Coupons in some product categories may be more impactful than others: one study found that coupons led to greater product trialing when promoting leading brands and categories that were popular, easy to store, had fewer products in the category (easier for customers to process less options), and were frequently on sale [55]. Another study found that while customized coupons led to increased purchases for both healthy and unhealthy products, they were more effective for unhealthy products [54].

Temporary Price Reductions

All eight studies that evaluated TPR detected associations with one or more consumer shopping behaviors, including purchase volume, impulse purchase volume, brand choice, and brand market share [58–65]. TPR may have a stronger impact on some outcomes compared to others: one study that assessed wine purchases in the UK found that TPR strongly influenced brand selection, somewhat influenced purchase volume, but did not influence purchase initiation [61].

Three articles assessed the impact of TPR in online retail [63–65]. Two out of three studies found that online price promotions were associated with increased purchases [63,64]; the third found no association [65]. One of the two studies that detected an association reported that because online purchases were delivered, barriers to stockpiling were eliminated, resulting in increased purchase volume compared to in traditional brick-and-mortar retail outlets [64]. The other reported that when a retailer with both online and brick-and-mortar retail outlets offered price promotions online, online sales increased, but sales in the brick-and-mortar stores decreased [63]. That study also found that high frequency of online promotions led to diminished effects over time [63].

Other Price Promotions

Thirteen articles on price promotions did not specify the type of price promotion studied or examined several types of price promotions together [6,8,50,66–75]. Many studies using panel data were unable to distinguish between types of price promotion used by customers. All studies identified positive associations between price promotions and one or more outcomes, including purchase volume, stockpiling purchase volume, purchase initiation, product trialing, and store choice. Within some studies, however, price promotions were positively associated with some outcomes and not others. For example, one study assessing Japanese market trends over time found that manufacturer expenditure on sales promotion was associated with an increase in total purchase volume but a decrease in manufacturer profits [66]. Another study found that price promotions led to short-term sales increases, but in more than half of cases, did not increase category revenue due to brand-switching (substitution) effects within the category [70].

Quantitative estimates on the impact of price promotions are difficult to compare because researchers used different outcome measures. Three studies, all using data from the Kantar Worldpanel, illustrate this challenge [6,8,69]. Nakamura et al. estimated that a 1% increase in price discount led to a sales uplift of 1.44% within a given category [6]. Smithson et al. found that approximately one-fifth of foods and beverages bought on price promotion were purchased in addition to what would be expected absent a price promotion, leading to an overall increase in food and drink purchase volume [8]. Revoredo-Giha et al. found that the presence of a price promotion increased spending between 2% and 10%, depending on the product category [69].

The effect of price promotions may differ across product categories and consumer characteristics. For example, one study found that while, price promotions did not, on average, affect beef sales, they did influence sales for certain cuts of meat and consumer groups (e.g., young families versus older adults) [68]. Another study found that price promotions were associated with increased soda sales across all levels of consumer education and retail formats, but the effect was weaker in neighborhoods with a higher proportion of residents with at least a post-secondary certificate or diploma [71].

Three studies compared differences in the impact of price promotion on healthy and unhealthy products [67,69,74]. Two of these studies found that purchase volume increased as price decreased for unhealthy foods but not for healthy foods [67,74]. Another, however, found that price promotions led to increases in total spending and spending by category for both healthy and unhealthy foods, though the effect was greater for less healthy foods [69]. Specifically, they found greater increases in spending for unhealthy categories such as confectionery (10%) and beverages (9%) and smaller increases for healthier categories such as fruits and vegetables (5%), grains (3%), and dairy (2%).

Perceived Importance of Price Promotions

Eight articles assessed consumer perceptions regarding the importance of price promotions in shaping their purchasing decisions [67,73,76–82]. Though the populations and contexts assessed varied across articles, all studies found that shoppers considered price promotions to be an important factor influencing their shopping behavior. Three of these studies assessed perceived importance of price promotions within specific cultural and religious contexts. In one study, Egyptian Muslim shoppers reported that TPR and bundled deals led them to engage in more stockpiling and spending, but other discount promotions considered not compliant with Shari'ah law, such as sweepstake draws and scratch-and-win promotions, did not shape their behavior [79]. In a study of Pakistani Muslim shoppers, participants reported that their intentions to purchase Halal products were shaped by price promotions [80]. Through interviews with "ethnic" shoppers in the UK, a final study found that participants reported diverse responses to price promotions, ranging from responsive to hostile, depending on the perceived "net worth" of the promotion [81].

3.2.2. Placement

Sixteen studies focused on how products were placed within stores, measuring visual attention, purchase volume, or spending as the primary outcomes [15,46,58,62,83–94]. Through slotting allowances and category management, manufacturers are able to secure placement in premium store locations, including on the endcap (i.e., end-of-aisle displays free from direct aisle-based competition), in the checkout aisle, and on freestanding displays. In 2012, an estimated 60% of products in stores were cross-promoted, meaning they are were displayed in secondary locations away from their "home" aisle [15]. Displays may be located anywhere in the store: approximately 42% of displays are located on the endcap, 28% in the aisle, 23% on the perimeter of the store, and 7% at the front of the store [15]. In an evaluation measuring shoppers' visual attention, 13% of all eye-fixations were drawn to in-store displays; of these, 44% were to endcaps, 34% to floor stands, 12% to in-line displays (i.e., gondola, or freestanding wire or metal shelving), and 10% to power wings (i.e., sidekick displays, or cardboard displays that attach to shelving) [15].

Endcaps

Five studies focused on placement in endcaps; all found significant positive effects on purchasing [46,83,85–87]. In a study of UK stores, endcap displays led to increased purchase volume for beer by 23.2%, for wine by 33.6%, for spirits by 46.1%, and for carbonated drinks by 51.7%; sales uplift was even greater for tea and coffee [85]. Two studies found that endcaps located at the rear of the store are more impactful than those at the front of the store [47,91]. In an experimental study in Australian grocery stores, placement of unhealthy products on rear endcap displays generated a 416% uplift in sales, while placement on front endcap displays generated a 346% uplift in sales [46]. Findings also suggest that endcaps are most impactful when located away from in-store sampling [87] and in stores without middle, perpendicular aisles [86].

Shelf Placement and Space

Category management and display fees can also affect where categories are placed within a store, and where individual products are placed on shelves (e.g., at eye-level for adult shoppers). Three experimental studies suggest that placement at the front of the store, in central aisles, at eye-level, and away from other popular categories can have positive effects on sales [88,91,92]. In one study, moving fruits and vegetables to a prominent location at the front of a grocery store led to an increase in sales volume and spending on fruits and vegetables [92]. In another, placement of dairy products in a central aisle was associated with increased product sales and purchase incidence, while placement next to popular categories had an "attention stealing" affect, leading to decreased sales [88]. In a laboratory-based study of college students, junk food items placed at eye-level received more visual attention than those on higher or lower shelves [91]. However, an observational study in New York City bodegas found no association between unhealthy beverage purchases and the placement of healthy products in prominent locations (i.e., water at eye-level and produce in at the front of the store) [89].

Total amount of dedicated shelf and display space (measured in feet) was associated with increased sales in two studies [84,90]. In one study, Minneapolis stores with more shelf space dedicated to fruits and vegetables had healthier purchases (i.e., more fruits and vegetables, more whole grains, and higher healthy eating index scores) [84]. Similarly, in a study of Hispanic shoppers in San Diego tiendas, each additional square foot of display space for fruits and vegetables was associated with a $0.02 increase in weekly amount spent on fruits and vegetables [90].

Other Placement Strategies

Four additional studies evaluated the impact of placement but did not specify how or where evaluated products were displayed [58,62,93,94]. All four studies found that presence of displays was positively associated with impulse purchase volume, spending, or brand choice. One of these studies was an industry report that assessed a multifaceted marketing campaign, however, and it is unclear what proportion of the sales uplift was attributed to placement [93].

3.2.3. Promotion

Sixteen articles focused on promotion [53,73,76,80,82,84,87,89,90,95–101]. Manufacturers use cooperative advertising and display fees to secure promotional signage, in-store sampling (i.e., taste tests), loudspeaker announcements, games, and other giveaways.

Signs

All three studies that measured the relationship between signs on shelf facings (called shelf-talkers or aisle violators) and purchase behavior focused on promoting healthy products; none detected a significant association [84,89,90]. In tiendas in San Diego, the number of signs promoting fruits and vegetables was not associated with fruit and vegetable purchases among Hispanic consumers [90]. In Minnesota stores, healthy advertising inside stores was not associated with purchasing, and, in fact, healthy advertising outside stores was associated with less healthy purchases [84]. In New York City bodegas, neither signs advertising water nor signs advertising sugar-sweetened beverages were associated with sugar-sweetened beverage purchases [89].

One study assessed "feature advertising" in two competing grocery stores, but did not describe components of "feature advertising" [73]. This study found that feature advertising led customers to choose to shop at the store with featured advertising over another store.

In-Store Sampling

In-store sampling was found to be associated with greater brand loyalty and purchase volume in three studies [53,87,99]. Several factors may moderate the impact of in-store sampling on purchases: studies suggest that benefits are maximized when the product being offered on sample matches the product displayed on the closest endcap [87,99]. One study also found a sales increase when in-store samples were offered close to the weekend compared to earlier in the week, when store personnel were present to offer the sample (24.3% increase compared to without store personnel present), when there was a sign promoting the product (90.8% increase compared to no sign), and when a commercial for the product is played on an in-store TV (36.3% increase compared to no commercial) [99].

Games, Giveaways and Limited-Time Offers

Findings on the impact of games, giveaways, and limited-time offers differed across studies [53,82,100]. In one study, customers reported that in-store games and lotteries led to greater customer loyalty and stronger relationships with promoted brands [53]. In another study, giveaways of collectible items increased the probability of brand choice and category purchase incidence, particularly when paired with a price discount, but did not change the purchase volume decision [100]. In a final study, both limited-time and membership deals were found to increase purchase incidence in an organic market [82].

Perceived Importance of Promotions

Seven articles assessed consumer perceptions regarding the importance of promotional activities in shaping their purchasing decisions [76,80,95–98,101]. Studies investigated different types of promotions and used different methods to assess customer perceptions, and found varying levels of perceived importance. Five studies found that consumers reported high levels of perceived importance of marketing on their attitudes toward purchasing [80,96–98,101]. Two studies, however, found promotional offers to be less persuasive: in a survey of Australian shoppers, 41% said they were influenced by promotional offers, but, in focus groups and interviews, many said that while promotional offers engaged them initially, trust and emotional connection to the brand was the primary driver of their purchase decisions [95]. In a survey of Vietnamese urban shoppers, participants described merchandise display and promotion as the least important factor from a list of seven factors influencing impulse purchase behavior [76].

3.2.4. Comparison of Marketing Healthy versus Unhealthy Products

As previously described, a small number of studies compared marketing of healthy versus unhealthy products [54,67,69,74,84,89,90]. Of these, four focused on price, three on placement, and three on promotion. Half of price-focused studies found that price promotions led to increased purchasing of unhealthy but not healthy products, [67,74] whereas the other half of studies found that while the effect was stronger for unhealthy products, price promotions led to increased purchasing of both healthy and unhealthy products. One of the three studies focused on placement found no association between prominent placement of healthy products and purchasing [89]. The other two studies, however, found that stores with more shelf and display space dedicated to fruits and vegetables had healthier sales [84,90]. Notably, both of these studies were cross-sectional and thus were unable to determine causality. Finally, none of the three studies focused on signs promoting healthy products detected a relationship with purchasing [84,89,90].

3.2.5. Comparison across Marketing Strategies

A small number of articles directly compared one retailer marketing strategy to another. Four of these asked participants to rank factors that shape their purchasing; in all four, participants reported that price promotions were the most or one of the most influential factors shaping their attitudes toward purchasing. Vietnamese shoppers reported that price promotions influenced their spontaneous purchase tendencies more than displays [76]. Taiwanese organic market shoppers reported that discounts and free giveaways impacted their shopping behavior more than membership or limited-time offers [82]. Two other studies focused on Muslim shoppers: in one [80], shoppers reported being equally influenced by Halal marketing promotions and pricing, while in the other [79], shoppers reported price discounts influenced their purchase intention more than giveaways, games, and in-store samples.

One study compared different types of price promotions, finding that sensitivity to coupons was greater than sensitivity to TPR [58]. The remaining studies quantitatively compared price promotions to either promotion or placement; results largely indicated that price promotions are more impactful than other types of marketing strategies [53,59,73,85]. Specifically, one study found that price was a stronger driver of stockpiling purchases than feature and display promotion [73]. Another found that a 20% TPR increased fair trade coffee sales more than providing information or a moral appeal [59]. Another study found that the effect size for endcap placement was equivalent to a price decrease for alcohol categories of between 4% and 9% per volume, and a price decrease for non-alcohol categories of between 22% and 62% per volume [85]. One study, however, found that price promotion and in-store sampling produced different benefits: in-store sampling helped nurture consumer loyalty more than coupons, but coupons resulted in more purchases [53].

3.2.6. Quality of Evidence Grading

On average, included studies received 65% of total possible stars (Appendix D). Only three of the 54 studies included in this review were of low-quality, having earned less than a third of all possible stars. The two categories in which studies most often earned zero stars were sample size ($n = 27$) and non-respondents ($n = 28$). Nearly half of the included articles omitted sample size calculations or justification; this was particularly common among studies using questionnaires or published in non-peer-reviewed sources. Only one study compared respondents and non-respondents or reported their response rate, though for 25 articles, this information was considered not applicable due to use of panel data. More than half of all studies earned the maximum number of stars in the assessment of outcome category by linking records or using an independent blind assessment to determine the outcome.

Table 2. Study design, marketing strategy, retailer format, country, study duration, data source, objectives, outcomes, and key findings for studies included in research Question 2 (n = 54).

Reference	Marketing Strategy	Retail Format	Country	Study Duration	Data Source	Objective	Outcome	Key Findings
Andorfer, et al. (2015) [59]	Price	Supermarket/ grocery store	Germany	5 mo (5 March, 2012–29 July 2012)	Scanner/panel data Customer surveys Direct observation	To identify how information, price, and moral considerations influence consumers' purchases of fair trade (FT) coffee products.	Purchase volume Purchase frequency	- A 20% TPR had a positive effect on coffee purchase volume when compared to the effects of information and moral appeal.
Arce-Urriza, et al. (2017) [65]	Price	Supermarket/ grocery store Online retailer	Spain	6 mo (15 May 2007–15 November 2007)	Scanner/panel data	To evaluate the differential effect of price promotions on brand choice when shopping at a grocery store's online outlet vs. brick-and-mortar store.	Brand choice	- Price promotions had a positive effect on purchases made in-person but not on purchases made online. - Frequent customers were more responsive to price promotions than infrequent customers.
Awan, et al. (2015) [80]	Price Promotion	Not specified	Pakistan	Not specified	Customer surveys	To identify which factors affect consumers' decisions to purchase Halal food.	Purchase attitude	- Customers were influenced by Halal marketing and branding practices (e.g., sales promotions and celebrity endorsements). - Customers were willing to spend considerable effort and money to purchase Halal food as a result of Halal marketing.
Aziz, et al. (2013) [101]	Promotion	Other (shopping mall)	Malaysia	Not specified	Customer surveys	To determine the relationships between factors, including Halal marketing, and intention to purchase Halal products.	Purchase attitude	- Halal marketing promotion was positively related to purchase intention.
Banks et al. (2016) [93]	Placement	Convenience store	UK	Not specified	Marketing data	To describe the impact of endcap placement and shelf-ready cases for cookies sales.	Purchase volume Spending Market share	- Marketing efforts led to an increase in shoppers' basket size (two-fold increase), spending (£3 increase), and market size (increased to £3.8bn) for cookies.
Bogomolova et al. (2019) [50]	Price	Supermarket/ grocery store	Australia	3 years (2 February 2012–31 December 2014)	Interviews/focus groups Loyalty card data	To assess reasons for first-time and impulse purchases	Product trialing Impulse purchasing	- The most common factor that prompted first-time brand purchases and impulse purchases was an item being placed on price promotion or having a special offer.

182

Table 2. *Cont.*

Reference	Marketing Strategy	Retail Format	Country	Study Duration	Data Source	Objective	Outcome	Key Findings
Breugelmans and Campo (2016) [63]	Price	Supermarket/ grocery store Online retailer	UK	78 weeks (July 2006–December 2007)	Scanner/panel data	To examine the cross-channel effects of price promotions (online vs. offline) on category purchase decisions.	Purchase incidence Purchase volume	- Price promotions had positive effects on purchasing decisions and degree of impact varied based on customer brand loyalty. - Promotions in one channel decreased category purchases in the other channel during the promotion period (online price promotions had a stronger impact on offline purchase decisions than vice versa). - High promotion frequency had negative effects on future promotion effectiveness.
Čábelková et al. (2015) [78]	Price	Supermarket/ grocery store	Czech Republic	2 months (October 2013–November 2013)	Customer surveys	To determine which activities are associated with customer store loyalty and differential effects by customer socio-demographic characteristics.	Customer loyalty	- Customer loyalty is linked to low prices and discount sales. - 44% of respondents said prices were one of the factors that compel them to make all their purchases in only one supermarket chain. - Probability of ranking prices and sales promotions as important factors was higher among older respondents and respondents who spent more monthly at supermarkets.
Caruso et al. (2018) [83]	Placement	Supermarket/ grocery store	Australia, New Zealand	56 hours (December 2008 and December 2015)	Direct observation	To assess how foot traffic and visual reach of endcaps differ by location.	Foot traffic Visual attention	- Back-of-store endcaps had 24% more foot traffic and 30% more visual reach than front-of-store endcaps.
Caspi et al. (2017) [84]	Placement Promotion	Dollar store Convenience store Other (pharmacy)	US	5 months (July 2014–November 2014)	Customer surveys Direct observation	To examine whether customers who shop at small/non-traditional food stores with more health promotions make healthier purchases.	Healthy eating index-2010 (HEI) score of products purchased	- Controlling for individual characteristics and store type, HEI scores for purchases were higher in stores with greater shelf space for fruits and vegetables. - Healthy advertisements on the store exterior were associated with lower purchase HEI scores. - The presence of interior healthy advertisements were not associated with purchase HEI scores.

Table 2. Cont.

Reference	Marketing Strategy	Retail Format	Country	Study Duration	Data Source	Objective	Outcome	Key Findings
Farrag (2012) [79]	Price	Supermarket/ grocery store	Egypt	Not specified	Interviews/focus groups	To measure to what extent compliance with Shariah moderates the relationship between sales promotion methods (price discount, product sampling, buy one get one free, sweepstakes/ lucky draws, scratch and win offers) of convenient products and consumer behaviors (product trial, stockpiling, spending more).	Purchase attitude	- Price discounts and buy-one-get-one were associated with self-reported stockpiling and spending more. - Price discounts had the strongest impact on consumer behavior (compared to sweepstakes/ lucky draw, scratch-and-win, free samples). - The relationship between price discounts and consumer behavior was moderated by Shariah law because some practices (e.g., scratch-and-win and sweepstake draws) were not compliant with Shariah law.
Felgate et al. (2012) [68]	Price	Supermarket/ grocery store	UK	86 weeks (29 May 2006–21 January 2008)	Scanner/panel data	To assess how supermarket loyalty card data can be used to analyze the effect of price promotions on spending.	Spending by product subgroup	- Promotions accounted for 14% of the variance in sales of beef. - While overall impact of promotion on sales of beef was insignificant, there was variability by cut of meat, customer group, and price promotions.
Fornari et al. (2013) [60]	Price	Supermarket/ grocery store	Italy	2011	Scanner/panel data	To assess the impact of different retailing-mix levers on private label market share.	Purchase volume	- Findings suggest partial support for price promotion increasing market share. - A significant presence on shelves, in width (increase in the number of product categories) and depth (increase in the number of SKUs in each product category) increased sales, suggesting that assortment is more important than price promotion.
Goić et al. (2011) [75]	Price	Supermarket/ grocery store	US	Not specified	Not specified	To investigate the effects of cross-market promotions (e.g., grocery store purchases that lead to price discounts for gas) on purchase volume and sales price.	Purchase volume Sales price	- Offering cross-market discounts on gas for grocery purchases led to an increase in both price and quantity of groceries purchased.

Table 2. *Cont.*

Reference	Marketing Strategy	Retail Format	Country	Study Duration	Data Source	Objective	Outcome	Key Findings
Guan et al. (2018) [54]	Price	Supermarket/grocery store	US	2 years (2003–2005)	Scanner/panel data	To compare the effects of individually-targeted coupons for less healthful and more healthful foods on consumer purchasing patterns.	Purchase volume	- Being exposed to coupons resulted in an increase in the rate of purchase as compared to those without coupons. - People responded more to targeted coupons than to untargeted coupons. - Targeted coupons significantly increased purchases of both healthy and less healthy items, with greater increases in the purchases of less healthy items.
Hong et al. (2016) [94]	Placement	Supermarket/grocery store	UK	Not specified	Scanner/panel data Direct observation	To examine whether the assortment or placement of one category affects purchase incidence in a different category that shares a common display space (e.g., frozen meals and ice cream).	Purchase incidence	- Consumers were less likely to purchase from a category of a given assortment when it was presented with another category assortment of greater variety and this effect was driven by the display proximity.
Huang et al. (2012) [57]	Price	Supermarket/grocery store	US	Not specified	Customer surveys Direct observation	To identify shopper trip-level and point-of-purchase-level drivers of unplanned consideration and purchase behavior.	Purchase incidenceImpulse purchases	- An impulse purchase was more likely if a shopper viewed fewer product shelf displays, stood closer to the shelf, and referenced external information.
Jamal et al. (2012) [81]	Price	Supermarket/grocery store	UK	Not specified	Interviews/focus groups	To investigate "ethnic" consumers' responses to different sales promotions.	Perceived importance for purchase decisions	- "Ethnic" customers reported a range of responses to sales promotion—some were responsive, some hostile—depending on the "net worth" of the sales promotion.
Johnson et al. (2013) [58]	PlacementPrice	Supermarket/grocery store	US	Not specified	Scanner/panel data	To examine how customized temporal discounts influence consumers' decisions to purchase products and overall profit of the retailers.	Purchase incidence Brand choice Profit	- The customization of discounts by time and value yielded an increase in profits of 18–40% relative to a model that optimizes the value of the discounts.
Kacen et al. (2012) [62]	Placement Price	Supermarket/grocery store	US	Not specified	Customer surveys	To assess the effect of retailing factors on the likelihood that a consumer will make an impulse purchase.	Impulse purchasing	- Products on sale and on display in a high-low pricing store increased the probability of an impulse buy to 7%. - A product had a 13.3% likelihood of being purchased if it was not on sale but a 17.6% likelihood if it was on sale. - A product had a 13.3% likelihood of being purchased if it was not on display, but a 20% likelihood if it was on display.

Table 2. Cont.

Reference	Marketing Strategy	Retail Format	Country	Study Duration	Data Source	Objective	Outcome	Key Findings
Kim et al. (2011) [66]	Price	Not specified	Japan	32 years (1976–2008)	Scanner/panel data Marketing data	To understand how changes among manufacturers in budget allocation from advertising to sales promotion affects sales volume and profitability.	Purchase volume profit	- Expenditure on sales promotion was associated with an increase in total volume sales but a decrease in profitability.
Leeflang et al. (2012) [70]	Price	Supermarket/ grocery store	Spain	1 year	Scanner/panel data	To determine the impact of price promotions in one category on the revenues of other categories.	Purchase volume Sales revenue	- Half of all price promotions expanded revenues for that category, especially for categories with deeper supported discounts. - There was a 61% probability that a price promotion affected sales of at least one other category. - Cross-promotional effects between categories more closely located in a store existed.
Levy and Gendel-Guterman (2012) [98]	Promotion	Supermarket/ grocery store	Not specified	Not specified	Customer surveys	To understand how consumer characteristics are correlated with advertising and the tendency to impulse buy store brands.	Impulse purchasing	- Advertising was positively correlated to the tendency to engage in impulse buying.
Liang et al. (2017) [82]	Promotion Price	Other (organic market)	Taiwan	2 month (2012)	Customer surveys	To understand organic food consumers' preferences for specific promotional programs (e.g., discounts, giveaways, limited time offers).	Purchase attitude	- Consumers preferred the programs in the discount category and the free giveaway category. - Limited time offers reduced purchase intention.
Mamiya et al. (2018) [71]	Price	Supermarket/ grocery store Convenience store Other (pharmacy)	Canada	6 years (January 2008–December 2013)	Scanner/panel data	To assess whether there was a differential impact of price discounting of soda on sales by store-neighborhood education.	Purchase volume	- Across all levels of education and types of store, discounting was positively associated with soda sales. - The modification of the effect of price discounting by education was most prominent in pharmacies, where the average log sales associated with discounting increased as education decreased.

Table 2. *Cont.*

Reference	Marketing Strategy	Retail Format	Country	Study Duration	Data Source	Objective	Outcome	Key Findings
Minnema et al. (2017) [100]	Promotion	Supermarket/ grocery store	Netherlands	20 weeks (2010)	Scanner/panel data	To examine the effectiveness of instant reward programs with bonus premiums (i.e., collectible giveaways).	Shopping tripsCategory purchase incidence Brand choice Purchase volume	- Instant giveaway of collectible premiums resulted in increased brand and category choice probability, but no change in purchase quantity. - Consumers were more likely to choose the promoted brand if it was promoted with both the bonus premium and price discount compared to when it was promoted with just a price discount.
Mortimer and Weeks (2011) [77]	Price	Supermarket/ grocery store	Australia	Not specified	Customer surveys	To examine how price information is differentially considered by men and women in an Australian grocery store and how this affects grocery shopping behavior.	Purchase attitude	- The mean score for how consumers rate the importance of promotional pricing on their shopping decisions was 4.41 out of 5. - Men considered price attributes of products and promotional tactics as being significantly lower in importance than did women.
Mussol et al. (2019) [53]	Promotion Price	Supermarket/ grocery store	France	Not specified	Customer surveys	To explore in-store sales promotions as a tool in developing in-store brand relationships with consumers.	Purchase attitude	- Samplings, in-store games, lotteries nurtured consumer loyalty and relationships with brands. - Price-based promotions should be used to trigger purchases, whereas non-monetary promotions should be used to nurture brand relationships.
Nakamura et al. (2014) [85]	Placement	Supermarket/ grocery store	UK	Not specified	Scanner/panel data	To estimate of the effect of end-of-aisle display on sales.	Purchase volume	- End-of-aisle display increased sales volumes by 23.2% for beer, 33.6% for wine, and 46.1% for spirits, by 51.7% for carbonated drinks, 73.5% for coffee, and 113.8% for tea. - The effect size was equivalent to a decrease in price of between 4% and 9% per volume for alcohol categories, and a decrease in price of between 22% and 62% per volume for non-alcohol categories.

187

Table 2. Cont.

Reference	Marketing Strategy	Retail Format	Country	Study Duration	Data Source	Objective	Outcome	Key Findings
Nakamura et al. (2015) [6]	Price	Supermarket/grocery store Convenience store Other (various)	UK	1 years (2010)	Scanner/panel data	To investigate if consumers are more responsive to promotions on less-healthy products; and if there are socioeconomic differences in food purchases in response to price promotions.	Purchase volume	- After controlling for the reference price, price discount rate, and brand-specific effects, the sales uplift arising from price promotions was larger in less-healthy than in healthier categories. - A 1% increase in the depth of price discount led to a sales uplift by 1.44% within a given category.
Nordfält and Lange (2013) [99]	Promotion	Supermarket/grocery store	Sweden	2 weeks (April 2008 and March 2009)	Scanner/Panel data Customer surveys	To investigate when and how in-store demonstrations work best.	Purchase volume	- In-store demonstrations increased sales, particularly when: closer to the weekend, the product was displayed next to the demonstration (235.07% increase), there was personnel offering the demonstration (24.31% increase), there was signage promoting the product (90.76% increase), and a commercial was run on an in-store TV (36.32%). - There was no significant change when in-store demonstrations were offered in a higher traffic area.
Osuna et al. (2016) [55]	Price	Supermarket/grocery store	Not specified	2 years (2008–2009)	Loyalty card data	To explore how targeted coupons influence the uptake of new category and brand purchases.	Coupon redemption Product trialing	- To entice customers to buy in new categories, coupon redemption rates were higher for leading brands and categories that are popular, easy to store, have a low number of SKUs, and are frequently on sale. - To increase incremental purchases, coupons should be in categories that have low purchase frequency and high number of SKUs.
Page et al. (2019) [86]	Placement	Supermarket/grocery store	Australia	24 hours	Direct observation	To explore the shopper traffic entering and exiting the middle aisle, and interaction with endcap promotions.	Shopper traffic Endcap use Basket size	- Overall use of endcaps in the store with a middle aisle was lower than that in the store with standard layout. - In a standard store, 2.2% of all observed shoppers were interacting with an endcap (48% at rear, 52% at front of store), while in the store with the middle aisle, 1.6%, (24% at the rear, 38% at the front, and 39% in the middle).

188

Table 2. Cont.

Reference	Marketing Strategy	Retail Format	Country	Study Duration	Data Source	Objective	Outcome	Key Findings
Panzone and Tiffin (2012) [61]	Price	Supermarket/grocery store Convenience store Other (liquor store)	England	Not specified	Customer surveys Receipts	To assess the impact of price promotions on wine on consumer purchases	Purchase volume Purchase initiation	- The presence of a discount was influential in determining what to buy (74% of the total impact of the discount), with a smaller effect on how much of a wine to buy (26% of the total impact), and no influence on interpurchase time. - Consumers primarily used discounts to determine the segment they will purchase from, and secondarily to purchase multiple units of the wine they had chosen.
Phillips et al. (2015) [87]	Placement Promotion	Supermarket/grocery store	US	3 days	Direct observation	To explore whether the effectiveness of an end-of-aisle display is weakened if there is a product demonstration occurring near the end-of-aisle.	Visual attention	- The presence of an in-store demonstration near the end-of-aisle affected shoppers' attention paid to the end-of-the-aisle. - The best way to attract attention to the end-of-aisle was not to have an in-store demonstration near it.
Phipps et al. (2010) [67]	Price	Supermarket/grocery store	US	Not specified	Scanner/panel data Interview/focus groups	To explore the associations of discounted prices on supermarket purchases of selected high-calorie foods and more healthful, low-calorie foods.	Purchase volume Purchase attitude	- Odds of purchasing on price promotion compared with off promotion was 2.4 for high-calorie products and 1.2 for low-calorie products. - Odds of purchasing on sale versus full price were higher for sweet snacks, grain-based snacks, and sugar-sweetened beverages. - Participants emphasized the lure of sale items and said they took advantage of sales to stock up.
Point of Purchase Advertising International (2012) [15]	Placement	Supermarket/grocery store	US	Not specified	Customer surveys Direct observation Other (store audit)	To investigate how shoppers are interacting with the in-store environment.	Purchase volume	- More than 1 in 6 purchases were made when a display with that brand was present in store.

Table 2. Cont.

Reference	Marketing Strategy	Retail Format	Country	Study Duration	Data Source	Objective	Outcome	Key Findings
Pozzi (2013) [64]	Price	Supermarket/ grocery store Online retailer	US	2 years (June 2004–June 2006)	Scanner/panel data	To assess if the introduction of e-commerce affects bulk purchase and stockpiling behavior by customers.	Purchase volume Impulse purchasing	- The share of expenditure on discounted items rose by 9–20% with the introduction of e-commerce. - Online shopping did not increase the likelihood of buying promoted items but positively impacted the amount customers bought when they bought promoted items. - The amount of purchasing increases as the amount of discount increases.
Ranjan (2018) [88]	Placement	Supermarket/ grocery store	US	8 months (1 May 2015–31 December 2015)	Scanner/panel data Loyalty card data Marketing data	To explore how category location, adjacencies, size and merchandizing determine consumers' category choices.	Spending Purchase volume	- Moving to a central (peripheral) position in the layout improved purchase quantity and purchase incidence. - There was an overall "attention-stealing" effect of having neighbors.
Revoredo-Giha (2015) [69]	Price	Supermarket/ grocery store Convenience store Other (various)	UK	2006–2013	Scanner/panel data	To analyze the overall effect of price promotions on consumers' food purchases.	Spending	- Price promotions had a positive effect on total household expenditure and expenditure by category across socioeconomic quintiles. - Consumers responded positively to price promotions on fruits, vegetables, soft drinks, juices, fats, and eggs.
Ruff et al. (2016) [89]	Placement Promotion	Convenience store	US	Not specified	Customer surveys Other (bag check)	To study how placement of products and signs in small convenience stores influence shopping behavior.	Purchase incidence	- Placement of water at eye-level and of produce in at the front of the store was not associated with sugar-sweetened beverage purchases. - Signs advertising water and sugar-sweetened beverages were not associated with sugar-sweetened beverage purchases.
Sanchez-Flack et al. (2017) [90]	Placement Promotion	Convenience store	US	1 years (2010)	Customer surveys Other (store audit)	To examine how product availability, placement, and promotion were associated with fruit and vegetable purchasing among Hispanic customers in San Diego County.	Purchase volume Spending	- Each additional square foot of display space dedicated to fruits and vegetables and each additional fresh fruits and vegetables display were associated with a $0.02 increase and $0.29 decrease, respectively, in fruit and vegetable purchasing.

Table 2. Cont.

Reference	Marketing Strategy	Retail Format	Country	Study Duration	Data Source	Objective	Outcome	Key Findings
Sano and Suzuki (2013) [72]	Price	Supermarket/grocery store	Japan	1 months (May 2009–June 2009)	Scanner/panel data Other (shopping path)	To determine the share of product categories that should be included on discount flyers.	Purchase volume	- Price promotion of items would likely increase sales, particularly in some categories like drinks and western deli. - Price promotion would be less effective where there are already a lot of discounts.
Seva et al. (2011) [94]	Placement	Supermarket/grocery store	Philippines	Not specified	Customer surveys Direct observation	To assess the effect of shelf position and product characteristics on the number and duration of eye fixations on a grocery shelf containing junk foods.	Visual attention	- Products placed at the top shelf received the highest attention from consumers as compared to the products placed on the other levels (the eye-level of majority of the subjects was in line with the top shelf). - Consumer attention decreased as the products' vertical position deviated from eye-level.
Singh (2013) [73]	Promotion Price	Supermarket/grocery store	US	Not specified	Scanner/panel data	To investigate how pricing and promotion in frequently purchased categories influenced consumer visits to competing multiproduct grocery stores.	Store choice	- Own-store and cross-store prices, and own-store and cross-store feature advertising in frequently purchased categories impacted consumers' choice. - For stockpiling categories, the own store feature activity (but not own store price) positively influenced consumer choice.
Smithson et al. (2015) [8]	Price	Supermarket/grocery store Convenience store Other (various)	UK	52 weeks (December 2004–December 2005)	Scanner/panel data	To explore the role that price promotions play in purchasing levels of high-sugar food and drinks.	Purchase volume Brand switching	- 1/5 of foods and beverages bought on price promotion were purchased in addition to what would be expected for a given category if the price promotion was not in place. - Price promotions led to short-term brand switching. - Price promotions led to an overall increase in take-home food and drink volumes.
Spanjaard (2014) [95]	Promotion	Supermarket/grocery store	Australia	Not specified	Customer surveys Direct observation Interviews/focus groups Other (diaries)	To understand which factors drive customer purchasing decisions.	Purchase attitude	- 41% of survey participants said they were influenced by promotional offers. - Trust and emotional connection the brand that are main purchasing decision drivers for customers.

Table 2. Cont.

Reference	Marketing Strategy	Retail Format	Country	Study Duration	Data Source	Objective	Outcome	Key Findings
Tacka (2019) [97]	Promotion	Not specified	US	5 days (19 September 2018–24 September 2018)	Customer surveys	To investigate the relationship between marketing activities (among other factors) and purchases of instant consumable snack foods	Purchase attitude	- Marketing activities were rated, on average, as being of "little importance" or "neither important nor unimportant," when purchasing an instant consumable snack food.
Talukdar and Lindsey (2013) [74]	Price	Supermarket/ grocery store	US	52 weeks (2003–2004)	Scanner/panel data Customer surveys	To predict the effects of price changes on consumers' food consumption behavior.	Purchase volume	- For healthy food, demand sensitivity was greater for a price increase than for a price decrease. - For unhealthy food, demand sensitivity was greater for a price decrease than a price increase.
Tan et al. (2018) [46]	Placement	Supermarket/ grocery store	Australia	Not specified	Scanner/panel data Direct observation	To compare the sales effectiveness of front versus back located end-of-aisle promotional displays in a supermarket.	Purchase volume	- Rear endcaps generated 416% sales uplift while front endcaps generated 346% sales uplift.
Tran (2019) [76]	Promotion Price	Supermarket/ grocery store	Vietnam	2 weeks	Customer surveys	To investigate factors that influence customers' impulse purchasing behavior.	Purchase attitude	- Sale promotion, presence of family and friends, emotion, merchandise display, money available and festival season accounted for 65.162% of impulse buying behavior.
Walmsley et al. (2018) [92]	Placement	Supermarket/ grocery store	England	170 weeks (January 2012–July 2017)	Scanner/panel data	To examine the effect of the store re-arrangements on purchasing of fruits and vegetables.	Purchase volume Spending	- The effect of the shop re-arrangement to make fruit and vegetables more prominent and moving the fruit and vegetable display to face the entrance led to an increase in sales and total dollars spent on fruits and vegetables.
Yildirim and Aydin (2012) [96]	Promotion	Supermarket/ grocery store	Turkey	10 days	Customer surveys	To assess the effect of supermarket announcements on customer behavior while shopping.	Purchase attitude	- Announcements related to price discounts, buy-one-get-one offers, membership deals, giveaways, and coupons were most desired and impactful announcements. - The most noticed type of announcement focused on price discounts.
Zhang (2017) [56]	Price	Online retailer	US	2 weeks (13 January 2014–26 January 2014)	Scanner/panel data	To evaluate the impact of coupons and informational nudges to customers identified through modeling on purchasing.	Purchase incidence	- Providing information and discounts to specific customers who are selected through modeling led to a higher conversion to purchase products.

4. Discussion

This review is the first to synthesize literature from academic and industry sources on the approaches that manufacturers use to shape retailer marketing strategies, and, in turn, consumer behavior and attitudes. More than half of the included studies focused on pricing; fewer articles assessed placement or promotion and many of these articles focused on purchase attitudes rather than behavior.

Findings suggest that all types of price promotions, including coupons, multi-buys, and TPR, shape purchasing behavior. Placement in premium store locations, such as on endcaps, and in-store samples are also effective drivers of sales. Other promotion activities, such as giveaways, games, and signs, may be less impactful. Notably, findings suggest that retailer marketing strategies may be less effective at driving sales for healthy foods and beverages [54,67,69,74,84,89,90]. Of the small number of studies that specifically considered sales of healthy products, the majority found that retailer marketing strategies, including signs and price promotions, were not associated with increased sales of healthy products. Two studies did find increases in healthy purchases, but effect sizes were smaller than for unhealthy products [54,69]. Previous reviews have similarly found that promotions of unhealthy products are more impactful than those for healthy products [4,9]. Studies of retailer- or investigator-driven interventions to specifically promote healthy purchases, however, were outside the scope of this study (these interventions are reviewed by Karpyn et al. in a paper published as part of this special issue) and may have identified retailer marketing strategies that effectively increase healthy purchases.

Findings regarding the impact of price promotions and product placement on consumer behavior are consistent with findings of previous reviews [3,9,20,21]. To the authors' knowledge, the review by Glanz et al. is the only study to also explore promotion; however, they did not identify any studies related to signage, and only one related to in-store sampling [21]. Several previous reviews, including Glanz et al., excluded studies in nontraditional retail settings, such as convenience and dollar stores and online retail. Findings from included studies of nontraditional retail formats suggest that retailer marketing strategies have similar effects across retail settings. One notable difference, however, is that consumers may be more likely take advantage of promotions in online retail by stockpiling, as they are not required to transport their purchases home themselves [64].

While only three studies were rated as "low quality," analytic rigor and rigor of data sources in included articles varied widely. Many articles from industry publications did not describe their analytic methods; thus, it was challenging to assess the quality of evidence of these articles. Additionally, while no studies listed conflicts of interest and many did not disclose funding sources, several were written by industry representatives and published in trade publications and may, therefore, have been more inclined to include findings that portrayed the companies favorably. A growing number of studies used store scanner and loyalty card data; these data sources, which provide large sample sizes and detailed sales information, should be used widely, particularly when paired with information on customer demographics. Several of the included studies occurred in controlled, laboratory settings; strategies that proved impactful in these settings, such as placement of products at eye-level, should be adapted and tested in real-world retail environments.

Study findings point to strategies that policymakers, public health practitioners, and retailers can use to ensure that retail environments promote healthy eating. Results suggest that policies and corporate practices that limit promotion of unhealthy products, rather than interventions to promote healthy products, may be needed to improve diet quality. Policies and practices can target each of the four TPPs identified in this study to curb promotion of unhealthy products. For example, policies could prohibit category captains from excluding competitors, or create healthy checkout aisles by prohibiting retailers from accepting stocking fees to display ultra-processed foods in checkout aisles. Considering SNAP is an important revenue stream for many US retailers, restrictions on promotion of unhealthy products could also be integrated into requirements for SNAP-authorized retailers [102].

4.1. Future Research Directions

Findings from this study highlight directions for future study. Research is needed to evaluate:

1. **Online and other nontraditional retail formats.** Eighty percent of included articles focused on retailer marketing strategies in grocery stores and supermarkets; other nontraditional retail formats such as dollar stores and online retailers should be assessed. Despite rapid proliferation of dollar stores in the past decade [103], they were assessed in only one of the included articles. Considering dollar stores are most common in rural and low-income communities, evaluations in dollar stores may provide insight into geographic and socioeconomic disparities in diet and food purchasing. In 2015, dollar stores represented two-thirds of new stores in designated "food deserts" [104]. Relatedly, online retail was the focus of only four of the included articles. While online grocery retail represented only 6.3% of total US grocery spending in 2019, [105] online sales are rapidly expanding, and due to concerns about COVID-19 transmission, are expected to grow more than 40% in 2020 [106].
2. **Distal consumer outcomes including consumption and health.** None of the included studies measured the impact of retailer marketing strategies on distal or long-term outcomes, such as diet quality or weight. Admittedly, it may be difficult to detect the impact of marketing strategies on health outcomes, especially because diet-related health outcomes are influenced by a multitude of environmental and biological factors. Dietary consumption, which has been linked to health outcomes in the public health literature, however, may be assessed. Analysis of these outcomes will require collection of different types of data, such as food frequency questionnaires or dietary recall surveys, coupled with objective purchase data. Dietary data collection methods, however, do have limitations (e.g., food frequency questionnaires may not be sensitive enough to detect small effect sizes, and dietary recalls are resource-intensive and subject to recall bias).
3. **Other outcomes of importance to retailers and manufacturers.** While this review excluded studies that did not measure consumer behavior or attitudes, the initial scan of titles and abstracts revealed few studies that assessed other outcomes of importance to industry, such as short- and long-term return on investment and customer lifetime value (i.e., the total profit a retailer makes from customers over their lifetime). Interventions that benefit public health, in order to be sustainable and acceptable to manufactures and retailers, must consider these outcomes.
4. **Differential impacts of retail practices on consumers by demographic characteristics.** Few studies compared how retailer marketing strategies affected different consumer segments, such as families with children, shoppers with low income, or shoppers who identify as racial or ethnic minorities. Insight into how certain populations may be disproportionately influenced or targeted by retailer marketing strategies can guide intervention efforts.
5. **Retailer marketing strategies that have the strongest impact on consumer behavior.** Only a small number of studies directly compared the impacts of different retailer marketing strategies, and most of these focused on perceived importance. Additional head-to-head comparison of retailer marketing strategies is needed to prioritize which components to include in future interventions.
6. **Trade promotion practices that have the strongest impact on retailer behavior.** Data on TPP are largely proprietary, and thus, research is limited on the amount manufacturers spend annually on TPP, which TPP are used most frequently, what proportion of retailer profit comes from TPP, and which TPP are the strongest drivers of retailer marketing. Additional research, potentially done in partnership with industry, is needed to understand these powerful market drivers.

4.2. Limitations

It is possible that different search terms or databases might have identified further studies. The quality of evidence grading tool was adapted from the Newcastle–Ottawa quality assessment scale, which was initially designed for case-control and cohort studies. Thus, it was challenging to assess quality of evidence for qualitative and observational studies, as well as industry reports and news articles, which provide few details on methods. Additionally, while study inclusion criteria were designed to capture studies from any country, only studies published in English were included. The majority of identified studies focused on the US and UK, and many countries were not represented in these findings. As a result, results may not be generalizable across countries and cultures.

5. Conclusions

This review finds evidence that by influencing retailer marketing strategies through TPP, manufacturers can shape consumer behavior and, ultimately, diets. The 74 studies included in this review suggest that TPP have a considerable effect on product placement, pricing, and promotion, and, in turn, on a range of customer outcomes, including purchase volume, spending, and attitudes. Findings point to a particularly strong relationship between price promotions and consumer behavior and differential impacts by product type and consumer characteristics. This review builds on previous work by synthesizing findings from recent studies and studies focused on non-traditional retail formats. Study findings provides valuable insight that can guide efforts by policymakers, public health practitioners, and food retailers to design retail environments that promote healthy eating. Public health practitioners and policymakers could consider policies that regulate promotion of unhealthy products by targeting each of the four TPPs identified in this study. Further investigation is warranted to determine the impact of retailer marketing on dietary outcomes and outcomes of importance to retailers. Further research is also needed in online and nontraditional retail settings.

Author Contributions: A.A.H. and C.L.P. were involved in conceptualizing this study, defining the methodology, conducting the literature search, analyzing findings, drafting and editing the manuscript, and funding acquisition. M.P., A.N.T., R.L.F. and A.J.M. were involved in conceptualizing the study, defining the methodology, and reviewing and editing the manuscript. All authors have read and agreed to the published version of the manuscript.

Funding: This research was supported by Healthy Eating Research, a national program of the Robert Wood Johnson Foundation. Training support for A.A.H. was provided through the Johns Hopkins Center for a Livable Future-Lerner Fellowship.

Acknowledgments: The authors would like to thank attendees of the January 2020 Healthy Retail Research Convening and the 2020 Healthy Eating Research Annual Meeting for their constructive feedback on research findings and conclusions. The authors would like to thank Megan Lott, Kirsten Arm and Mary Story from Healthy Eating Research for their project support.

Conflicts of Interest: The authors declare no conflict of interest. The funders commissioned research on this topic but had no role in the design of the study; in the collection, analyses, or interpretation of data; in the writing of the manuscript; or in the decision to publish the results.

Appendix A

Food and Beverage Retail Formats *:

- **Supermarkets:** A food retailer with greater than 9000 square feet of selling space and at least $2 million in annual sales. Non-food sales must account for 15% or less of total store sales (e.g., Kroger, Safeway).
- **Drug stores:** Drug stores feature prescription-based pharmacies but generate at least 20% of their total sales from other categories, including general merchandise and food (e.g., Rite-Aid, CVS).
- **Mass merchandisers:** Large department stores that sell primarily general merchandise and nonperishables but also carry a limited assortment of grocery products (e.g., K-Mart, Target).
- **Supercenters:** Also known as hypermarkets and superstores, supercenters are hybrid stores that combine mass merchandisers with full supermarkets (e.g., Walmart Supercenter, Fred Meyer).
- **Convenience and corner stores:** Convenience stores typically sell gasoline, general merchandise, alcohol and tobacco, and a limited selection of staple and ready-to-eat, prepared foods (e.g., 7-Eleven, Exxon).

- **Dollar stores:** Dollar stores typically emphasize low prices (many products cost $1) and offer little in the way of customer service. Traditionally, they focused on staple consumer goods and other nonfood items but, have increasingly offered food (e.g., Dollar Tree, Dollar General).
- **Club stores:** Also referred to as warehouse or volume stores, these are large-format outlets that specialize in selling food and selected general merchandise in bulk for relatively low prices, per unit. Consumers need paid memberships to shop at them (e.g., Costco, Sam's Club).
- **Online retailers:** Retailers with an ecommerce presence, providing grocery click-and-collect or delivery services. These retailers can take any brick-and-mortar format (i.e., convenience stores, supermarkets, and mass merchandisers can all be online retailers).
- **Other:** Includes military commissaries, hospitals, and other food service providers, as well as direct-to-consumer food outlets such as farmers markets and community-supported agriculture.

* Definitions adapted from Volpe R, Kuhns A, and Jaenicke T. 2017. Store Formats and Patterns in Household Grocery Purchases, EIB-167, U.S. Department of Agriculture, Economic Research Service.

Appendix B

Search Terms

Research Question 1 Search String

((("Food" OR "Beverage")
AND ("Manufacturer *" OR "Distributor *" OR "Supplier *" OR "Processor *" OR "grower *" OR "trade association *" OR "producer *" OR "industry" OR "company")
AND ("Category captain *" OR "Category management" OR "Cooperative advertising" OR "Cooperative marketing" OR "dealer aid *" OR "fee *" OR "In-kind remuneration" OR "Pay-to-stay" OR "pouring right *" OR "Promotional allowance *" OR "Slotting" OR "Trade promotion" OR "Trade spend")
AND ("Grocer *" OR "Grocery store *" OR "Supermarket *" OR "Food store *" OR "Online grocer *" OR "Superstore *" OR "Warehouse *" OR "Club store *" OR "Convenience store *" OR "Food retailer *" OR "Food outlet *" OR "pharmac *" OR "corner store *" OR "discount store *" OR "dollar store *")
NOT "pharmaceutical *"

Research Question 2 Search String

((("Food" OR "Beverage")
AND ("Manufacturer *" OR "Distributor *" OR "Supplier *" OR "Processor *" OR "grower *" OR "trade association *" OR "producer *" OR "industry" OR "company") OR ("Grocer *" OR "Grocery store *" OR "Supermarket *" OR "Food store *" OR "Online grocer * " OR "Superstore *" OR "Warehouse *" OR "Club store *" OR "Convenience store *" OR "Food retailer *" OR "Food outlet *" OR "pharmac *" OR "corner store *" OR "discount store *" OR "dollar store *"))
AND ("Category captain *" OR "Category management" OR "Cooperative advertising" OR "Cooperative marketing" OR "dealer aid *" OR "fee *" OR "In-kind remuneration" OR "Pay-to-stay" OR "pouring right *" OR "Promotional allowance *" OR "Slotting" OR "Trade promotion" OR "Trade spend" OR "Buy-one-get-one" OR "buy one get one" OR "Circular *" OR "Coupon *" OR "Cross Promotion *" OR "Discount *" OR "Display *" OR "endcap" OR "Feature and display" OR "Incentive *" OR "In-store sampl" OR "loss leader *" OR "Placement" OR "POINT-of-sale advertis *" OR "Price Promotion *" OR "Rollback *" OR "Sales Promotion *" OR "Sign *" OR "Shipper *" OR "Shelf talker *" OR "Temporary price reduction *" OR "Two-for-one" OR "two for one")
AND ("Customer" OR "Shopper" OR "Consumer")
AND ("Behavior" OR "Preference" OR "Demand" OR "Consumption" OR "Choice" OR "decision" OR "purchas *" OR "attitude *" OR "willingness to pay")
NOT ("pharmaceutical *")

Appendix C

Table A1. Newcastle–Ottawa quality scale adapted grading criteria.

Selection (max of 5 stars)	(1) Representativeness of the sample:	(a) Truly representative of the average in the target population [1] (e.g., all subjects or random sampling)	*
		(b) Somewhat representative of the average in the target population [1] (e.g., nonrandom sampling)	*
		(c) Selected group of users	No stars
		(d) No description of the sampling strategy	No stars
	(2) Sample size:	(a) Justified and satisfactory	*
		(b) Not justified	No stars
	(3) Non-respondents:	(a) Comparability between respondents' and non-respondents' characteristics is established, and the response rate is satisfactory	*
		(b) The response rate is unsatisfactory, or the comparability between respondents and non-respondents is unsatisfactory	No stars
		(c) No description of the response rate or the characteristics of the responders and the non-responders	No stars
		(d) Not applicable (e.g., aggregate sales data)	NA
	(4) Ascertainment of risk factor:	(a) Built into dataset	**
		(b) Built into study design	**
		(c) Self-reported/-stated	*
		(d) No information disclosed	No stars
Comparability (max of 2 stars)	(1) The subjects in different outcome groups are comparable, based on the study design or analysis. Confounding factors are controlled	(a) The study controls for the most important factor (e.g., income/SES)	*
		(b) The study controls for any additional factor (e.g., age, gender, household size, race)	*
		(c) Not applicable (e.g., there is no comparison group)	NA
Outcome (max of 3 stars)	(1) Assessment of the outcome:	(a) Independent blind assessment	**
		(b) Record linkage	**
		(c) Self reports	*
		(d) No description	No stars
	(2) Statistical test:	(a) The statistical test used to analyze the data is clearly described and appropriate, and the measurement of the association is presented, including confidence intervals and the probability level (p value)	*
		(b) The statistical test is not appropriate, not described or incomplete	No stars

[1] "Target population" defined based on authors' definition of their "target population." The Newcastle–Ottawa quality scale assigns studies composite quality scores by awarding up to nine stars. A study can be awarded a maximum of one star (*) in the categories of: representativeness of the sample, sample size, non-respondents, and statistical test. A maximum of two stars (**) can be awarded in the categories of: ascertainment of risk factor, comparability, and assessment of outcome.

Appendix D

Table A2. Quality assessment of the included studies using the Newcastle–Ottawa quality scale ($n = 54$).

Reference	Selection				Comparability	Outcome		Overall Score
	Representativeness of the Sample	Sample Size	Non-Respondents	Ascertainment of Risk Factor	Are Confounding Factors Controlled	Assessment of Outcome	Statistical Test	
Andorfer et al. (2015)	0	1	0	2	1	1	1	6/10
Arce-Urriza et al. (2017)	1	1	NA	2	NA	2	1	7/7
Awan et al. (2015)	1	0	0	1	NA	1	1	4/8
Aziz et al. (2013)	0	0	0	1	0	1	1	3/10 *
Banks et al. (2016)	0	0	NA	1	NA	1	0	2/7 *
Bogomolova et al. (2019)	1	1	NA	1	2	1	1	7/9
Breugelmans and Campo (2016)	1	1	NA	2	1	2	1	8/9
Čábelková et al. (2015)	1	1	0	1	2	1	1	7/10
Huang et al. (2012)	1	0	0	2	2	2	1	8/10
Caruso et al. (2018)	1	1	0	2	0	2	1	7/10
Caspi et al. (2017)	1	0	0	1	1	1	1	5/10
Farrag (2012)	0	0	0	2	0	1	1	4/10
Felgate et al. (2012)	1	1	NA	2	0	2	1	7/9
Fornari et al. (2013)	1	0	NA	2	NA	2	1	6/7
Goić et al. (2011)	0	0	NA	2	NA	0	1	3/7
Guan et al. (2018)	1	1	0	2	2	1	1	8/10
Hong et al. (2016)	1	1	NA	2	1	2	1	8/9
Jamal et al. (2012)	1	1	0	1	NA	1	0	4/8
Johnson et al. (2013)	1	0	0	2	NA	2	1	6/8
Kacen et al. (2012)	1	0	NA	2	2	1	1	7/9
Kim et al. (2011)	1	1	NA	2	NA	2	1	7/7
Leeflang et al. (2012)	0	0	NA	2	NA	2	1	5/7
Levy and Gendel-Guterman (2012)	1	1	0	1	2	2	1	7/10
Liang et al. (2017)	1	1	NA	2	0	2	1	7/9
Mamiya et al. (2018)	1	1	NA	2	2	2	1	9/9
Minnema et al. (2017)	1	1	0	2	2	2	1	9/10
Mortimer and Weeks (2011)	1	1	0	2	1	1	1	7/10

Table A2. *Cont.*

Reference	Selection				Comparability	Outcome		Overall Score *
	Representativeness of the Sample	Sample Size	Non-Respondents	Ascertainment of Risk Factor	Are Confounding Factors Controlled	Assessment of Outcome	Statistical Test	
Mussol et al. (2019)	1	0	0	2	1	1	1	6/10
Nakamura et al. (2015)	1	1	0	2	1	2	1	8/10
Nakamura et al. (2014)	1	0	NA	2	NA	2	1	6/7
Nordfält and Lange (2013)	1	0	NA	2	NA	2	1	6/7
Osuna et al. (2016)	1	0	NA	2	1	2	1	7/9
Page et al. (2019)	1	0	NA	2	2	2	1	8/9
Panzone and Tiffin (2012)	1	1	0	1	0	1	1	5/10
Phillips et al. (2015)	1	0	NA	2	1	2	1	7/9
Phipps et al (2010)	0	0	0	2	1	2	1	6/10
Point of Purchase Advertising International (2012)	1	1	0	2	0	2	0	6/10
Pozzi (2013)	1	1	NA	2	2	2	1	9/9
Ranjan (2018)	1	0	NA	2	1	2	1	7/9
Revoredo-Giha (2015)	1	1	0	2	1	2	1	8/10
Ruff et al. (2016)	1	0	0	2	2	1	1	7/10
Sanchez-Flack et al. (2017)	1	1	1	2	2	1	1	9/10
Sano and Suzuki (2013)	0	0	NA	2	NA	2	1	5/9
Seva et al. (2011)	0	0	0	2	0	2	1	5/10
Singh (2013)	1	0	0	2	2	2	1	8/10
Smithson et al. (2015)	1	1	0	2	2	2	1	9/10
Spanjaard (2014)	1	1	0	1	NA	1	NA	4/7
Tacka (2019)	1	0	0	1	0	1	1	4/10
Talukdar and Lindsey (2013)	1	0	NA	2	2	2	1	8/9
Tan et al. (2018)	1	0	NA	2	1	2	1	7/9
Tran (2019)	0	0	0	1	0	1	1	3/10 *
Walmsley et al. (2018)	1	1	NA	2	0	2	1	7/9
Yildirim and Aydin (2012)	1	1	0	2	1	1	1	7/10
Zhang (2017)	1	1	NA	2	2	2	1	9/9

* Indicates low quality.

References

1. Willett, W.C.; Koplan, J.P.; Nugent, R.; Dusenbury, C.; Puska, P.; Gaziano, T.A. Prevention of Chronic Disease by Means of Diet and Lifestyle Changes. In *Disease Control Priorities in Developing Countries*; Jamison, D.T., Breman, J.G., Measham, A.R., Alleyne, G., Claeson, M., Evans, D.B., Jha, P., Mills, A., Musgrove, P., Eds.; World Bank: Washington, DC, USA, 2006; ISBN 978-0-8213-6179-5.
2. Riesenberg, D.; Backholer, K.; Zorbas, C.; Sacks, G.; Paix, A.; Marshall, J.; Blake, M.R.; Bennett, R.; Peeters, A.; Cameron, A.J. Price Promotions by Food Category and Product Healthiness in an Australian Supermarket Chain, 2017–2018. *Am. J. Public Health* **2019**, *109*, 1434–1439. [CrossRef] [PubMed]
3. Bennett, R.; Zorbas, C.; Huse, O.; Peeters, A.; Cameron, A.J.; Sacks, G.; Backholer, K. Prevalence of healthy and unhealthy food and beverage price promotions and their potential influence on shopper purchasing behaviour: A systematic review of the literature. *Obes Rev.* **2019**. [CrossRef] [PubMed]
4. Ravensbergen, E.A.; Waterlander, W.E.; Kroeze, W.; Steenhuis, I.H. Healthy or unhealthy on sale? A cross-sectional study on the proportion of healthy and unhealthy foods promoted through flyer advertising by supermarkets in the Netherlands. *BMC Public Health* **2015**, *15*, 470. [CrossRef] [PubMed]
5. Zorbas, C.; Gilham, B.; Boelsen-Robinson, T.; Blake, M.R.; Peeters, A.; Cameron, A.J.; Wu, J.H.; Backholer, K. The frequency and magnitude of price-promoted beverages available for sale in Australian supermarkets. *Aust. N. Z. J. Public Health* **2019**, *43*, 346–351. [CrossRef]
6. Nakamura, R.; Suhrcke, M.; Jebb, S.A.; Pechey, R.; Almiron-Roig, E.; Marteau, T.M. Price promotions on healthier compared with less healthy foods: A hierarchical regression analysis of the impact on sales and social patterning of responses to promotions in Great Britain. *Am. J. Clin. Nutr.* **2015**, *101*, 808–816. [CrossRef]
7. López, A.; Seligman, H.K. Online Grocery Store Coupons and Unhealthy Foods, United States. *Prev. Chronic Dis.* **2014**, *11*. [CrossRef]
8. Smithson, M.; Kirk, J.; Capelin, C. Sugar reduction: The evidence for action Annexe 4: An analysis of the role of price promotions on the household purchases of food and drinks high in sugar. A research project for Public Health England conducted by Kantar Worldpanel; London. 2015. Available online: https://assets.publishing.service.gov.uk/government/uploads/system/uploads/attachment_data/file/470175/Annexe_4._Analysis_of_price_promotions.pdf (accessed on 6 October 2020).
9. Martin, L.; Bauld, L.; Angus, K. *Rapid Evidence Review: The Impact of Promotions on High Fat, Sugar and Salt (HFSS) Food and Drink on Consumer Purchasing and Consumption Behaviour and the Effectiveness of Retail Environment Interventions*; NHS Health Scotland: Edinburgh, UK, 2017.
10. Hales, C.M.; Carroll, M.D.; Fryar, C.D.; Ogden, C.L. Prevalence of obesity and severe obesity among adults: United States, 2017–2018. NCHS Data Brief 2020. Available online: https://www.cdc.gov/nchs/data/databriefs/db360-h.pdf (accessed on 6 October 2020).
11. Grier, S.A.; Kumanyika, S.K. The Context for Choice: Health Implications of Targeted Food and Beverage Marketing to African Americans. *Am. J. Public Health* **2008**, *98*, 1616–1629. [CrossRef]
12. Moran, A.J.; Musicus, A.; Findling, M.T.G.; Brissette, I.F.; Lowenfels, A.A.; Subramanian, S.; Roberto, C.A. Increases in Sugary Drink Marketing During Supplemental Nutrition Assistance Program Benefit Issuance in New York. *Am. J. Prev. Med.* **2018**, *55*, 55–62. [CrossRef]
13. Lang, T.; Heasman, M. *Food Wars: The Global Battle for Mouths, Minds and Markets*, 2nd ed.; Routledge Earthscan: London, UK, 2015.
14. Mancino, L.; Guthrie, J.F.; Ver Ploeg, M.; Lin, B. *Nutritional Quality of Foods Acquired by Americans: Findings from USDA's National Household Food Acquisition and Purchase Survey*; U.S. Department of Agriculture Economic Research Service: Washington, DC, USA, 2018.
15. 2012 Shopper Engagement Study Media Topline Report. 2012. Available online: http://ww1.prweb.com/prfiles/2012/05/08/9489590/Media-Topline-Final.pdf (accessed on 6 October 2020).
16. Cohen, D.A.; Lesser, L.I. Obesity prevention at the point of purchase. *Obes. Rev.* **2016**, *17*, 389–396. [CrossRef]
17. Rivlin, G. *Rigged: Supermarket Shelves for Sale*; Center for Science in the Public Interest: Washington, DC, USA, 2016.
18. Kotler, P.; Armstrong, G. *Principles of Marketing*, 17th ed.; Pearson: London, UK, 2017.
19. The Path to Efficient Trade Promotions; Nielsen. 2015. Available online: https://www.nielsen.com/us/en/insights/report/2015/the-path-to-efficient-trade-promotions/ (accessed on 6 October 2020).

20. Backholer, K.; Sacks, G.; Cameron, A.J. Food and Beverage Price Promotions: An Untapped Policy Target for Improving Population Diets and Health. *Curr. Nutr. Rep.* **2019**, *8*, 250–255. [CrossRef]
21. Glanz, K.; Bader, M.D.M.; Iyer, S. Retail grocery store marketing strategies and obesity: An integrative review. *Am. J. Prev. Med.* **2012**, *42*, 503–512. [CrossRef] [PubMed]
22. Welch, V.; Petticrew, M.; Tugwell, P.; Moher, D.; O'Neill, J.; Waters, E.; White, H.; PRISMA-Equity Bellagio group. PRISMA-Equity 2012 extension: Reporting guidelines for systematic reviews with a focus on health equity. *PLoS Med.* **2012**, *9*. [CrossRef] [PubMed]
23. Modesti, P.A.; Reboldi, G.; Cappuccio, F.P.; Agyemang, C.; Remuzzi, G.; Rapi, S.; Perruolo, E.; Parati, G.; ESH Working Group on CV Risk in Low Resource Settings. Panethnic differences in blood pressure in Europe: A systematic review and meta-analysis. *PLoS ONE* **2016**, *11*, e0147601. [CrossRef] [PubMed]
24. Takahashi, N.; Hashizume, M. A systematic review of the influence of occupational organophosphate pesticides exposure on neurological impairment. *BMJ Open* **2014**, *4*, e004798. [CrossRef]
25. Achrol, R.S. Slotting allowances: A time series analysis of aggregate effects over three decades. *J. Acad. Mark. Sci.* **2012**, *40*, 673–694. [CrossRef]
26. Ayala, G.X.; D'Angelo, H.; Gittelsohn, J.; Horton, L.; Ribisl, K.; Sindberg, L.S.; Olson, C.; Kharmats, A.; Laska, M.N. Who is behind the stocking of energy-dense foods and beverages in small stores? The importance of food and beverage distributors. *Public Health Nutr.* **2017**, *20*, 3333–3342. [CrossRef]
27. Dhar, S.K.; Hoch, S.J.; Kumar, N. Effective category management depends on the role of the category. *J. Retail.* **2001**, *77*, 165–184. [CrossRef]
28. Efthymiou, N. Shelved Cases. *Mark. Week* **2003**, *26*, 43–44.
29. Feig, B. Notes From Orlando. *Frozen Food Age* **2002**, *51*, 18.
30. Gomez, M.I.; Maratou, L.M.; Just, D.R. Factors Affecting the Allocation of Trade Promotions in the U.S. Food Distribution System. *Rev. Agric. Econ.* **2007**, *29*, 119–140. [CrossRef]
31. Guissoni, A.; Consoli, M.; Rodrigues, J. Is Category Management in Small Supermarket Worth the Effort? *Rev. Adm. Empresas* **2013**, *53*, 592–603. [CrossRef]
32. Hamilton, S.F. Slotting Allowances as a Facilitating Practice by Food Processors in Wholesale Grocery Markets: Profitability and Welfare Effects. *Am. J. Agric. Econ.* **2003**, *85*, 797. [CrossRef]
33. Henry, J.A.; Guthrie, J.C.; McLeod, G.F.H. A Model of Supermarket Pricing Behaviour. *Asian J. Bus. Res.* **2015**, *5*, 44–57. [CrossRef]
34. Hingley, M.K. Power Imbalance in UK Agri-Food Supply Channels: Learning to Live with the Supermarkets? *J. Mark. Manag.* **2005**, *21*, 63–88. [CrossRef]
35. Hyvonen, S.; Lindblom, A.; Olkkonen, R.; Ollila, P. Exploring the effects of manufacturers' influence strategies and control on category performance in the grocery goods sector. *Int. Rev. Retail Distrib. Consum. Res.* **2010**, *20*, 311–333. [CrossRef]
36. Laska, M.N.; Sindberg, L.S.; Ayala, G.X.; D'Angelo, H.; Horton, L.A.; Ribisl, K.M.; Kharmats, A.; Olson, C.; Gittelsohn, J. Agreements between small food store retailers and their suppliers: Incentivizing unhealthy foods and beverages in four urban settings. *Food Pol.* **2018**, *79*, 324–330. [CrossRef]
37. Major, M. Charting new territory. *Progress. Groc.* **2005**, *84*, 104–108.
38. Martinelli, E.; Marchi, G. Enabling and Inhibiting Factors in Adoption of Electronic-Reverse Auctions: A Longitudinal Case Study in Grocery Retailing. *Int. Rev. Retail Distrib. Consum. Res.* **2007**, *17*, 203–218. [CrossRef]
39. Silveira, P.D.; Marreiros, C.G. Shopper Centric Category Management in Convenience Stores: A Qualitative Study. In Proceedings of the BE-ci 2016 International Conference on Business and Economics, Selangor, Malaysia, 21–23 September 2016; pp. 327–338. Available online: https://www.europeanproceedings.com/files/data/article/47/1416/article_47_1416_pdf_100.pdf (accessed on 6 October 2020).
40. Stanton, J.L.; Herbst, K.C. Slotting allowances: Short-term gains and long-term negative effects on retailers and consumers. *Int. J. Retail Distrib. Manag.* **2006**, *34*, 187–197. [CrossRef]
41. Urbanski, A. Captains of your fate? *Progress. Groc.* **2002**, *81*, 28.
42. Food makers must prove their worth to the new "marketing aristocrats". *Mark. News* **1988**, *22*, 23-23.
43. Category management is working at Giant. *Chain Store Age* **1997**, *73*, 56.
44. Managing for profits. *Beverage Ind.* **1997**, *88*, 20.

45. Federal Trade Commission. Slotting Allowances in the Retail Grocery Industry: Selected Case Studies in Five Product Categories; 2003. Available online: https://www.ftc.gov/sites/default/files/documents/reports/use-slotting-allowances-retail-grocery-industry/slottingallowancerpt031114.pdf (accessed on 6 October 2020).
46. Tan, P.J.; Corsi, A.; Cohen, J.; Sharp, A.; Lockshin, L.; Caruso, W.; Bogomolova, S. Assessing the sales effectiveness of differently located endcaps in a supermarket. *J. Retail. Consum. Serv.* **2018**, *43*, 200–208. [CrossRef]
47. Gomez, M.I.; Rao, V.R. Market power and trade promotions in US supermarkets. *Br. Food J.* **2009**, *111*, 866–877. [CrossRef]
48. Taillie, L.S.; Ng, S.W.; Xue, Y.; Harding, M. Deal or no deal? The prevalence and nutritional quality of price promotions among U.S. food and beverage purchases. *Appetite* **2017**, *117*, 365–372. [CrossRef]
49. Price, R.K.; Livingstone, M.B.; Burns, A.A.; Furey, S.; McMahon-Beattie, U.; Holywood, L.E. What foods are Northern Ireland supermarkets promoting? A content analysis of supermarket online. *Proc. Nutr. Soc.* **2017**, *76*. [CrossRef]
50. Bogomolova, S.; Dunn, S.; Trinh, G.; Taylor, J.; Volpe, R.J. Price promotion landscape in the US and UK: Depicting retail practice to inform future research agenda. *J. Retail. Consum. Serv.* **2015**, *25*, 1–11. [CrossRef]
51. Coker, T.; Rumgay, H.; Whiteside, E.; Rosenberg, G.; Vohra, J. *Paying the Price: New Evidence on the Link between Price Promotions, Purchasing of Less Healthy Food and Drink, and Overweight and Obesity in Great Britain*; Cancer Research: Oxford, UK, 2019.
52. Inmar Inc 2017 Marks the Demise of Print-at-Home Coupons as Digital Redemption Climbs 67%. Available online: https://www.inmar.com/blog/press/2017-marks-demise-print-home-coupons-digital-redemption-climbs-67 (accessed on 8 January 2020).
53. Mussol, S.; Aurier, P.; de Lanauze, G.S. Developing in-store brand strategies and relational expression through sales promotions. *J. Retail. Consum. Serv.* **2019**, *47*, 241–250. [CrossRef]
54. Guan, X.; Atlas, S.A.; Vadiveloo, M. Targeted retail coupons influence category-level food purchases over 2-years. *Int. J. Behav. Nutr. Phys. Act.* **2018**, *15*, 111. [CrossRef]
55. Osuna, I.; González, J.; Capizzani, M. Which categories and brands to promote with targeted coupons to reward and to develop customers in supermarkets. *J. Retail.* **2016**, *92*, 236–251. [CrossRef]
56. Zhang, N. Essays on Nudging Customers' Behaviors: Evidence from Online Grocery Shopping and Crowdfunding. Ph.D. Thesis, Purdue University, West Lafayette, IN, USA, 2017.
57. Huang, Y.; Hui, S.; Inman, J.; Suher, J. Capturing the "First Moment of Truth": Understanding Point-of-Purchase Drivers of Unplanned Consideration and Purchase. Available online: https://www.msi.orghttps://www.msi.org/reports/capturing-the-first-moment-of-truth-understanding-point-of-purchase-drivers (accessed on 13 May 2020).
58. Johnson, J.; Tellis, G.J.; Ip, E.H. To Whom, When, and How Much to Discount? A Constrained Optimization of Customized Temporal Discounts. *J. Retail.* **2013**, *89*, 361–373. [CrossRef]
59. Andorfer, V.A.; Liebe, U. Do information, price, or morals influence ethical consumption? A natural field experiment and customer survey on the purchase of Fair Trade coffee. *Soc. Sci. Res.* **2015**, *52*, 330–350. [CrossRef] [PubMed]
60. Fornari, E.; Fornari, D.; Grandi, S.; Menegatti, M. The influence of retailing -mix levers on private label market share: The case of the Italian FMCG market. *J. Retail. Consum. Serv.* **2013**, *20*, 617–624. [CrossRef]
61. Panzone, L.; Tiffin, R. The Impact of Price Promotions on Producer Strategies in Markets With Large Product Heterogeneity. *AGRIBUSINESS* **2012**, *28*, 421–439. [CrossRef]
62. Kacen, J.J.; Hess, J.D.; Walker, D. Spontaneous selection: The influence of product and retailing factors on consumer impulse purchases. *J. Retail. Consum. Serv.* **2012**, *19*, 578–588. [CrossRef]
63. Breugelmans, E.; Campo, K. Cross-Channel Effects of Price Promotions: An Empirical Analysis of the Multi-Channel Grocery Retail Sector. *J. Retail.* **2016**, *92*, 333–351. [CrossRef]
64. Pozzi, A. E-commerce as a stockpiling technology: Implications for consumer savings. *Int. J. Ind. Organ.* **2013**, *31*, 677–689. [CrossRef]
65. Arce-Urriza, M.; Cebollada, J.; Fernanda Tarira, M. The effect of price promotions on consumer shopping behavior across online and offline channels: Differences between frequent and non-frequent shoppers. *Inf. Syst. E-Bus. Manag.* **2017**, *15*. [CrossRef]
66. Kim, C.; Xu, Y.; Hyde, K.F. Advertising versus Sales Promotion: An Examination of the Japanese Food Industry, 1976-2008. *J. Glob. Sch. Mark. Sci.* **2011**, *21*, 193–200. [CrossRef]

67. Phipps, E.J.; Kumanyika, S.K.; Stites, S.D.; Singletary, S.B.; Cooblall, C.; DiSantis, K.I. Buying Food on Sale: A Mixed Methods Study With Shoppers at an Urban Supermarket, Philadelphia, Pennsylvania, 2010–2012. *Prev. Chronic Dis.* **2014**, 11. [CrossRef] [PubMed]
68. Felgate, M.; Fearne, A.; DiFalco, S.; Martinez, M.G. Using supermarket loyalty card data to analyse the impact of promotions. *Int. J. Mark. Res.* **2012**, *54*, 221–240. [CrossRef]
69. Revoredo-Giha, C.; Akaichi, F.; Leat, P.M.K. Retailers' Promotions: What Role Do They Play in Household Food Purchases by Degree of Food Access in Scotland? Available online: https://ageconsearch.umn.edu/record/189695 (accessed on 13 May 2020).
70. Leeflang, P.S.H.; Parreño-Selva, J. Cross-category demand effects of price promotions. *J. Acad. Mark. Sci.* **2012**, *40*, 572–586. [CrossRef] [PubMed]
71. Mamiya, H.; Moodie, E.E.M.; Ma, Y.; Buckeridge, D.L. Susceptibility to price discounting of soda by neighbourhood educational status: An ecological analysis of disparities in soda consumption using point-of-purchase transaction data in Montreal, Canada. *Int. J. Epidemiol.* **2018**, *47*, 1877–1886. [CrossRef]
72. Sano, N.; Suzuki, T. Evaluation of Discount Effects Using Poisson Regression Based on Interaction Effects Between Bargain Scale and Product Category. In Proceedings of the 2013 IEEE 13th International Conference on Data Mining Workshops; Institute of Electrical and Electronics Engineers (IEEE), Dallas, TX, USA, 7–10 December 2013; pp. 234–241.
73. Singh, S. *Consumer Information Search and Choice in Retail Markets*; ProQuest Information & Learning: Cambridge, UK, 2013.
74. Talukdar, D.; Lindsey, C. To Buy or Not to Buy: Consumers' Demand Response Patterns for Healthy versus Unhealthy Food. *J. Mark.* **2013**. [CrossRef]
75. Goic, M.; Jerath, K.; Srinivasan, K. Cross-Market Discounts. *Mark. Sci.* **2011**, *30*, 134–148. [CrossRef]
76. Tran, T.-T. Factors affecting the impulse shopping intention of Vietnamese people: An application case in Ho Chi Minh City. *Int. J. Adv. Appl. Sci.* **2019**, *6*, 65–74. [CrossRef]
77. Mortimer, G.S.; Weeks, C.S. Grocery product pricing and Australian supermarket consumers: Gender differences in perceived importance levels. *Int. Rev. Retail Distrib. Consum. Res.* **2011**, *21*, 361–373. [CrossRef]
78. Čábelková, I.; Pogorilyak, B.; Strielkowski, W.; Stříteský, V. Customer Store Loyalty Determinants: A Case of the Czech Republic. *Dlsu Bus. Econ. Rev.* **2015**, *25*, 28–44.
79. Farrag, D.A. Impact of Shari'ah on Consumers' Behavior Toward Sales Promotion Tools: Focus on Egyptian Convenience Products. *J. Food Prod. Mark.* **2017**, *23*, 533–552. [CrossRef]
80. Awan, H.M.; Siddiquei, A.N.; Haider, Z. Factors affecting Halal purchase intention-evidence from Pakistan's Halal food sector. *Manag. Res. Rev.* **2015**, *38*, 640–660. [CrossRef]
81. Jamal, A.; Peattie, S.; Peattie, K. Ethnic minority consumers' responses to sales promotion sinthe packaged food market. *J. Retail. Consum. Serv.* **2012**, *19*, 98–108. [CrossRef]
82. Liang, A.R.-D.; Yang, W.; Chen, D.-J.; Chung, Y.-F. The effect of sales promotions on consumers' organic food response An application of logistic regression model. *Br. Food J.* **2017**, *119*, 1247–1262. [CrossRef]
83. Caruso, W.; Corsi, A.M.; Bogomolova, S.; Cohen, J.; Sharp, A.; Lockshin, L.; Tan, P.J. The Real Estate Value Of Supermarket Endcaps Why Location In-Store Matters. *J. Advert. Res.* **2018**, *58*, 177–188. [CrossRef]
84. Caspi, C.E.; Lenk, K.; Pelletier, J.E.; Barnes, T.L.; Harnack, L.; Erickson, D.J.; Laska, M.N. Association between store food environment and customer purchases in small grocery stores, gas-marts, pharmacies and dollar stores. *Int. J. Behav. Nutr. Phys. Act.* **2017**, 14. [CrossRef]
85. Nakamura, R.; Pechey, R.; Suhrcke, M.; Jebb, S.A.; Marteau, T.M. Sales impact of displaying alcoholic and non-alcoholic beverages in end-of-aisle locations: An observational study. *Soc. Sci. Med.* **2014**, *108*, 68–73. [CrossRef]
86. Page, B.; Trinh, G.; Bogomolova, S. Comparing two supermarket layouts: The effect of a middle aisle on basket size, spend, trip duration and endcap use. *J. Retail. Consum. Serv.* **2019**, *47*, 49–56. [CrossRef]
87. Phillips, M.; Parsons, A.G.; Wilkinson, H.J.; Ballantine, P.W. Competing for attention with in-store promotions. *J. Retail. Consum. Serv.* **2015**, *26*, 141–146. [CrossRef]
88. Ranjan, B. *Studying Shopping Decisions and Layout Planning in Physical Retail Settings*; ProQuest Information & Learning: Cambridge, UK, 2018.
89. Ruff, R.R.; Akhund, A.; Adjoian, T. Small Convenience Stores and the Local Food Environment: An Analysis of Resident Shopping Behavior Using Multilevel Modeling. *Am. J. Health Promot.* **2016**, *30*, 172–180. [CrossRef]

90. Sanchez-Flack, J.; Pickrel, J.L.; Belch, G.; Lin, S.-F.; Anderson, C.A.M.; Martinez, M.E.; Arredondo, E.M.; Ayala, G.X. Examination of the Relationship between In-Store Environmental Factors and Fruit and Vegetable Purchasing among Hispanics. *Int. J. Env. Res. Public Health* **2017**, 14. [CrossRef]
91. Seva, R.R.; Go, K.; Garcia, K.; Grindulo, W. Predictive Model of Attention in Viewing Selected Grocery Products. *Dlsu Bus. Econ. Rev.* **2011**, *21*, 97–110.
92. Walmsley, R.; Jenkinson, D.; Saunders, I.; Howard, T.; Oyebode, O. Choice architecture modifies fruit and vegetable purchasing in a university campus grocery store: Time series modelling of a natural experiment. *BMC Public Health* **2018**, *18*, 1149. [CrossRef] [PubMed]
93. Banks, S. Tap into the treat trends. *Conv. Store* **2016**, 57–60.
94. Hong, S.; Misra, K.; Vilcassim, N. The Perils of Category Management: The Effect of Product Assortment on Multicategory Purchase Incidence. *J. Mark.* **2016**, *80*, 34–52. [CrossRef]
95. Spanjaard, D.; Young, L.; Freeman, L. Emotions in supermarket brand choice: A multi-method approach. *Qual. Mark. Res. Int. J.* **2014**, *17*, 209–224. [CrossRef]
96. Yildirim, Y.; Aydin, O. Investigation of the effects of discount announcements on consumers' purchase decisions: A case study in supermarket. *Procedia Soc. Behav. Sci.* **2012**, *62*, 1235–1244. [CrossRef]
97. Tacka, R.C. *Consumer Impulsivity and Attitude: A Quantitative study of Instant Consumable Snack Food Purchases*; ProQuest Information & Learning: Cambridge, UK, 2019.
98. Levy, S.; Gendel-Guterman, H. Does advertising matter to store brand purchase intention? A conceptual framework. *J. Prod. Brand Manag. St. Barbar.* **2012**, *21*, 89–97. [CrossRef]
99. Nordfält, J.; Lange, F. In-store demonstrations as a promotion tool. *J. Retail. Consum. Serv.* **2013**, *20*, 20–25. [CrossRef]
100. Minnema, A.; Bijmolt, T.H.A.; Non, M.C. The impact of instant reward programs and bonus premiums on consumer purchase behavior. *Int. J. Res. Mark.* **2017**, *34*, 194–211. [CrossRef]
101. Aziz, Y.; Chok, N. The Role of Halal Awareness, Halal Certification, and Marketing Components in Determining Halal Purchase Intention Among Non-Muslims in Malaysia: A Structural Equation Modeling Approach:: Vol 25, No 1. *J. Int. Food Agribus. Mark.* **2012**, 25. [CrossRef]
102. United States Department of Agriculture SNAP Retailer Data: 2019 Year End Summary; 2019. Available online: https://fns-prod.azureedge.net/sites/default/files/resource-files/2019-SNAP-Retailer-Management-Year-End-Summary.pdf (accessed on 18 May 2020).
103. Donahue, M.; Mitchell, S. *Dollar Stores Are Targeting Struggling Urban Neighborhoods and Small Towns. One Community Is Showing How to Fight Back*; Institute for Local Self-Reliance: Washington, DC, USA, 2018. Available online: https://ilsr.org/dollar-stores-target-cities-towns-one-fights-back/ (accessed on 6 October 2020).
104. Dollar Stores Are Taking Over the Grocery Business, and It's Bad News for Public Health and Local Economies. Available online: https://civileats.com/2018/12/17/dollar-stores-are-taking-over-the-grocery-business-and-its-bad-news-for-public-health-and-local-economies/ (accessed on 18 May 2020).
105. 2019 Ecommerce in Review: U.S. Online Grocery Sales. Available online: https://www.digitalcommerce360.com/2019/12/24/2019-ecommerce-in-review-online-grocery-sales/ (accessed on 18 May 2020).
106. Redman, R. Online Grocery Sales to Grow 40% in 2020. Available online: https://www.supermarketnews.com/online-retail/online-grocery-sales-grow-40-2020 (accessed on 18 May 2020).

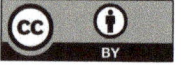

© 2020 by the authors. Licensee MDPI, Basel, Switzerland. This article is an open access article distributed under the terms and conditions of the Creative Commons Attribution (CC BY) license (http://creativecommons.org/licenses/by/4.0/).

MDPI
St. Alban-Anlage 66
4052 Basel
Switzerland
Tel. +41 61 683 77 34
Fax +41 61 302 89 18
www.mdpi.com

International Journal of Environmental Research and Public Health Editorial Office
E-mail: ijerph@mdpi.com
www.mdpi.com/journal/ijerph

www.ingramcontent.com/pod-product-compliance
Lightning Source LLC
LaVergne TN
LVHW070747100526
838202LV00013B/1322